The Gut Microbiome

Editor

EAMONN M.M. QUIGLEY

GASTROENTEROLOGY CLINICS OF NORTH AMERICA

www.gastro.theclinics.com

March 2017 • Volume 46 • Number 1

ELSEVIER

1600 John F. Kennedy Boulevard • Suite 1800 • Philadelphia, Pennsylvania, 19103-2899
http://www.theclinics.com

GASTROENTEROLOGY CLINICS OF NORTH AMERICA Volume 46, Number 1
March 2017 ISSN 0889-8553, ISBN-13: 978-0-323-50978-7

Editor: Kerry Holland
Developmental Editor: Alison Swety

Gastroenterology Clinics of North America (ISSN 0889-8553) is published quarterly by Elsevier Inc., 360 Park Avenue South, New York, NY 10010-1710. Months of issue are March, June, September, and December. Business and Editorial Offices: 1600 John F. Kennedy Blvd., Suite 1800, Philadelphia, PA 19103-2899. Customer Service Office: 6277 Sea Harbor Drive, Orlando, FL 32887-4800. Periodicals postage paid at New York, NY and additional mailing offices. Subscription prices are $330.00 per year (US individuals), $100.00 per year (US students), $616.00 per year (US institutions), $361.00 per year (Canadian individuals), $220.00 per year (Canadian students), $756.00 per year (Canadian institutions), $458.00 per year (international individuals), $220.00 per year (international students), and $756.00 per year (international institutions). Foreign air speed delivery is included in all *Clinics* subscription prices. All prices are subject to change without notice. **POSTMASTER:** Send address changes to *Gastroenterology Clinics of North America*, Elsevier Health Sciences Division, Subscription Customer Service, 3251 Riverport Lane, Maryland Heights, MO 63043. **Telephone: 1-800-654-2452 (U.S. and Canada); 314-447-8871 (outside U.S. and Canada). Fax: 314-447-8029. E-mail: journalscustomerservice-usa@elsevier.com (for print support); journalsonlinesupport-usa@elsevier.com (for online support).**

Reprints. For copies of 100 or more, of articles in this publication, please contact the Commercial Reprints Department, Elsevier Inc., 360 Part Avenue South, New York, New York 10010-1710. Tel. 212-633-3874, Fax: 212-633-3820, E-mail: reprints@elsevier.com.

Gastroenterology Clinics of North America is also published in Italian by Il Pensiero Scientifico Editore, Rome, Italy; and in Portuguese by Interlivros Edicoes Ltda., Rua Commandante Coelho 1085, 21250 Cordovil, Rio de Janeiro, Brazil.

Gastroenterology Clinics of North America is covered in *MEDLINE/PubMed (Index Medicus), Excerpta Medica, Current Contents/Clinical Medicine, Science Citation Index, ISI/BIOMED,* and *BIOSIS.*

Contributors

EDITOR

EAMONN M.M. QUIGLEY, MD, FRCP, FACP, MACG, FRCPI
Chief, Division of Gastroenterology and Hepatology, Lynda K. and David M. Underwood Center for Digestive Disorders, Houston Methodist Hospital, Professor of Medicine, Weill Cornell Medical College, Houston, Texas

AUTHORS

CHATHUR ACHARYA, MBBS
Division of General Internal Medicine, Virginia Commonwealth University, Richmond, Virginia

JASMOHAN S. BAJAJ, MD, MS
Associate Professor, Division of Gastroenterology, Hepatology, and Nutrition, McGuire VA Medical Center, Virginia Commonwealth University, Richmond, Virginia

JOHN F. CRYAN, PhD
APC Microbiome Institute, Department of Anatomy and Neuroscience, University College Cork, Cork, Ireland

PÁRAIC Ó CUÍV, PhD
The University of Queensland Diamantina Institute, The University of Queensland, Translational Research Institute, Brisbane, Queensland, Australia

TIMOTHY G. DINAN, MD, PhD
APC Microbiome Institute, Professor, Department of Psychiatry and Neurobehavioural Science, University College Cork, Cork, Ireland

BURKHARDT FLEMER, Dipl. Ing. (FH), PhD
School of Microbiology & APC Microbiome Institute, University College Cork, Cork, Ireland

JEFFREY S. GERBER, MD, PhD
Division of Infectious Diseases, Department of Pediatrics, The Children's Hospital of Philadelphia, Assistant Professor of Pediatrics and Epidemiology, University of Pennsylvania School of Medicine, Philadelphia, Pennsylvania

UDAY C. GHOSHAL, MD, DNB, DM, FACG, RFF
Professor, Department of Gastroenterology, Sanjay Gandhi Postgraduate Institute of Medical Sciences, Lucknow, India

UJJALA GHOSHAL, MD
Professor, Department of Microbiology, Sanjay Gandhi Postgraduate Institute of Medical Sciences, Lucknow, India

DAVID GROEGER, PhD
Alimentary Health Pharma Davos, Davos Platz, Switzerland

RICHARD H. HUNT, MB, FRCP, FRCP Ed, FRCPC
Division of Gastroenterology and Farncombe Family Digestive Health Research Institute, Professor Emeritus, McMaster University, Hamilton, Ontario, Canada

LIZA KONNIKOVA, MD, PhD
Department of Pediatric and Newborn Medicine, Attending Neonatologist, Brigham and Women's Hospital, Instructor in Pediatrics, Harvard Medical School, Boston, Massachusetts

JIA V. LI, PhD
Section of Biomolecular Medicine, Division of Computational & Systems Medicine, Department of Surgery & Cancer, Faculty of Medicine, Imperial College London, London, United Kingdom

JULIAN R. MARCHESI, PhD
Section of Biomolecular Medicine, Division of Computational and Systems Medicine, Department of Surgery and Cancer, Faculty of Medicine, Divison of Digestive Diseases, Department of Surgery and Cancer, Faculty of Medicine, Department of Surgery and Cancer, Centre for Digestive and Gut Health, Imperial College London, London, United Kingdom; School of Biosciences, Cardiff University, Cardiff, United Kingdom

MARK MORRISON, PhD
The University of Queensland Diamantina Institute, The University of Queensland, Translational Research Institute, Brisbane, Queensland, Australia

NIDA MURTAZA, MTech
The University of Queensland Diamantina Institute, The University of Queensland, Translational Research Institute, Brisbane, Queensland, Australia

PAUL W. O'TOOLE, BA (Mod.), PhD
School of Microbiology & APC Microbiome Institute, University College Cork, Cork, Ireland

LIAM O'MAHONY, PhD
Swiss Institute of Allergy and Asthma Research, University of Zurich, Davos Platz, Switzerland

EAMONN M.M. QUIGLEY, MD, FRCP, FACP, MACG, FRCPI
Chief, Division of Gastroenterology and Hepatology, Lynda K. and David M. Underwood Center for Digestive Disorders, Houston Methodist Hospital, Professor of Medicine, Weill Cornell Medical College, Houston, Texas

YEHUDA RINGEL, MD, AGAF, FACG
Professor, Department of Gastroenterology, Rabin Medical Center, Petach Tikva, Israel; School of Medicine, University of North Carolina at Chapel Hill, Chapel Hill, North Carolina

FERGUS SHANAHAN, MD, DSc
Department of Medicine, APC Microbiome Institute, University College Cork, National University of Ireland, Ireland

DONAL SHEEHAN, MB
Department of Medicine, APC Microbiome Institute, University College Cork, National University of Ireland, Ireland

MICHAEL A. SILVERMAN, MD, PhD
Division of Infectious Diseases, Department of Pediatrics, The Children's Hospital of Philadelphia, Assistant Professor of Pediatrics, Perelman School of Medicine, University of Pennsylvania, Philadelphia, Pennsylvania

SYLWIA SMOLINSKA, PhD
Department of Clinical Immunology, Wroclaw Medical University, Wroclaw, Poland

CHRISTINA M. SURAWICZ, MD
Professor of Medicine, Division of Gastroenterology, Department of Medicine, University of Washington, Seattle, Washington

JONATHAN SWANN, PhD
Section of Biomolecular Medicine, Division of Computational & Systems Medicine, Department of Surgery & Cancer, Faculty of Medicine, Imperial College London, London, United Kingdom

STEPHEN M. VINDIGNI, MD, MPH
Gastroenterology Fellow, Division of Gastroenterology, Department of Medicine, School of Medicine, University of Washington, Seattle, Washington

MOHAMMAD YAGHOOBI, MD, MSc (Epi), FRCPC
Division of Gastroenterology and Farncombe Family Digestive Health Research Institute, Assistant Professor, McMaster University, Hamilton, Ontario, Canada

Contents

Preface   xiii

Eamonn M.M. Quigley

Basic Definitions and Concepts: Organization of the Gut Microbiome   1

Eamonn M.M. Quigley

New claims are frequently made for a role for the microbiome in a disease or disorder previously considered remote from the gut. The microbiome has been linked to such seemingly unrelated entities as depression, anorexia nervosa, autism, Parkinson disease, allergy, and asthma. Although many of these proposals have been based on animal studies, explorations of the microbiome in human disease continue to proliferate, facilitated by technologies that provide a detailed assessment of the microbial inhabitants of our gastrointestinal tract and their biological activities and metabolic products. With these technologies come new terminologies, which are identified in this article.

From Culture to High-Throughput Sequencing and Beyond: A Layperson's Guide to the "Omics" and Diagnostic Potential of the Microbiome   9

Paul W. O'Toole and Burkhardt Flemer

Detailed knowledge of the community of organisms in the gut has become possible in recent years because of the development of culture-independent methods. Largely based on latest DNA sequencing platforms, it is now possible to establish the composition of the microbiota and the repertoire of biochemical functions it encodes. Variations in either or both of these parameters have been linked to intestinal and extraintestinal disease. This article summarizes how these methods are applied, with special reference to gastroenterology, and describes the achievements and future potential of microbiota analysis as a diagnostic tool.

Biology of the Microbiome 1: Interactions with the Host Immune Response   19

Sylwia Smolinska, David Groeger, and Liam O'Mahony

The intestinal immune system is intimately connected with the vast diversity of microbes present within the gut and the diversity of food components that are consumed daily. The discovery of novel molecular mechanisms, which mediate host-microbe-nutrient communication, have highlighted the important roles played by microbes and dietary factors in influencing mucosal immune responses. Dendritic cells, epithelial cells, innate lymphoid cells, T regulatory cells, effector lymphocytes, natural killer T cells, and B cells can all be influenced by the microbiome. Many of the mechanisms being described are bacterial strain or metabolite specific.

Biology of the Microbiome 2: Metabolic Role   37

Jia V. Li, Jonathan Swann, and Julian R. Marchesi

The human microbiome is a new frontier in biology and one that is helping to define what it is to be human. Recently, we have begun to understand that the "communication" between the host and its microbiome is via a metabolic superhighway. By interrogating and understanding the molecules involved we may start to know who the main players are, and how we can modulate them and the mechanisms of health and disease.

Diet and the Microbiome   49

Nida Murtaza, Páraic Ó Cuív, and Mark Morrison

The gut microbiota provides a range of ecologic, metabolic, and immunomodulatory functions relevant to health and well-being. The gut microbiota not only responds quickly to changes in diet, but this dynamic equilibrium may be managed to prevent and/or treat acute and chronic diseases. This article provides a working definition of the term "microbiome" and uses two examples of dietary interventions for the treatment of large bowel conditions to emphasize the links between diet and microbiome. There remains a need to develop a better functional understanding of the microbiota, if its management for clinical utility is to be fully realized.

Impact of Antibiotics on Necrotizing Enterocolitis and Antibiotic-Associated Diarrhea   61

Michael A. Silverman, Liza Konnikova, and Jeffrey S. Gerber

Antibiotic treatment alters the composition and metabolic function of the intestinal microbiota. These alterations may contribute to the pathogenesis of necrotizing enterocolitis (NEC) and antibiotic-associated diarrhea (AAD). Recent studies are beginning to unravel the contribution of specific groups of microbes and their metabolic pathways to these diseases. Probiotics or other microbiota-targeted therapies may provide effect strategies to prevent and treat NEC and AAD.

The Microbiome-Gut-Brain Axis in Health and Disease   77

Timothy G. Dinan and John F. Cryan

Gut microbes are capable of producing most neurotransmitters found in the human brain. Evidence is accumulating to support the view that gut microbes influence central neurochemistry and behavior. Irritable bowel syndrome is regarded as the prototypic disorder of the brain-gut-microbiota axis that can be responsive to probiotic therapy. Translational studies indicate that certain bacteria may have an impact on stress responses and cognitive functioning. Manipulating the gut microbiota with psychobiotics, prebiotics, or even antibiotics offers a novel approach to altering brain function and treating gut-brain axis disorders, such as depression and autism.

The Gut Microbiome in Irritable Bowel Syndrome and Other Functional Bowel Disorders   91

Yehuda Ringel

Emerging data from epidemiologic, microbiome, and physiology research in patients with functional bowel disorders (FBDs) provide evidence for a linkage between alterations in the intestinal microbiota and FBDs. However, currently most of the data is based on association studies, and the causality role of the microbiota in these disorders is not established. Growing evidence for compositional changes and the increasing recognition of the association between the intestinal microbiota and gut-brain functions that are relevant to the pathophysiology and/or clinical symptoms of FBDs have led to increased interest in manipulating the intestinal microbiota for the treatment of these disorders.

Small Intestinal Bacterial Overgrowth and Other Intestinal Disorders   103
Uday C. Ghoshal and Ujjala Ghoshal

Gut microbiota is the largest organ of the human body. Although growth of bacteria more than 10^5 colony forming unit (CFU) per milliliter in culture of upper gut aspirate is used to diagnosis small intestinal bacterial overgrowth (SIBO), 10^3 CFU or more is being considered to suggest the diagnosis, particularly if colonic type bacteria are present in the upper gut. Although neither very sensitive nor specific, hydrogen breath tests are widely used to diagnose SIBO. Rifaximin is the best treatment for SIBO due to its broad spectrum, lack of systemic absorption, and safety profile.

The Esophageal and Gastric Microbiome in Health and Disease   121
Richard H. Hunt and Mohammad Yaghoobi

The esophagus and stomach are host to their own population of bacteria, which differs in health and disease. *Helicobacter pylori* uniquely colonizes only gastric mucosa, but an increasing number of bacteria is now isolated from the gastric juice and gastric mucosa, including *Lactobacillus*. The presence of *H pylori* alters populations of other gastric bacteria with a marked reduction in diversity. Alterations in intragastric acidity may be the cause or the consequence of changes in the microbial populations of the stomach. Esophageal inflammation is associated with an altered microbiota in gastroesophageal reflux disease, Barrett's esophagus, eosinophilic esophagitis, and cancer.

The Gut Microbiota in Inflammatory Bowel Disease   143
Donal Sheehan and Fergus Shanahan

Genes, bacteria, and immunity contribute to the pathogenesis of inflammatory bowel disease. Most genetic risk relates to defective sensing of microbes and their metabolites or defective regulation of the host response to the microbiota. Because the composition of the microbiota shapes the developing immune system and is determined in early life, the prospect of therapeutic manipulation of the microbiota in adulthood after the onset of disease is questionable. However, the microbiota may be a marker of risk and a modifier of disease activity and a contributor to extraintestinal manifestations and associations in some patients with inflammatory bowel disease.

Gut Microbiota and Complications of Liver Disease   155
Chathur Acharya and Jasmohan S. Bajaj

Chronic liver disease, cirrhosis, and its complications are epidemic worldwide. Most complications are mediated through a dysfunctional gut-liver axis. New techniques have made culture-independent analysis of the gut microbiome widespread. With insight into an unfavorable microbiome (dysbiosis) and how it affects liver disease, investigators have discovered new targets to potentially improve outcomes. Dysbiosis is associated with endotoxemia and propagates liver injury due to nonalcoholic steatohepatitis and alcohol. The composition and functionality of the microbiome changes with the development of cirrhosis, decompensation, and with treatments for these conditions. Gut microbiota can be used to predict clinically relevant outcomes in cirrhosis.

Fecal Microbiota Transplantation   171

Stephen M. Vindigni and Christina M. Surawicz

Fecal microbiota transplantation (FMT) is the transfer of stool from a healthy donor into the colon of a patient whose disease is a result of an altered microbiome, with the goal of restoring the normal microbiota and thus curing the disease. The most effective and well-studied indication for FMT is recurrent *Clostridium difficile* infection. At this time, there is insufficient evidence to recommend FMT for other gastrointestinal diseases, but studies are under way. There is also insufficient evidence to recommend FMT for nongastrointestinal diseases at this time. The field is rapidly emerging.

Index   187

GASTROENTEROLOGY CLINICS OF NORTH AMERICA

FORTHCOMING ISSUES

June 2017
Liver Pathology
Jay H. Lefkowitch, *Editor*

September 2017
Crohn's Disease
Edward V. Loftus, *Editor*

December 2017
Complementary and Alternative Medicine in Inflammatory Bowel Disease
Ali Keshavarzian and Ece A. Mutlu, *Editors*

RECENT ISSUES

December 2016
Obesity and Gastroenterology
Octavia Pickett-Blakely and Linda A. Lee, *Editors*

September 2016
Gastrointestinal Neoplasia
Paul J. Limburg and Dan A. Dixon, *Editors*

June 2016
Women's Health in Gastroenterology
Laurel R. Fisher, *Editor*

Preface

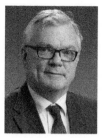

Eamonn M.M. Quigley, MD, FRCP, FACP, MACG, FRCPI
Editor

Such has been the volume of new information on the topic of gastrointestinal bacteria in health and disease over the past decade that the practicing gastroenterologist can be forgiven if he or she finds the topic inaccessible and often incomprehensible. This field of biomedical science has, indeed, developed a new vocabulary and introduced at an alarming pace new techniques for the assessment of the members of our gastrointestinal microbial populations, their functions, and their interaction with us in health and disease. This issue attempts to provide an update on the field as it relates to gastrointestinal health and disease and, in so doing, introduces the technologies that facilitate this field of study, places the many exciting discoveries achieved in the laboratory in a clinical context, and clinically assesses the question that every clinician asks: what are the diagnostic, prognostic, and therapeutic implications of the microbiome in gastrointestinal practice?

Eamonn M.M. Quigley, MD, FRCP, FACP, MACG, FRCPI
Division of Gastroenterology and Hepatology
Lynda K. and David M. Underwood
Center for Digestive Disorders
Houston Methodist Hospital and
Weill Cornell Medical College
6550 Fannin Street, SM 1201
Houston, TX 77030, USA

E-mail address:
equigley@tmhs.org

Gastroenterol Clin N Am 46 (2017) xiii
http://dx.doi.org/10.1016/j.gtc.2016.12.001
0889-8553/17/© 2016 Published by Elsevier Inc.

gastro.theclinics.com

Basic Definitions and Concepts: Organization of the Gut Microbiome

 CrossMark

Eamonn M.M. Quigley, MD, FRCP, MACG, FRCPI

KEYWORDS

• Microbiome • Microbiota • Enterotypes • Gastrointestinal function

KEY POINTS

- New claims are frequently made for a role for the microbiome in a disease or disorder previously considered remote from the gut, not to mention its bacterial population.
- The microbiome has been linked to such seemingly unrelated entities as depression, anorexia nervosa, autism, Parkinson disease, allergy, and asthma.
- Although many of these proposals have been based on animal studies, explorations of the microbiome in human disease continue to proliferate, facilitated by the availability of a variety of technologies that rapidly and with ever-increasing economy provide a detailed assessment of the microbial inhabitants of our gastrointestinal tract, their biological activities, and metabolic products.
- With these technologies come new terminology, such as microbiota, microbiome, metagenomics, and metabonomics, which are identified in this article.

To the busy clinician the tsunami of information that hits his or her desk or computer on a daily basis relating to the science and clinical implications of the microbiome has become simply overwhelming. Not a day goes by without a new claim for a role for the microbiome in a disease or disorder previously considered remote from the gut, not to mention its bacterial population. Thus, the microbiome has been liked to such seemingly unrelated entities as depression,[1,2] anorexia nervosa,[3] autism,[4–6] Parkinson disease,[7–9] allergy, and asthma.[10–12] Although many of these proposals have been based on animal studies, explorations of the microbiome in human disease continue to proliferate, facilitated by the availability of a variety of technologies that rapidly and with ever-increasing economy provide a detailed assessment of the microbial inhabitants of our gastrointestinal tract and their biological activities and metabolic products.[13–16] With these technologies comes a new terminology:

> *Microbiota* is the assemblage of microorganisms (bacteria, archaea, or lower eukaryotes) present in a defined environment, such as the gastrointestinal tract.

Division of Gastroenterology and Hepatology, Lynda K and David M Underwood Center for Digestive Disorders, Houston Methodist Hospital, Weill Cornell Medical College, 6550 Fannin Street, SM 1001, Houston, TX 77030, USA
E-mail address: equigley@tmhs.org

Gastroenterol Clin N Am 46 (2017) 1–8
http://dx.doi.org/10.1016/j.gtc.2016.09.002
gastro.theclinics.com

Microbiome is the full complement of microbes (bacteria, viruses, fungi, and proto-zoa) and their genes and genomes (though strictly speaking different, the terms *microbiome* and *microbiota* are often used interchangeably).

Metagenomics is the study of the gene content and encoded functional attributes of the gut microbiome in healthy humans.

Metabonomics is the quantitative measurement of the multiparametric (time related) metabolic responses of complex systems to a pathophysiologic stimulus or genetic modification, often used synonymously with *metabolomics.*

The term *flora,* which dates from the time when bacteria were included in the plant kingdom, has now been largely abandoned and replaced by *microbiota.* Although the focus of the review is on the possible role of the microbiota in gastrointestinal diseases and disorders, one must first briefly review what is known of the microbiota in health.[17]

THE MICROBIOME IN HEALTH: DEVELOPMENT, INFLUENCES, AND FUNCTIONS

Much of what we know of the composition and functions of the normal gut microbiota comes from large national or multinational consortia.[18–22] Although the microbiome of each individual is quite distinct at the level of individual bacterial strains, data from a European consortium indicated that, at a higher level of organization, some general patterns can be identified across populations.[19,20] They identified 3 broad groupings (enterotypes) driven by the predominance of certain species: *Prevotella, Bacteroides,* and *Ruminococcus.* Enterotype prevalence seemed independent of age, body mass index, or geographic location but might have been driven by differing dietary habits.[20]

Although the delineation of the full range of normal variations in the composition of the gut microbiota within and between individuals continues to be defined, certain trends have emerged. Traditionally, it was thought that the intestinal tract is sterile at birth; new evidence indicates that the colonization of the infant's gut may commence in utero from the placenta.[23,24] However, the balance of evidence indicates that most of the infant's microbiome is acquired from the mother during birth and continues to be populated through feeding and other contacts.[25–29] Several factors influence the microbiome over these critical early months and years of life[25–28]: mode of delivery (vaginal birth vs cesarean delivery),[29–32] diet (breast milk vs formula),[27,33,34] geography,[35] and exposure to antibiotics.[36] By 2 to 3 years of age, the child's microbiota has come to closely resemble that of an adult in terms of composition[17,37,38]; some further evolution through to adolescence has, however, recently been reported.[39] Thereafter, the microbiota is thought to remain relatively stable[35] until old age when changes are seen, possibly related to alterations in digestive physiology and diet[40–42]; further longitudinal studies are required to more precisely define age-related changes in adults.

Several factors influence the composition of the microbiota in health and must be accounted for in the interpretation of findings in disease. Foremost among these is diet.[43] General characteristics of the diet (total calories, highly processed vs vegetable and fruit based)[20,35,44,45] as well as the relative concentrations of specific components, such as carbohydrate,[46–48] protein,[49] fat,[50,51] fiber,[51–53] and vitamins,[54,55] have all been shown to influence the composition of the microbiota. It has been assumed that diet-related changes reflect the long-term effects of a particular dietary pattern over a lifetime[20,35,42,56]; it is now evident that relatively acute, albeit drastic, changes in dietary habit may also result in shifts in microbial populations.[56] All of these observations are highly relevant to the study of gastrointestinal diseases given the restrictions that gut ill health per se may impose on eating patterns and of the propensity for individuals afflicted by gastrointestinal symptoms to alter their diet, sometimes drastically, in an attempt to alleviate these same symptoms.[47,48,57,58]

Other factors that may independently influence the structure of the microbiome (in the short- and long-term) include antibiotic use,[59–61] acid suppression,[62,63] and cultural and geographic factors.[35,64] It is now apparent that other prescription drugs, such as metformin, may also influence microbiota architecture.[65,66] It has been postulated (and supported by some evidence) that antibiotic and other exposures during the early years of life, when the microbiome is in evolution, may be especially deleterious and could result in metabolic and inflammatory disorders later in life.[60,67,68] Two recent population-based studies from the Netherlands and Belgium have emphasized the influence of diet, medications, smoking habit, and disease state on the composition of the gut microbiome in adults.[21,22] The last observation is especially noteworthy; studies of the microbiome in disease states have assumed, for the most part, that the relationship is unidirectional, that is, that an altered microbiome causes the disease. This approach fails to consider the alternative possibility: that the disease alters the microbiome, as exemplified by the impact of inflammatory processes on the microbiome.[69,70]

A detailed exploration of the many proven and postulated functions of the gut microbiome is beyond the scope of this review; the reader is referred to several excellent reviews for a detailed discussion.[17,37,71–77] Suffice it to say that a vast amount of laboratory and clinical research has already provided abundant justification for the gut microbiota to be considered "the forgotten organ."[77] Experiments in germ-free animals have convinced us that an intact microbiome is essential for the development and function of many, if not all, of the components of an intact gastrointestinal tract: the mucosa- or, gut-associated immune system (mucosa-associated lymphoid tissue or gut-associated lymphoid tissue), immunologic tolerance, epithelial and barrier function, motility, and vascularity. The resident commensal microbiota continues to contribute to such homeostatic functions during life as pathogen exclusion, immunomodulation, upregulation of cytoprotective genes, prevention and regulation of apoptosis, and maintenance of barrier function.[17,71,75]

The sophistication of the relationship between the microbiota and its host is elegantly illustrated by the manner in which the immune system of the gut differentiates between friend and foe when it encounters bacteria.[78] Various phenomena operative at the level of the intestinal epithelium lead to the recognition (tolerance) of commensals as friend and differentiate them from pathogens (foe): the masking or modification of microbial-associated molecular patterns that are usually recognized by pattern recognition receptors, such as Toll-like receptors,[79] the preferential induction of regulatory T cells resulting in the production of the antiinflammatory cytokine, interleukin 10,[80] and the associated inhibition of the nuclear factor kappa-light-chain-enhancer of activated B cells inflammatory pathway.[81]

The metabolic functions of the microbiome continue to be revealed and are now seen to extend well beyond its long-recognized ability to salvage unabsorbed dietary sugars and convert them into short-chain fatty acids; synthesize nutrients and vitamins, such as folate and vitamin K; deconjugate bile salts[82]; and metabolize dietary xenobiotics as well as an expanding list of commonly used drugs.[76] Thus, metabolic products of the microbiome, including neurotransmitters and neuromodulators, impact not just on the enteric neuromodulatory apparatus[83–86] but also seem capable of influencing the development and function of the central nervous system,[5,6,8,9,87–91] thereby, leading to the concept of the microbiota-gut-brain axis.[77,83,92,93]

REFERENCES

1. Jiang H, Ling Z, Zhang Y, et al. Altered fecal microbiota composition in patients with major depressive disorder. Brain Behav Immun 2015;48:186–94.
2. Zheng P, Zeng B, Zhou C, et al. Gut microbiome remodeling induces depressive-like behaviors through a pathway mediated by the host's metabolism. Mol Psychiatry 2016;21(6):786–96.
3. Kleiman SC, Watson HJ, Bulik-Sullivan EC, et al. The intestinal microbiota in acute anorexia nervosa and during renourishment: relationship to depression, anxiety, and eating disorder psychopathology. Psychosom Med 2015;77:969–81.
4. Mangiola F, Ianiro G, Franceschi F, et al. Gut microbiota in autism and mood disorders. World J Gastroenterol 2016;22:361–8.
5. Desbonnet L, Clarke G, Shanahan F, et al. Microbiota is essential for social development in the mouse. Mol Psychiatry 2014;19:146–8.
6. Desbonnet L, Clarke G, Traplin A, et al. Gut microbiota depletion from early adolescence in mice: implications for brain and behaviour. Brain Behav Immun 2015;48:165–73.
7. Scheperjans F, Aho V, Pereira PAB, et al. Gut microbiota are related to Parkinson's disease and clinical phenotype. Mov Disord 2015;30:350–8.
8. Mulak A, Bonaz B. Brain-gut-microbiota axis in Parkinson's disease. World J Gastroenterol 2015;21:10609–20.
9. Felice VD, Quigley EM, Sullivan AM, et al. Microbiota-gut-brain signalling in Parkinson's disease: implications for non-motor symptoms. Parkinsonism Relat Disord 2016;27:1–8.
10. Riiser A. The human microbiome, asthma, and allergy. Allergy Asthma Clin Immunol 2015;11:35.
11. Fujimura KE, Lynch SV. Microbiota in allergy and asthma and the emerging relationship with the gut microbiome. Cell Host Microbe 2015;17:592–602.
12. Huang YJ, Boushey HA. The microbiome in asthma. J Allergy Clin Immunol 2015; 135:25–30.
13. Claesson MJ, O'Toole PW. Evaluating the latest high-throughput molecular techniques for the exploration of microbial gut communities. Gut Microbes 2010;1: 277–8.
14. Tottey W, Denonfoux J, Jaziri F, et al. The human gut chip "HuGChip", an explorative phylogenetic microarray for determining gut microbiome diversity at family level. PLoS One 2013;8:e62544.
15. Wang WL, Xu SY, Ren ZG, et al. Application of metagenomics in the human gut microbiome. World J Gastroenterol 2015;21:803–14.
16. Kim Y, Koh I, Rho M. Deciphering the human microbiome using next-generation sequencing data and bioinformatics approaches. Methods 2015;79–80:52–9.
17. Sekirov I, Russell SL, Antunes LC, et al. Gut microbiota in health and disease. Physiol Rev 2010;90:859–904.
18. NIH HMP Working Group, Peterson J, Garges S, Giovanni M, et al. The NIH Human Microbiome Project. Genome Res 2009;19:2317–23.
19. Qin J, Li R, Raes J, et al. A human gut microbial gene catalogue established by metagenomic sequencing. Nature 2010;464:59–65.
20. Arumugam M, Raes J, Pelletier E, et al. Enterotypes of the human gut microbiome. Nature 2011;473:174–80.
21. Zhernakova A, Kurilshikov A, Bonder MJ, et al. Population-based metagenomics analysis reveals markers for gut microbiome composition and diversity. Science 2016;352:565–9.

22. Falony G, Joossens M, Vieira-Silva S, et al. Population-level analysis of gut microbiome variation. Science 2016;352:560–4.
23. Collado MC, Rautava S, Aakko J, et al. Human gut colonisation may be initiated in utero by distinct microbial communities in the placenta and amniotic fluid. Sci Rep 2016;6:23129.
24. Aagaard K, Ma J, Antony KM, et al. The placenta harbors a unique microbiome. Sci Transl Med 2014;6:237ra65.
25. Palmer C, Bik EM, DiGiulio DB, et al. Development of the human infant intestinal microbiota. PLoS Biol 2007;5:1556–73.
26. Koenig JE, Spor A, Scalfone N, et al. Succession of microbial consortia in the developing infant gut microbiome. Proc Natl Acad Sci U S A 2011;108:4578–85.
27. Marques TM, Wall R, Ross RP, et al. Programming infant gut microbiota: influence of dietary and environmental factors. Curr Opin Biotechnol 2010;21:149–56.
28. Fouhy F, Ross RP, Fitzgerald GF, et al. Composition of the early intestinal microbiota: knowledge, knowledge gaps and the use of high-throughput sequencing to address these gaps. Gut Microbes 2012;3(4):1–18.
29. Dominguez-Bello MG, Costello EK, Contreras M, et al. Delivery mode shapes the acquisition and structure of the initial microbiota across multiple body habitats in newborns. Proc Natl Acad Sci U S A 2010;107:11971–5.
30. Jakobsson HE, Abrahamsson TR, Jenmalm MC, et al. Decreased gut microbiota diversity, delayed Bacteroidetes colonisation and reduced Th1 responses in infants delivered by caesarean section. Gut 2014;63:559–66.
31. Dogra S, Sakwinska O, Soh SE, et al, GUSTO Study Group. Dynamics of infant gut microbiota are influenced by delivery mode and gestational duration and are associated with subsequent adiposity. MBio 2015;6 [pii:e02419–14].
32. Dominguez-Bello MG, De Jesus-Laboy KM, Shen N, et al. Partial restoration of the microbiota of cesarean-born infants via vaginal microbial transfer. Nat Med 2016;22:250–3.
33. Cong X, Xu W, Janton S, et al. Gut microbiome developmental patterns in early life of preterm infants: impacts of feeding and gender. PLoS One 2016;11: e0152751.
34. Bäckhed F, Roswall J, Peng Y, et al. Dynamics and stabilization of the human gut microbiome during the first year of life. Cell Host Microbe 2015;17:690–703.
35. Yatsunenko T, Rey FE, Manary MJ, et al. Human gut microbiome viewed across age and geography. Nature 2012;486:222–7.
36. Vangay P, Ward T, Gerber JS, et al. Antibiotics, pediatric dysbiosis, and disease. Cell Host Microbe 2015;17:553–64.
37. Clemente JC, Ursell LK, Parfrey LW, et al. The impact of the gut microbiota on human health: an integrative view. Cell 2012;148:1258–70.
38. O'Toole PW, Claesson MJ. Gut microbiota: changes throughout the lifespan from infancy to elderly. Int Dairy J 2010;20:281–91.
39. Hollister EB, Riehle K, Luna RA, et al. Structure and function of the healthy preadolescent pediatric gut microbiome. Microbiome 2015;3:36.
40. Mariat D, Firmesse O, Levenez F, et al. The Firmicutes/Bacteroidetes ratio of the human microbiota changes with age. BMC Microbiol 2009;9:123.
41. Ley RE, Lozupone CA, Hamady M, et al. Worlds within worlds: evolution of the vertebrate gut microbiota. Nat Rev Microbiol 2008;6:776–8.
42. Claesson MJ, Jeffery IB, Conde S, et al. Gut microbiota composition correlates with diet and health in the elderly. Nature 2012;488:178–84.
43. Doré J, Blottière H. The influence of diet on the gut microbiota and its consequences for health. Curr Opin Biotechnol 2015;32:195–9.

44. Smith MI, Yatsunenko T, Manary MJ, et al. Gut microbiomes of Malawian twin pairs discordant for kwashiorkor. Science 2013;339:548–54.
45. Subramanian S, Huq S, Yatsunenko T, et al. Persistent gut microbiota immaturity in malnourished Bangladeshi children. Nature 2014;510:417–21.
46. Sonnenburg ED, Sonnenburg JL. Starving our microbial self: the deleterious consequences of a diet deficient in microbiota-accessible carbohydrates. Cell Metab 2014;20:779–86.
47. Kashyap PC, Marcobal A, Ursell LK, et al. Complex interactions among diet, gastrointestinal transit, and gut microbiota in humanized mice. Gastroenterology 2013;144:967–77.
48. McIntosh K, Reed DE, Schneider T, et al. FODMAPs alter symptoms and the metabolome of patients with IBS: a randomised controlled trial. Gut 2016. [Epub ahead of print].
49. Clarke SF, Murphy EF, O'Sullivan O, et al. Exercise and associated dietary extremes impact on gut microbial diversity. Gut 2014;63:1913–20.
50. Hildebrandt MA, Hoffmann C, Sherrill-Mix SA, et al. High-fat diet determines the composition of the murine gut microbiome independently of obesity. Gastroenterology 2009;137:1716–24.
51. Heinritz SN, Weiss E, Eklund M, et al. Intestinal microbiota and microbial metabolites are changed in a pig model fed a high-fat/low-fiber or a low-fat/high-fiber diet. PLoS One 2016;11:e0154329.
52. Kovatcheva-Datchary P, Nilsson A, Akrami R, et al. Dietary fiber-induced improvement in glucose metabolism is associated with increased abundance of Prevotella. Cell Metab 2015;22:971–82.
53. Sonnenburg ED, Smits SA, Tikhonov M, et al. Diet-induced extinctions in the gut microbiota compound over generations. Nature 2016;529:212–5.
54. Degnan PH, Taga ME, Goodman AL. Vitamin B12 as a modulator of gut microbial ecology. Cell Metab 2014;20:769–78.
55. Degnan PH, Barry NA, Mok KC, et al. Human gut microbes use multiple transporters to distinguish vitamin B_{12} analogs and compete in the gut. Cell Host Microbe 2014;15:47–57.
56. Wu GD, Chen J, Hoffmann C, et al. Linking long-term dietary patterns with gut microbial enterotypes. Science 2011;334:105–8.
57. Halmos EP, Christophersen CT, Bird AR, et al. Diets that differ in their FODMAP content alter the colonic luminal microenvironment. Gut 2015;64:93–100.
58. Bonder MJ, Tigchelaar EF, Cai X, et al. The influence of a short-term gluten-free diet on the human gut microbiome. Genome Med 2016;8:45.
59. Robinson CJ, Young VB. Antibiotic administration alters the community structure of the gastrointestinal microbiota. Gut Microbes 2010;1:279–84.
60. Modi SR, Collins JJ, Relman DA. Antibiotics and the gut microbiota. J Clin Invest 2014;124:4212–8.
61. Blaser MJ. Antibiotic use and its consequences for the normal microbiome. Science 2016;352:544–5.
62. Jackson MA, Goodrich JK, Maxan ME, et al. Proton pump inhibitors alter the composition of the gut microbiota. Gut 2016;65:749–56.
63. Freedberg DE, Toussaint NC, Chen SP, et al. Proton pump inhibitors alter specific taxa in the human gastrointestinal microbiome: a crossover trial. Gastroenterology 2015;149:883–5.
64. Wu GD, Compher C, Chen EZ, et al. Comparative metabolomics in vegans and omnivores reveal constraints on diet-dependent gut microbiota metabolite production. Gut 2016;65:63–72.

65. Devkota S. Prescription drugs obscure microbiome analyses. Science 2016;351: 452–3.
66. Forslund K, Hildebrand F, Nielsen T, et al. Disentangling type 2 diabetes and metformin treatment signatures in the human gut microbiota. Nature 2015;528:262–6.
67. Cho I, Yamanishi S, Cox L, et al. Antibiotics in early life alter the murine colonic microbiome and adiposity. Nature 2012;488:621–6.
68. Cox LM, Yamanishi S, Sohn J, et al. Altering the intestinal microbiota during a critical developmental window has lasting metabolic consequences. Cell 2014;158: 705–21.
69. Elinav E, Strowig T, Kau AL, et al. NLRP6 inflammasome regulates colonic microbial ecology and risk for colitis. Cell 2011;145:745–57.
70. Levy M, Thaiss CA, Zeevi D, et al. Microbiota-modulated metabolites shape the intestinal microenvironment by regulating NLRP6 inflammasome signaling. Cell 2015;163:1428–43.
71. O'Hara AM, Shanahan F. The gut flora as a forgotten organ. EMBO Rep 2006;7: 688–93.
72. Patel RM, Lin PW. Developmental biology of gut-probiotic interaction. Gut Microbes 2010;1:186–95.
73. Kau AL, Ahern PP, Griffin NW, et al. Human nutrition, the gut microbiome and the immune system. Nature 2011;474:327–36.
74. Turnbaugh PJ, Gordon JI. The core gut microbiome, energy balance and obesity. J Physiol 2009;587:4153–8.
75. Surana NK, Kasper DL. Deciphering the tête-à-tête between the microbiota and the immune system. J Clin Invest 2014;124:4197–203.
76. Carmody RN, Turnbaugh PJ. Host-microbial interactions in the metabolism of therapeutic and diet-derived xenobiotics. J Clin Invest 2014;124:4173–81.
77. Mayer EA, Tillisch K, Gupta A. Gut/brain axis and the microbiota. J Clin Invest 2015;125:926–38.
78. Medzhitov R. Origin and physiological roles of inflammation. Nature 2008;452: 428–35.
79. Lebeer S, Vanderleyden J, De Keersmaecker SC. Host interactions of probiotic bacterial surface molecules: comparison with commensals and pathogens. Nat Rev Microbiol 2010;8:171–84.
80. Neish AS, Gewirtz AT, Zeng H, et al. Prokaryotic regulation of epithelial responses by inhibition of IκB-α ubiquitination. Science 2000;289:1560–3.
81. O'Mahony C, Scully P, O'Mahony D, et al. Commensal-induced regulatory T cells mediate protection against pathogen-stimulated NF-kappaB activation. PLoS Pathog 2008;4:e1000112.
82. Jones BV, Begley M, Hill C, et al. Functional and comparative metagenomic analysis of bile salt hydrolase activity in the human gut microbiome. Proc Natl Acad Sci U S A 2008;105:13580–5.
83. Forsythe P, Kunze W, Bienenstock J. Moody microbes or fecal phrenology: what do we know about the microbiota-gut-brain axis? BMC Med 2016;14:58.
84. Savidge TC. Epigenetic regulation of enteric neurotransmission by gut bacteria. Front Cell Neurosci 2016;9:503.
85. Kabouridis PS, Lasrado R, McCallum S, et al. The gut microbiota keeps enteric glial cells on the move; prospective roles of the gut epithelium and immune system. Gut Microbes 2015;6:398–403.
86. Dey N, Wagner VE, Blanton LV, et al. Regulators of gut motility revealed by a gnotobiotic model of diet-microbiome interactions related to travel. Cell 2015; 163:95–107.

87. Heijtz RD, Wang S, Anuar F, et al. Normal gut microbiota modulates brain development and behavior. Proc Natl Acad Sci U S A 2011;108:3047–52.
88. Neufeld KM, Kang N, Bienenstock J, et al. Reduced anxiety-like behavior and central neurochemical change in germ-free mice. Neurogastroenterol Motil 2011;23:255–64.
89. Bravo JA, Forsythe P, Chew MV, et al. Ingestion of Lactobacillus strain regulates emotional behavior and central GABA receptor expression in a mouse via the vagus nerve. Proc Natl Acad Sci U S A 2011;108:16050–5.
90. Yarandi SS, Peterson DA, Treisman GJ, et al. Modulatory effects of gut microbiota on the central nervous system: how gut could play a role in neuropsychiatric health and diseases. J Neurogastroenterol Motil 2016;22:201–12.
91. De Palma G, Blennerhassett P, Lu J, et al. Microbiota and host determinants of behavioural phenotype in maternally separated mice. Nat Commun 2015;6:7735.
92. Cryan JF, O'Mahony SM. The microbiome-gut-brain axis: from bowel to behavior. Neurogastroenterol Motil 2011;23:187–92.
93. De Palma G, Collins SM, Bercik P, et al. The microbiota-gut-brain axis in gastrointestinal disorders: stressed bugs, stressed brain or both? J Physiol 2014;592:2989–97.

From Culture to High-Throughput Sequencing and Beyond

A Layperson's Guide to the "Omics" and Diagnostic Potential of the Microbiome

Paul W. O'Toole, BA (Mod.), PhD*, Burkhardt Flemer, Dipl. Ing. (FH), PhD

KEYWORDS

- Microbiota • Microbiome • Gastrointestinal disease • Metagenome • FMT

KEY POINTS

- Sequence-based microbiota analyses provide fast and forensically detailed insights.
- Costs are becoming more affordable, but true metagenomic sequencing is still prohibitively expensive for routine application.
- Contrary to earlier impressions, a majority of intestinal bacteria can be cultured in the laboratory, but their fastidious nature makes it challenging.
- Alterations in microbiota composition already show promise as biomarkers for colorectal cancer (CRC), obesity, metabolic disease, and irritable bowel syndrome.

INTRODUCTION

Studies of the community of bacteria in the human intestine have had a major impact on gastroenterology research in the last decade. As summarized elsewhere in this issue, it is now appreciated that altered microbial communities in the gut are associated with a broad range of functional gastrointestinal disorders as well as being increasingly linked to extraintestinal diseases. It is important to point out that, at the time of writing, there are no examples other than *Clostridium difficile*–associated diarrhea (CDAD) where an altered microbiota is responsible for a disease and where the disease can be cured by restoring a normal microbiota. There is mounting evidence, however, for microbiota involvement in obesity, inflammatory bowel disease (IBD), irritable bowel syndrome, type 2 diabetes mellitus, and metabolic syndrome, and many microbiome start-up companies are scrambling to develop first-to-market

School of Microbiology & APC Microbiome Institute, University College Cork, Room 447, Food Science Building, Cork T12 Y337, Ireland
* Corresponding author.
E-mail address: pwotoole@ucc.ie

Gastroenterol Clin N Am 46 (2017) 9–17
http://dx.doi.org/10.1016/j.gtc.2016.09.003
0889-8553/17/© 2016 Elsevier Inc. All rights reserved.

therapeutics based on these conditions. The practicing gastroenterologist, therefore, benefits from an understanding of how the microbiota is studied and what the data mean. Microbiota profiling and microbiome-based diagnostics, however, will soon reach routine clinical application, because even if altered microbiota compositions do not ultimately prove responsible for the named or other diseases, the respective microbiota changes are being validated as novel biomarkers for disease risk. The purpose of this review is, therefore, to explain how microbiota composition and function are analyzed, to outline the scale of the technical and infrastructural investment required to start microbiota analysis from scratch, to convey the powers and limits of microbiota analysis by culture-dependent and independent analysis, and finally to show the potential for clinical application of microbiome analysis to identify disease risk.

SAMPLE TYPES, COLLECTION, TRANSPORT, AND STORAGE

Many studies of the gut microbiota/gut microbiome actually examine the fecal microbiota. The main reason for this is that it is difficult to collect luminal samples or mucosal biopsies from healthy people because they would be required to undergo colonoscopy, a request that usually does not receive ethical approval. So although it is well established that the fecal microbiota is different from that of intestinal mucosa,[1–3] analysis of fecal samples is a pragmatic and widely accepted compromise in many studies. Mucosal samples still provide interesting and uniquely informative data when available, such as jejunoscopy in small volunteer studies of probiotic effect on host gene transcription,[4] rectal biopsies offering microbiome-based diagnostic potential in pediatric Crohn disease,[5] and the presence of bacterial biofilms in right-sided colorectal biopsy tissue.[6] If designing a microbiome study of a clinical syndrome for the first time, it is prudent to include relevant mucosal biopsy samples if possible.

Mucosal biopsy samples may be conveniently collected during colonoscopy or bowel surgery; polyps are typically too small to allow microbiota analysis in addition to routine histology requirements.[2] Fecal samples can be collected by subjects in their own homes using a range of commercial kits that overcome the objectionable nature of this task for a majority of subjects. The authors endeavor to have the stool sample brought to the research laboratory for DNA extraction within 3 hours, without freezing, because freezing has modest but detectable effects on apparent microbiota composition.[7–10]

If a microbiome study is conducted in a single facility or geographic center, freezing samples at $-80°C$ as they are collected over time is a convenient way to bulk them and process them in batches. For studies that involve multiple clinical centers and sending samples to a single processing laboratory, the authors and other investigators have validated a commercial transport medium, which has a negligible effect on microbiota composition, providing an alternative to shipping samples on dry ice.[11,12] These samples can be processed, however, for nucleic acid extraction only and currently appear unsuitable for analyses, such as metabolomics, which would still be possible with frozen whole stool.

CULTURE-BASED ANALYSIS OF THE GUT MICROBIOME

An often-stated advantage of culture-independent microbiota analysis is that it solves the problem of the supposed unculturability of up to 70% of the microbiota. Studies featuring engraftment of human microbes to mice via a culture step[13] and several recent exhaustive bacteriologic culture studies,[14,15] however, have shown that it is possible to culture more than 95% of microbiota members present at more than

0.1% relative abundance. These were essentially targeted studies, where the goal was to capture as much of the phylogenetic diversity of the microbiota as possible. Other studies have pragmatically focused on culturing of sufficient microbiota diversity to allow laboratory isolates to be blended in an artificial stool cocktail that effectively replaced whole feces in fecal microbiota transplantation (FMT) to successfully treat CDAD.[16] Bacteriologic culture of fastidious anaerobic organisms is an undertaking for specialist laboratories, requiring anaerobic cabinets, dedicated gas equipment, and a level of operating skill surpassing that required for routine bacteriologic analysis in the clinic. Achieving comprehensive species coverage is also time consuming and expensive; 1 recent study used 33 different culture media.[15] Whether or not this investment is feasible or worthwhile depends on the value to the investigator of recovering microbial taxa from the condition of interest. Fecal collection from the donor must be accomplished quickly and the stool must be moved into an anaerobic device for transport to the anaerobic cabinet in the laboratory. Whether or not the sample is made into a suspension and frozen and in what cryoprotectant requires consideration.

The significant advantage of culture-based studies is that the cultured organisms become available for biological studies and potential exploitation as therapeutics. Examples of cultured gut commensals include *Faecalibacterium prausnitzii*, which was identified as being depleted in the microbiota of IBD patients[17] and is being developed as a therapeutic,[18] and *Eubacterium hallii*, which is less abundant in subjects with metabolic syndrome but is restored during an FMT[19] that provides some restoration of insulin sensitivity. Successful culture of fastidious anaerobes will add to the increasing commercial interest in exploiting the microbiome for novel therapeutics, evidenced by the numbers of new start-up companies in this area.[20]

DNA EXTRACTION METHODS

Choosing an appropriate DNA extraction technique is critical for successful analysis of microbial ecosystems using next-generation sequencing workflows. To achieve optimal cell disruption, particularly of archaeal and gram-positive bacterial cell walls, a mechanical lysis step needs to be included in the protocol.[21] This usually involves the addition of glass or silica beads of various sizes (0.1 mm, 1 mm, and 4–5 mm) to fecal samples and homogenizing them with a bead-beater device. Different extraction methods can lead to different sequencing results,[22] so it is thus important to use the same protocol for all samples in a study. The International Human Microbiome Standards project (http://www.microbiome-standards.org/) aims to define the best extraction method for fecal samples. The outcome will be important for the research community because it will provide valid recommendations for standardized protocols, which are a prerequisite for applying outcomes to clinical settings. Many different extraction methods are currently available and several companies sell nucleic acid extraction kits optimized for various sample types, such as stool, saliva, tissue, or skin. The general principles for extraction of nucleic acids from such different tissue types are similar but, for example, stool contains many polymerase chain reaction (PCR) inhibitors that are effectively removed with dedicated commercial products.

MICROBIOTA COMPOSITION DETERMINATION

The simplest and cheapest way to study the microbiota is to generate a list of the bacteria present by sequencing a pool of amplicons generated by a PCR reaction targeting a region of the 16S ribosomal RNA gene. This gene is present in all cells (including in mammalian cells where it is called 18S) and it encodes an RNA strand that forms part of the ribosome involved in transcript binding to initiate translation. An adaptation of the protocol is to hybridize the amplicon pool to a chip bearing oligonucleotides specific for individual bacterial taxa, and this protocol seems to yield substantially similar data to amplicon sequencing,[23] although it is more laborious and it is slower throughput compared with current sequencing technologies. Most investigators use the same universal primers for all samples, purify the PCR product, and perform a second index PCR with a primer pair featuring a unique barcode identifier in the primer for each sample. These amplicons are then purified and mixed in equimolar amounts for sequencing on a massively parallel instrument.

A vast array of 16S amplification primers and protocols for amplicon sequencing have been developed in multiple laboratories over the past decade, often accompanying changes in the dominant sequencing platform[24] and the read-length available. For a new user investigating the microbiome in a clinical context, there is a bewildering choice of protocols available. For a detailed technical analysis of current options and protocol recommendations, readers are referred to an excellent study by Gohl and colleagues[25] and an imminent publication from the International Human Microbiome Standards project (http://www.microbiome-standards.org/).

Currently the most popular sequencing platform is probably the Illumina MiSeq (Illumina, San Diego, California, USA), which offers 2 × 300 base pair paired end reads and a run cost for 384 samples that brings the pure sequencing cost to below €10 per sample. This platform was recently used in a demonstration of how microbiome analysis can be accelerated to a 48-hour test.[26] In practice, in the authors' laboratory, 285 samples per run is not exceeded, and the per-sample cost does not include reagent, primer, and staff costs for amplicon preparation. Nevertheless, compared with 10 years ago and the original pyrosequencing protocols, this is a huge cost improvement.

No amplicon sequencing methods are completely free of bias and the best solution is to apply shotgun metagenomics sequencing (discussed later). This is a more challenging prospect for new users because the per-sample cost may be 20 to 30 times higher than amplicon sequencing, the data sets are much larger, and current significant data storage and analysis present challenges.

MICROBIOME FUNCTION

16S ribosomal RNA (rRNA) amplicon sequencing only provides a census of the bacteria in an ecosystem. Despite recent efforts to (predictively) link the results obtained through 16S rRNA sequencing to functional properties of the microbiota,[27] this approach only provides an approximation of the functional potential. First, the conventional sequence similarity cutoff of 97% used to group sequencing reads into operational taxonomic units (OTUs) leads to loss of actual diversity. Thus, differences in genetic content between species[28] grouped in the same OTU are missed using this approach. Furthermore, many genomic differences may be present even between members of the same bacterial species; for example, pks^+ *Escherichia coli* harbors a pathogenicity island that is implicated in the development of CRC[29] but 16S rRNA amplicon sequencing is not able to distinguish between commensal and pathogenic *E coli*. Thus, detailed studies of the functions associated with distinct microbiota types (the microbiome) necessarily use metagenomics shotgun sequencing, that is, sequencing of the whole DNA content of a bacterial ecosystem. Thus researchers were able to define typical functional profiles associated with health and disease.[30–32] Although metagenomics shotgun sequencing provides finer resolution information on the microbial ecosystem, the costs associated with such an analysis prohibit its use in routine diagnostic settings. Similarly, the study of all expressed genes in an ecosystem, metatranscriptomics, is too expensive to be carried out routinely for diagnostic purposes. Moreover, computational requirements for processing meta-transcriptomic and metagenomic shotgun sequencing data are significantly higher than those for 16S rRNA amplicon sequencing, making the availability of powerful servers a prerequisite for such an analysis.

COMPUTATIONAL APPROACHES AND REQUIREMENTS FOR NEW USERS

A typical pipeline for the analysis of 16S rRNA amplicon sequencing data from the Illumina MiSeq sequencing platform starts with demultiplexing of the raw sequences. Sequences are assigned to individual samples based on multiplex barcode identifiers introduced during library preparation. This is followed by a quality filtering step and merging of paired-end sequencing reads to form single reads. Primer-binding sites, which are largely uninformative for taxonomic classification, are removed. Then, in open-reference OTU picking, the reads are clustered into OTUs, usually at 97% sequence similarity roughly representing bacterial species. Chimeras (artifacts of PCR) must be removed, for example, by searching against a curated 16S rRNA database (eg, Gold database available at https://gold.jgi.doe.gov/) and finally an OTU table is obtained by mapping the original reads to representative OTU sequences. In closed-reference OTU picking, sequencing reads are directly mapped onto an existing database of OTUs, such as Greengenes.[33] Classification of OTUs, usually to the bacterial genus, is achieved by searching against 16S rRNA catalogs, such as Ribosomal Database Project or Greengenes.[33,34] The OTU table and classification form the basis for statistical analysis using, for example, the open-source statistical programming language R[35] or commercially available programs, such as SPSS.

Contemporary software, such as Mothur,[36] QIIME,[37] or Usearch,[38] combine all these sequence processing steps in 1 package and, therefore, are a good starting point for newcomers to microbiota analysis. Illumina also provides an in-house sequence analysis platform BaseSpace through the cloud. Finally DADA2 has recently been provided as an R-based pipeline, which can be used to perform all of the above steps, including biostatistical analyses on a normal laptop.[39] Recent developments in 16S rRNA amplicon sequencing data analysis pipelines make it possible to analyze the data associated with, for example, Illumina MiSeq platforms on a laptop computer, so some degree of autonomy from servers and mainframes is possible for parts of the analysis process.

DIAGNOSTIC POTENTIAL

Although many studies have reported significant microbiota composition differences between healthy and disease states, considerable overlap is usually also present, which requires identification of the most distinguishing organisms to use the microbiota for diagnostic purposes.[5] Moreover, in the gastroenterology context, abundance differences of single microbial organisms found at mucosal sites are often not detected in fecal samples[2,5] indicating that fecal microbiota at least partially fails to reflect relevant differences. Consequentially, fecal microbiota from a new-onset IBD case-control population could not be used to reliably predict disease (area under the curve [AUC] of 0.66) whereas microbiota associated with ileal and rectal biopsies performed well as a predictor (AUC 0.85 and AUC 0.78, respectively).[5] Tests carried out with fecal microbiota from children suffering from IBD for 34.8 months on average, however, obtained much higher sensitivity (80.3%) and specificity (69.7%). In pediatric IBD cases, this represents a powerful tool because doctors are usually reluctant to recommend colonoscopy for children.[40] The composition of the (fecal) microbiota has been assessed in several studies for its potential to serve as a noninvasive means to detect CRC. Consistent increase in the abundance of bacterial taxa, such as *Peptostreptococcus stomatis, Parvimonas micra, Porphyromonas* spp, and *Fusobacterium nucleatum*, has been observed in fecal samples from individuals with CRC.[32,41–44] Zeller and colleagues[32] identified 22 metagenomic microbial markers for the detection of CRC (AUC 0.84), including possibly oral pathogens that were most discriminative in this model. Baxter and colleagues[41] reported, however, that the abundance of these taxa did not contribute much to their model of detecting CRC with both fecal immune test and fecal microbiota because of their high correlation with the results of the fecal immune test. But overall the potential of the microbiota to complement existing noninvasive tests for better early detection, particularly of adenomas (AUC increase from 0.639 to 0.755) was highlighted in this study.[41] Yu and colleagues[44] identified 2 genes in a metagenomics data set, which could be quantified by quantitative PCR and reached an AUC of 0.84 for the detection of CRC, including stage I and stage II cancers.

Other diseases where the potential for microbiota-based diagnosis is encouraging include obesity, where individuals with a low gene count are less likely to respond well to intervention[45]; type 2 diabetes mellitus, where particular taxa are enriched[46]; and irritable bowel syndrome in which only a subset of patients has an altered microbiota.[47] Continued research is expected to identify other syndromes for which intestinal microbiota may be profiled as a predictive biomarker.

SUMMARY

Microbiome analysis is an exciting addition to the gastroenterologist's armory that is moving from being an interesting research method to offering potential for routine application. Microbiome research is still a young discipline, and the most groundbreaking discoveries are still being replicated, but research-active gastroenterologists can expect to either generate or evaluate microbiota data in coming years, and analysis of this data may also enter into the clinic soon. For research applications, a newcomer to the field should establish collaborations with an established practitioner and import a functional biological and bioinformatics pipeline en masse but still pay attention to the technical pitfalls highlighted in this review.

ACKNOWLEDGMENTS

This work was supported, in part, by Science Foundation Ireland through a Centre award to the APC Microbiome Institute (SFI/12/RC/2273).

REFERENCES

1. Eckburg PB, Bik EM, Bernstein CN, et al. Diversity of the human intestinal microbial flora. Science 2005;308(5728):1635–8.
2. Flemer B, Lynch DB, Brown JM, et al. Tumour-associated and non-tumour-associated microbiota in colorectal cancer. Gut 2016. [Epub ahead of print].
3. Zoetendal EG, von Wright A, Vilpponen-Salmela T, et al. Mucosa-associated bacteria in the human gastrointestinal tract are uniformly distributed along the colon and differ from the community recovered from feces. Appl Environ Microbiol 2002;68(7):3401–7.
4. van Baarlen P, Troost FJ, van Hemert S, et al. Differential NF-kappaB pathways induction by Lactobacillus plantarum in the duodenum of healthy humans correlating with immune tolerance. Proc Natl Acad Sci U S A 2009; 106(7):2371–6.

5. Gevers D, Kugathasan S, Denson LA, et al. The treatment-naive microbiome in new-onset Crohn's disease. Cell Host Microbe 2014;15(3):382–92.
6. Dejea CM, Wick EC, Hechenbleikner EM, et al. Microbiota organization is a distinct feature of proximal colorectal cancers. Proc Natl Acad Sci U S A 2014; 111(51):18321–6.
7. Bahl MI, Bergstrom A, Licht TR. Freezing fecal samples prior to DNA extraction affects the Firmicutes to Bacteroidetes ratio determined by downstream quantitative PCR analysis. FEMS Microbiol Lett 2012;329(2):193–7.
8. Dominianni C, Wu J, Hayes RB, et al. Comparison of methods for fecal microbiome biospecimen collection. BMC Microbiol 2014;14:103.
9. Voigt AY, Costea PI, Kultima JR, et al. Temporal and technical variability of human gut metagenomes. Genome Biol 2015;16:73.
10. Fouhy F, Deane J, Rea MC, et al. The effects of freezing on faecal microbiota as determined using MiSeq sequencing and culture-based investigations. PLoS One 2015;10(3):e0119355.
11. Hill CJ, Brown JR, Lynch DB, et al. Effect of room temperature transport vials on DNA quality and phylogenetic composition of faecal microbiota of elderly adults and infants. Microbiome 2016;4(1):19.
12. Choo JM, Leong LE, Rogers GB. Sample storage conditions significantly influence faecal microbiome profiles. Sci Rep 2015;5:16350.
13. Faith JJ, Ahern PP, Ridaura VK, et al. Identifying gut microbe-host phenotype relationships using combinatorial communities in gnotobiotic mice. Sci Transl Med 2014;6(220):220ra211.
14. Browne HP, Forster SC, Anonye BO, et al. Culturing of 'unculturable' human microbiota reveals novel taxa and extensive sporulation. Nature 2016;533(7604): 543–6.
15. Lau JT, Whelan FJ, Herath I, et al. Capturing the diversity of the human gut microbiota through culture-enriched molecular profiling. Genome Med 2016;8(1):72.
16. Petrof EO, Gloor GB, Vanner SJ, et al. Stool substitute transplant therapy for the eradication of Clostridium difficile infection: 'RePOOPulating' the gut. Microbiome 2013;1(1):3.
17. Manichanh C, Rigottier-Gois L, Bonnaud E, et al. Reduced diversity of faecal microbiota in Crohn's disease revealed by a metagenomic approach. Gut 2006; 55(2):205–11.
18. Quevrain E, Maubert MA, Michon C, et al. Identification of an anti-inflammatory protein from Faecalibacterium prausnitzii, a commensal bacterium deficient in Crohn's disease. Gut 2016;65(3):415–25.
19. Vrieze A, Van Nood E, Holleman F, et al. Transfer of intestinal microbiota from lean donors increases insulin sensitivity in individuals with metabolic syndrome. Gastroenterology 2012;143(4):913–6.e7.
20. Olle B. Medicines from microbiota. Nat Biotechnol 2013;31(4):309–15.
21. Salonen A, Nikkila J, Jalanka-Tuovinen J, et al. Comparative analysis of fecal DNA extraction methods with phylogenetic microarray: effective recovery of bacterial and archaeal DNA using mechanical cell lysis. J Microbiol Methods 2010; 81(2):127–34.
22. Wesolowska-Andersen A, Bahl MI, Carvalho V, et al. Choice of bacterial DNA extraction method from fecal material influences community structure as evaluated by metagenomic analysis. Microbiome 2014;2:19.
23. Claesson MJ, O'Sullivan O, Wang Q, et al. Comparative analysis of pyrosequencing and a phylogenetic microarray for exploring microbial community structures in the human distal intestine. PLoS One 2009;4(8):e6669.

24. Claesson MJ, Wang Q, O'Sullivan O, et al. Comparison of two next-generation sequencing technologies for resolving highly complex microbiota composition using tandem variable 16S rRNA gene regions. Nucleic Acids Res 2010; 38(22):e200.

25. Gohl DM, Vangay P, Garbe J, et al. Systematic improvement of amplicon marker gene methods for increased accuracy in microbiome studies. Nat Biotechnol 2016;34(9):942–9.

26. Quinn RA, Navas-Molina JA, Hyde ER, et al. From sample to Multi-Omics conclusions in under 48 Hours. mSystems 2016;1(2):e00038-16.

27. Langille MG, Zaneveld J, Caporaso JG, et al. Predictive functional profiling of microbial communities using 16S rRNA marker gene sequences. Nat Biotechnol 2013;31(9):814–21.

28. Sun Z, Harris HM, McCann A, et al. Expanding the biotechnology potential of lactobacilli through comparative genomics of 213 strains and associated genera. Nat Commun 2015;6:8322.

29. Arthur JC, Perez-Chanona E, Muhlbauer M, et al. Intestinal inflammation targets cancer-inducing activity of the microbiota. Science 2012;338(6103):120–3.

30. Consortium HMP. A framework for human microbiome research. Nature 2012; 486(7402):215–21.

31. Qin J, Li R, Raes J, et al. A human gut microbial gene catalogue established by metagenomic sequencing. Nature 2010;464(7285):59–65.

32. Zeller G, Tap J, Voigt AY, et al. Potential of fecal microbiota for early-stage detection of colorectal cancer. Mol Syst Biol 2014;10:766.

33. DeSantis TZ, Hugenholtz P, Larsen N, et al. Greengenes, a chimera-checked 16S rRNA gene database and workbench compatible with ARB. Appl Environ Microbiol 2006;72(7):5069–72.

34. Cole JR, Wang Q, Fish JA, et al. Ribosomal Database Project: data and tools for high throughput rRNA analysis. Nucleic Acids Res 2014;42(Database issue): D633–42.

35. R Development Core Team. R: A language and environment for statistical computing. Vienna (Austria): R Foundation for Statistical Computing; 2013.

36. Schloss PD, Westcott SL, Ryabin T, et al. Introducing mothur: open-source, platform-independent, community-supported software for describing and comparing microbial communities. Appl Environ Microbiol 2009;75(23):7537–41.

37. Caporaso JG, Kuczynski J, Stombaugh J, et al. QIIME allows analysis of high-throughput community sequencing data. Nat Methods 2010;7(5):335–6.

38. Edgar RC. Search and clustering orders of magnitude faster than BLAST. Bioinformatics 2010;26(19):2460–1.

39. Callahan BJ, McMurdie PJ, Rosen MJ, et al. DADA2: High-resolution sample inference from Illumina amplicon data. Nat Methods 2016;13(7):581–3.

40. Papa E, Docktor M, Smillie C, et al. Non-invasive mapping of the gastrointestinal microbiota identifies children with inflammatory bowel disease. PLoS One 2012; 7(6):e39242.

41. Baxter NT, Ruffin MT, Rogers MA, et al. Microbiota-based model improves the sensitivity of fecal immunochemical test for detecting colonic lesions. Genome Med 2016;8(1):37.

42. Zackular JP, Rogers MA, Ruffin MT, et al. The Human Gut Microbiome as a Screening Tool for Colorectal Cancer. Cancer Prev Res (Phila) 2014;7(11): 1112–21.

43. Nakatsu G, Li X, Zhou H, et al. Gut mucosal microbiome across stages of colorectal carcinogenesis. Nat Commun 2015;6:8727.

44. Yu J, Feng Q, Wong SH, et al. Metagenomic analysis of faecal microbiome as a tool towards targeted non-invasive biomarkers for colorectal cancer. Gut 2015. [Epub ahead of print].

45. Le Chatelier E, Nielsen T, Qin J, et al. Richness of human gut microbiome correlates with metabolic markers. Nature 2013;500(7464):541–6.

46. Pedersen HK, Gudmundsdottir V, Nielsen HB, et al. Human gut microbes impact host serum metabolome and insulin sensitivity. Nature 2016;535(7612):376–81.

47. Jeffery IB, O'Toole PW, Ohman L, et al. An irritable bowel syndrome subtype defined by species-specific alterations in faecal microbiota. Gut 2012;61: 997–1006.

Biology of the Microbiome 1

Interactions with the Host Immune Response

Sylwia Smolinska, PhD[a], David Groeger, PhD[b],
Liam O'Mahony, PhD[c],*

KEYWORDS

- Microbiome • Innate immune system • Adaptive immune system • SCFA
- Histamine

KEY POINTS

- Highly sophisticated cellular and molecular networks need to be constantly coordinated in order to tolerate the presence of many diverse bacteria on mucosal surfaces.
- Different types of bacteria induce different immune responses, and these effects are strain specific.
- Bacterial metabolism of dietary factors generates metabolites, which have significant effects on host immune responses.
- More accurate endotyping of patients with inflammatory disorders may be assisted by determining the composition and metabolic activity of an individual's microbiome.
- Novel therapeutics directly targeting microbiome activities may be considered as complementary to existing drugs for treatment of inflammatory disorders.

INTRODUCTION

The mammalian gastrointestinal tract is a highly evolved system specialized to perform the essential functions of nutrient digestion, absorption, and waste disposal. The intestinal mucosal immune system must maintain intestinal integrity in the presence of a vast quantity of external or foreign antigens, such as food proteins and the microbiome. The

L. O'Mahony is a consultant to Alimentary Health Ltd and has received research funding from GSK. D. Groeger is an employee of AHPD. S. Smolinska has no conflicts of interest.

Financial support and sponsorship: The authors are supported by Swiss National Foundation grants (project numbers: CRSII3_154488, 310030_144219, 310030_127356, and 310030_144219), Allergiestiftung Ulrich Müller-Gierok, European Union Marie Curie grants, and by the Polish National Science Centre (grant number 2012/04/M/NZ6/00355).

[a] Department of Clinical Immunology, Wroclaw Medical University, Chalubinskiego 5, Wroclaw 50-368, Poland; [b] Alimentary Health Pharma Davos, Obere Strasse 22, Davos Platz 7270, Switzerland; [c] Molecular Immunology, Swiss Institute of Allergy and Asthma Research, University of Zurich, Obere Strasse 22, Davos Platz 7270, Switzerland
* Corresponding author.
E-mail address: liam.omahony@siaf.uzh.ch

ability to tolerate a wide range of bacterial antigens is a unique feature of the mucosal system that is not seen with the systemic immune system. Tolerance to food and microbial antigens at mucosal surfaces is not a passive process. Highly sophisticated cellular and molecular networks need to be constantly coordinated in order to tolerate the presence of many diverse bacteria, and protective immune responses to potential pathogens must be maintained and induced on demand. Expression of pattern recognition receptors (PRRs) allows the immune system to discriminate between commensal and harmful microbes. Inappropriate immune responses to bacterial or dietary antigens is a significant component in several intestinal pathologies, including inflammatory bowel disease, irritable bowel syndrome, and food allergies.[1,2]

The balance between immune tolerance and inflammation is regulated in part by the crosstalk between innate and adaptive immune cells and the intestinal microbiota. Disrupted communication between the microbiome and the host due to altered microbiome composition and/or metabolism is thought to negatively influence intestinal immune homeostatic networks.[3] This negative influence can be clearly seen in mice bred under germ-free or sterile conditions, whereby mucosal tolerance mechanisms do not fully develop; these mice display increased allergic sensitization to food antigens.[4] The deliberate modification of microbial species and their metabolism has led to the probiotic and prebiotic concepts.[5] Probiotics can be defined as live microorganisms that, when administered in adequate amounts, confer a health benefit on the host. Notably, the definition of a probiotic does not differentiate between the wide range of potential health benefits; it is clear that not all probiotics will influence the immune system in the same way. Prebiotics can be defined as selectively fermented ingredients that allow specific changes, both in the composition and/or activity in the gastrointestinal microflora, that confer benefits on host well-being and health. As with the probiotic definition, not all prebiotics will have the same effect on immunologic functions. The combination of probiotics and prebiotics is termed synbiotics.

The mucosal immune system is classified as organized or diffuse gut-associated lymphoid tissues (GALTs). The organized GALT includes Peyer patches, mesenteric lymph nodes, and solitary lymphoid follicles in the gut wall where antigen uptake, processing, and presentation occur. In contrast, diffuse GALT is a nonorganized system whereby individual cells, such as intraepithelial lymphocytes, are dispersed throughout the gut. Finally, epithelial cells themselves provide a barrier to antigen translocation and actively participate as sensors of luminal bacterial activity.

INNATE IMMUNE SYSTEM

The innate immune system is composed of many different cell types, and these cells are often the first cells to come into contact with intestinal microbes and their metabolic products.

Dendritic Cells

Intestinal dendritic cells are located within specific intestinal lymphoid tissues, collectively termed GALTs, or diffusely distributed throughout the intestinal lamina propria.[6] Dendritic cells are very important cells that act as sensors of microbial ligands through activation of innate immune receptors (eg, toll-like receptors [TLRs] and c-type lectin receptors). For example, a *Lactobacillus rhamnosus* bacterial strain is recognized by dendritic cell TLR-2 and Dendritic Cell-Specific Intercellular adhesion molecule-3-Grabbing Non-integrin.[7] The signaling pathways triggered by bacterial-derived molecules allow for changes in dendritic cell phenotypes and cytokine secretion, which polarize the subsequent adaptive T-cell immune response into T helper 1 (T_H1), T_H2,

T_H9, T_H17, T_H22, or T regulatory cells (T regs). Thus, appropriate dendritic cell recognition of microbial factors is key to the integration of microbial and/or host metabolism with immune functions (**Fig. 1**).

Metabolism of vitamin A to retinoic acid is a key immunomodulatory activity associated with intestinal dendritic cells.[8] Certain, but not all, intestinal microbes can induce retinoic acid metabolism by human dendritic cells in vitro and by murine CD103[+] dendritic cells within the small intestine lamina propria.[9,10] In contrast, *Helicobacter pylori* infection severely disrupted gastric retinoic acid biosynthesis, which could impair dendritic cell retinoic acid signaling and may contribute to disease progression.[11] In addition to vitamin A metabolism, induction of another dendritic cell metabolic enzyme, heme oxygenase-1, was shown to be required for induction of mucosal T regs within mesenteric lymph nodes by *Lactobacillus rhamnosus*.[12]

The influence of the microbiota on innate immune cells has been shown to affect the host response to cancer therapy. For example, germ-free mice and mice that are treated with antibiotics both show a diminished response to immunotherapy by CpG oligonucleotides and chemotherapy owing to the impaired function of myeloid-derived cells in the tumor microenvironment.[13] Furthermore, bifidobacteria enhance immunity to tumors through the augmentation of dendritic-cell function leading to better control of implanted syngeneic tumors by CD8-expressing T cells.[14] These studies

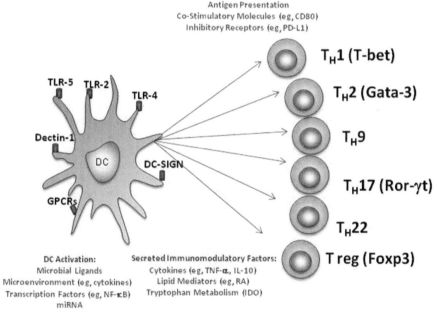

Fig. 1. Dendritic cell activation by microbes polarizes the adaptive immune response. Dendritic cells recognize microbial components and metabolites via PRRs (eg, toll-like receptors [TLRs], Nucleotide-binding oligomerization domain [NOD]) and GPCRs (eg, histamine receptor 2). Following activation, dendritic cells present antigen, alter cell surface expression of costimulatory or inhibitory molecules, and release mediators, such as cytokines or metabolites, which shape the subsequent adaptive immune response. DC, dendritic cell; GPCR, G protein-coupled receptor; IDO, Indoleamine-pyrrole 2,3-dioxygenase; IL, interleukin; NF-κB, nuclear factor kappa-light-chain-enhancer of activated B cells; PD-L1, Programmed death-ligand 1; RA, retinoic acid; TNF-α, tumor necrosis factor alpha.

open up a fascinating avenue of research whereby specific members of the micro-biome may promote antitumor innate immune responses that are required for cancer therapies to be successful.

Macrophages

Macrophages are professional myeloid phagocytes and are highly specialized in removal of host cellular debris, foreign substances, microbes, and cancer cells. Myeloid cells modulate important pathways, such as interleukin 22 (IL-22) production by innate lymphoid cells (ILCs), which induces the production of epithelial regenerating islet-derived protein 3 (RegIII)β and RegIIIγ, antimicrobial peptides that are important for maintaining a spatial separation between most commensal bacteria and the intestinal epithelial layer; this modulation is also pivotal for the local containment of commensals.[15–17] Local concentrations of microbiota-derived metabolites, as well as systemic levels of microbial products, seem to drive myeloid-cell differentiation and function through PRR signaling. Indeed, these microbiota-driven alterations in the myeloid-cell pool greatly influence the susceptibility of the host to a variety of disorders, which range from infection to allergy and asthma.[18–20] Intestinal microbial colonization drives the continuous replenishment of macrophages in the intestinal mucosa by monocytes that express C-C chemokine receptor type 2.[21] Microbial sensing by myeloid cells within the lamina propria provides regulatory signals that are crucial for the maintenance of commensal mutualism and the initiation of inflammatory responses in the host.[22]

Innate Lymphoid Cells

ILCs, a recently discovered lymphocyte branch of the innate immune system, develop normally in the absence of the microbiota; but the proper functioning of ILCs depend on commensal microbial colonization.[23–26] Similarly to T lymphocytes, which are classified according to their cytokine secretion and transcription factor expression, ILCs have been classified as ILC1, ILC2, and ILC3. Most studies that examine the influence of the microbiota on ILCs have focused on ILC3. The importance of ILC3 cells in host-microbiota interactions became clear when their depletion and the resulting abrogation of IL-22 production was shown to produce a loss of bacterial containment in the intestine.[16] However, other studies have reported elevated secretion of IL-22 by ILCs in the absence of the microbiota, whereas further studies have documented the abrogation of IL-22 secretion using antibiotics.[27] One part of this response, which may be important, is flagellin sensing by CD103$^+$ myeloid cells that drives IL-23-mediated production of IL-22 by ILCs.[28] In addition, the presentation of microbial antigens by ILC3s limits commensal-specific T-cell responses, which maintain tolerance to commensal bacteria.[29,30] An equally important microbiota-instructed function of ILCs is their communication with epithelial cells. Microbiota-induced IL-22 production by ILC3s induces expression of the enzyme fucosyltransferase 2 (galactoside 2-α-L-fucosyltransferase 2) and fucosylation of surface proteins by intestinal epithelial cells, which is required for host defense against enteric pathogens.[31] Indeed, this pathway may function to promote the growth of beneficial members of the microbiota and contribute to the maintenance of a stable community of microorganisms, as during the starvation associated with intestinal infection, the shedding of fucosylated proteins into the intestinal lumen serves as a source of energy for commensal bacteria.[32] The microbiota might also influence the activity of the other ILC subsets, such as ILC2s, which are activated by epithelial cell–derived IL-25 produced in a microbiota-dependent manner.[33]

Epithelial Cells

Although not classically considered to be bona fide members of the innate immune system, intestinal epithelial cells are equipped with an extensive repertoire of innate immune receptors. However, the most important job of the epithelial cell is nutrient absorption. Pathogen infection can reduce epithelial cell digestive enzyme activity; but this detrimental effect can be reversed by certain commensal microbes, possibly via modulation of mucosal inflammatory responses.[34,35] In addition to their absorptive function, epithelial cells form a mucosal barrier that protects host tissue from damaging agents such as luminal pathogens and toxic products. One protective barrier mechanism is the production and secretion of antimicrobial peptides, such as defensins and cathelicidins. Gut microbes have been shown to differentially regulate defensin expression and protein secretion, which is influenced by local inflammatory mediators.[36] Metabolites from the microbiome induce epithelial cell inflammasome signaling resulting in IL-18 secretion and antimicrobial peptide production.[37] Interestingly, host genetic deficiency in this pathway results in dysbiosis; this dysbiotic microbiome can hijack the microbiome of wild-type animals. Autophagy is an important adaptive response to stress, which promotes cell survival and is required for maintenance of the epithelial barrier. Several bifidobacteria have been recently described that promote autophagy in an intestinal cell line.[38] The mucous layer coating the gastrointestinal tract is an important barrier component, and gut bacteria have been shown to promote mucin production by goblet cells in the intestine. Recently, a protein called p40 from a lactobacillus strain was demonstrated to be sufficient for stimulation of mucin production through transactivation of the epithelial epidermal growth factor receptor.[39]

Excessive epithelial cell responses to microbial ligands result in local inflammatory responses, which disrupt the epithelial barrier. The presence of certain microbes can actually protect the epithelial cells and dampen the epithelial cell cytokine and chemokine responses.[40–42] However, not all chemokine responses are impacted to the same extent by every bacterial strain; a single bacterial strain may reduce expression of certain chemokines, while increasing the expression of others. For example, *Bifidobacterium bifidum* PRL2010 suppresses CCL22 expression but enhances CCL19 expression, suggesting that strain-specific and chemokine-specific responses are induced by gut bacteria.[43]

The PRR nucleotide-binding oligomerization domain-containing protein 2 (NOD2), which is highly expressed in the Paneth cells of the small intestine, is activated by microbial peptidoglycans present within the gut and generates a cellular response that includes the secretion of cytokines, the induction of autophagy, intracellular vesicle trafficking, epithelial regeneration, and the production of antimicrobial peptides, thereby influencing epithelial health and the composition of the microbiota.[44–46] Epithelial cell NOD1 expression is important for both the C-C motif chemokine 20–mediated generation of isolated lymphoid follicles in the intestine and control of bacterial colonization.[47] NOD1 is one of the important sensors that regulates the communication between the host and microorganisms through the production of inflammasome-mediated IL-18 and the downstream expression of antimicrobial peptides, and it also controls the secretion of mucus by goblet cells.[48]

ADAPTIVE IMMUNE SYSTEM

The adaptive immune system receives polarizing signals from the innate cells to expand an appropriately controlled lymphocyte response to bacterial and metabolic factors.

T Lymphocytes

The beneficial effects of microbiome interactions with the host immune response against diseases, such as allergy or colitis, are often associated with enhancement of T reg cells.[49,50] The main mechanisms underpinning T reg cell effects include production of inhibitory cytokines (IL-10, transforming growth factor [TGF]-β. and IL-35), effector cells cytolysis (via secretion of granzymes A and B), direct targeting of dentritic cells via inhibitory programmed cell death protein 1 and cytotoxic T-lymphocyte-associated protein 4 cell surface molecules, and metabolic disruption of effector cells (CD25, cAMP, adenosine, CD39, and CD73) and T reg cells that are induced by bacteria can have systemic antiinflammatory functions.[51] The relative contribution of individual members or defined communities within the gut microbiota in the accumulation and functional maturation of T reg cells in the intestine is starting to be documented. Clostridia strains that fall within clusters IV, XIVa, and XVIII seem to have a strong capacity for inducing the accumulation of T reg cells in the colon.[52,53] Clostridia from this cluster also stimulate ILC3s to produce IL-22, which helps to reinforce the epithelial barrier and reduces the permeability of the intestine to dietary proteins. Mice colonized by a microbiota that includes Clostridia display a suppressed response to food allergens.[54] Many other commensal microbes, such as *Bifidobacterium longum*, *Lactobacillus reuteri*, and *Lactobacillus murinus*, have been also shown to increase the proportion of T reg cells in mice.[55–59] Notably, consumption of *B longum* 35624 by healthy human volunteers resulted in an increased proportion of FOXP3 T reg cells in peripheral blood, whereas administration of this probiotic to patients with psoriasis, chronic fatigue syndrome, or ulcerative colitis consistently resulted in reduced levels of serum proinflammatory biomarkers, such as C- reactive protein, possibly mediated by increased numbers of T reg cells.[10,60]

Crosstalk between innate and adaptive cells to microbial signals promotes immune homeostasis in the intestine, including the induction of T regs. A recent study has revealed how complicated this crosstalk can be. Microbial signals sensed by intestinal macrophages resulted in IL-1β secretion, and this IL-1β promoted granulocyte macrophage colony-stimulating factor (GM-CSF) release by local ILC3 cells. ILC3-derived GM-CSF then triggers dendritic cell and macrophage secretion of retinoic acid and IL-10, which, in turn, promotes the induction and expansion of T regs. Disturbance of this crosstalk significantly altered mucosal immune effector functions, resulting in impaired oral tolerance to dietary antigens.[61] Interestingly, more severe allergic responses to food allergen challenge was observed in gnotobiotic mice reconstituted with microbes from allergic animals.[62] In this animal model, allergic responses were associated with a decreased abundance of Firmicutes and increased abundance of Proteobacteria. In contrast, Proteobacteria seemed to be less abundant in infants with atopic symptoms, which was hypothesized to be related to the lipopolysaccharide (LPS) incorporated into the bacteria cell wall. LPS drives T_H1 polarization by enhancing IL-12 secretion, which may dampen T_H2-dominant responses in atopic individuals. Collectively, there is considerable overlap between the responses of T reg cells to many (but not all) microbes present within the gut, which indicates that different cellular and molecular pathways supporting T reg generation and survival converge in the intestine. The induction and maintenance of T reg cells might be a common and crucial mechanism for maintaining the homeostatic and beneficial relationship between the microbiota and the host.

T_H17 cells secrete IL-17 that protects mucosal cells from infection, but exaggerated activity of this cell subset induces tissue inflammation. It was recently shown that the gut microbiota induces dendritic cells and macrophages to produce IL-1β and IL-6, which both drive T_H17 differentiation and arthritis.[63] The number of T_H17 cells in the intestines varies widely between animal facilities, even in genetically identical mice that have been reared in specific pathogen-free conditions, and often reflects whether mice have been colonized with segmented filamentous bacteria (SFB), and SFB also promote fucosylation of the epithelium through the activation of ILC3 cells.[31,64] On the other hand, gut-derived commensal bacteria have also been shown to suppress T_H17 responses both through direct and indirect mechanisms. $T_H17/IL-17$ activity can be suppressed by inducing T reg and/or T_H1 cell subsets, by induction of IL-27 production, which suppress the generation of IL-17 and induce IL-10 or by stimulation of TLR-9 on T_H17 cells.[65] These data suggest that the commensal microbiota is important for inducing both proinflammatory and regulatory responses in order to rapidly clear infections and minimize inflammation-associated tissue damage.

Natural Killer T Cells

Natural killer T (NKT) cells are central mediators of intestinal inflammation; pathogenic NKT cell activation is mediated by $CD1d^+$ bone-marrow-derived cells, whereas $CD1d^+$ epithelial cells protect against intestinal inflammation.[66] It has been shown that NKT cells can be influenced by the gut microbiome, and microbial lipid antigens may directly activate NKT cells.[67,68] Recently a healthy human volunteer study showed that the combination of xylo-oligosaccharide with Bifidobacterium animalis reduced CD16/56 expression on NKT cells.[69] However, the functional consequences of altered NKT cell activation by the microbiome in humans remain to be determined.

B Cells

B lymphocytes have an essential role in humoral immune responses via their secretion of antigen-specific antibodies. In addition, B cells can limit aggressive immune reactivity. B cells regulate immune responses mainly via IL-10, which has been shown in experimental models of infection, allergic inflammation, and tolerance.[70] Indeed, the gut microbiota is important in driving the differentiation of IL-10–producing B regulatory cells.[63]

B cell–dependent modulation of the microbiome was shown in immunoglobulin A (IgA)–deficient mice. IgA-deficient mice had persistent intestinal colonization with γ-Proteobacteria that cause sustained intestinal inflammation and increased susceptibility to neonatal and adult models of intestinal injury. The group also identified an IgA-dependent mechanism responsible for the maturation of the intestinal microbiota in mice.[71] Recently another group showed that the number of gut-homing IgG+ and IgA+ B cells was significantly higher in infants compared with adults. This finding suggests that activation of naïve B cells in the gut overlaps with the establishment of the gut microbiota in humans.[72] Oral administration of Lactobacillus gasseri SBT2055 (LG2055) induced IgA production and increased the number of IgA+ cells in Peyer patches and in the lamina propria. Combined stimulation of B cells with B-cell activating factor and LG2055 enhanced the induction of IgA production. Clostridia-induced T reg cells support the production of IgA in the intestine, which contributes to increased diversity of the microbiota and, in particular, of Clostridia.[73] Communication between B cells and other cell types is important for IgA production, as the secretion of lymphotoxin-α (also known as tumor necrosis factor-β) by ILC3s is crucial for the production of B-cell IgA and for microbiota homeostasis in the intestine.[74] In the absence of IgA, the commensal bacterium Bacteroides thetaiotaomicron, which typically does not trigger inflammation in the human gut, expresses high levels of gene products that are involved in the metabolism of nitric oxide and elicits proinflammatory signals in the host.[75] IgA that has undergone affinity maturation through somatic hypermutation binds to and selects for particular components of the microbiota, which leads to an increase in the diversity of the microbial community and enhances mutualism between the microbiota and the host.[73] Consistent with this observation, people who are deficient in IgA have more bacteria from taxa with potentially inflammatory properties.[76] Mice that are deficient in T cells owing to a lack of T-cell antigen receptor chains β and δ, as well as those that lack T follicular cells and the T-cell-dependent IgA pathway owing to T-cell-specific inactivation of the gene Bcl6 in CD4+ T cells, retain an IgA-mediated response that is specific to antigens from commensal bacteria, indicating that T-cell–independent B-cell IgA production is directed at the microbiota.[77] However, this response is characterized largely by the low-affinity binding of IgA to antigens that are shared by multiple species of bacteria.[78] Thus, B-cell–derived IgA plays an important role in host defense against mucosally transmitted pathogens, controls the adherence of commensal bacteria to epithelial cells, and neutralizes bacterial toxins to maintain homeostasis at the mucosal surfaces.[79]

BACTERIAL FACTORS THAT INFLUENCE MUCOSAL IMMUNE RESPONSES

Bacterial cell wall components and metabolites from the microbiome have been associated with immunoregulatory effects within the gut mucosa. For example, major histocompatibility complex II–dependent presentation of segmented filamentous bacterial antigens by intestinal CD11c$^+$ dendritic cells promotes the local induction of T_H17 lymphocytes.[64] In addition, capsular polysaccharide A (PSA) from *Bacteroides fragilis* has been shown to interact directly with mouse plasmacytoid dendritic cells via TLR-2. PSA-exposed plasmacytoid dendritic cells express molecules involved in protection against colitis and stimulated CD4$^+$ cells to secrete IL-10.[80] *B fragilis* boosts the production of IL-10 by T reg cells of the colon, and this activity is mediated by polysaccharide A70 from the bacterium's capsule.[81] Outer-membrane vesicles containing PSA that are released by *B fragilis* might also be taken up by dendritic cells of the intestine to stimulate their production of IL-10 through TLR-2 signaling. The IL-10 from these dendritic cells might then induce T reg cells to also produce IL-10. Similarly, an exopolysaccharide from *Bacillus subtilis* prevents gut inflammation stimulated by *Citrobacter rodentium*, which depends on TLR-4 and MyD88 signaling.[82]

The production of short-chain fatty acids (SCFA) occurs in the colon following microbiome fermentation of dietary fibers, and SCFAs can also be consumed in certain foods, such as butter.[83] SCFAs are an important energy source for colonocytes and regulate the assembly and organization of tight junctions. Abnormalities in the production of these metabolites (due to dietary factors and/or dysbiosis) might play a role in the pathogenesis of type 2 diabetes, obesity, inflammatory bowel disease, colorectal cancer, and allergies.[84] SCFAs can modulate epithelial barrier function, production of antimicrobial peptides, and secretion of proinflammatory mediators.[85,86] Among the SCFA, butyrate seems to be more potent than acetate or propionate in inducing immunomodulatory effects. Butyrate influences the activity of histone deacetylases (HDAC), which is responsible for decreasing dendritic cell IL-12 and IL-6 cytokine secretion and allows dendritic cells to promote T reg cells. Propionate can also contribute to the induction of T-cell FOXP3 expression by dendritic cells, whereas acetate does not have this activity possibly because of the lack of HDAC activity.[87] Butyrate also inhibits intestinal macrophage HDAC.[88] Another recent study has confirmed and extended the observation that butyrate promotes dendritic cell regulatory activity resulting in the induction of T reg cells and IL-10–secreting T cells. These effects were mediated by the g protein–coupled receptor GPR109a on colonic dendritic cells and macrophages.[89] In contrast, butyrate has also been shown to promote IL-23 secretion by murine dendritic cells, which may promote T_H17 responses under certain circumstances.[90] In addition to dendritic cells, direct effects on lymphocytes can also be mediated by SCFA, such as acetate, propionate, butyrate, and n-butyrate. Oral administration of a mixture of 17 Clostridia strains to mice attenuated the severity of colitis and allergic diarrhea in a T reg-TGF-β–dependent mechanism. This process is most likely due to SCFA produced by the Clostridia strains.[52,91] In addition to GPR109a, GPR43 is also a receptor for SCFAs. GPR43 signaling ameliorates diseases, such as colitis, inflammatory arthritis, and allergic airway diseases.[91,92] GPR43 is expressed by neutrophils and eosinophils, and GPR43 expression on colonic inducible T reg cells is associated with their expansion and IL-10 secretion. As already described earlier for dendritic cells, SCFAs inhibit HDAC activity also in lymphocytes enhancing histone H3 acetylation in the promoter and conserved noncoding sequence regions of the *Foxp3* locus.[91,93]

As bacterial metabolism of nondigestible fibers results in SCFA production, several studies have examined the influence of fiber consumption on immune responses. Mice fed a low-fiber diet before nasal sensitization with house dust mite extract developed higher local T_H2 responses within the lung, associated with increased mucus and goblet cell hyperplasia. In parallel, the composition of the microbiome changed, with increased Erysipelotrichaceae in the low-fiber group, whereas a high-fiber diet promoted Bacteroidaceae and Bifidobacteriaceae.[92] The high-fiber diet increased circulating levels of SCFA, and administration of the SCFA propionate enhanced generation of macrophage and dendritic cell precursors from the bone marrow. Subsequently the presence of dendritic cells with high phagocytic capacity in lung tissue was noted, associated with an impaired ability to induce T_H2 effector cell functions. These effects were shown to depend on GPR41 but not GPR43. In another allergic asthma mouse model, dietary fiber intake significantly influenced clinical symptoms, eosinophil infiltration, goblet cell metaplasia, serum allergen-specific IgE levels, as well as T_H2 cytokines in the nose and lung, which was paralleled by increased Bacteroidetes and Actinobacteria, with reduced abundance of Firmicutes and Proteobacteria in fecal samples.[94]

Microbial fermentation of amino acids results in the secretion of biogenic amines within the gut. For example, microbial decarboxylation of histidine generates histamine. Four host histamine receptors have been described (H1R–H4R), and histamine-induced immune effects depend on the type of receptor expressed by a specific cell.[95] The H2R has been shown to exert regulatory effects in multiple models, and histamine triggering of H2R on dendritic cells results in suppressed dendritic cell activation to microbial ligands.[96] Interestingly, mucosal histamine levels are increased in patients with irritable bowel syndrome and inflammatory bowel disease; but the cellular sources of histamine in these patients is not well described.[97] However, it was recently shown that patients with inflammatory bowel disease do display dysregulated expression of histamine receptors, with diminished antiinflammatory effects associated with H2R signaling.[98] Administration of a histamine-secreting *Lactobacillus* strain to mice resulted in rapid weight loss and influenced Peyer patch cytokine secretion, which was exaggerated in H2R-deficient animals.[99] In a separate study, the suppression of intestinal inflammation by a *Lactobacillus reuteri* strain was shown to depend on histamine secretion by the bacterium and its activation of H2R.[100] Recently, it was shown that histamine-secreting microbes are increased in the gut microbiome of adult patients with asthma, and histamine from these microbes may contribute to the effector responses in patients with atopic asthma.[101] Histamine-secreting *Escherichia coli*, *Lactobacillus vaginalis*, and *Morganella morganii* strains were isolated from the gut microbiome of these patients with asthma.

Thus, dietary intake of substrates required for microbial metabolism and generation of immunoregulatory compounds is essential. These data highlight the connection between nutrition, microbiome, and immune health (**Fig. 2**).

MICROBIOME EFFECTS EARLY IN LIFE

The timing of bacterial colonization early in life is thought to be important for appropriate immune education, and the transmission of microbes from the mother to the fetus during pregnancy and birth is being better described. Cultures of meconium have shown diverse groups of gram-positive and gram-negative bacteria, possibly not all derived after delivery. The development of the gut microbiome is a dynamic process, and early colonization with Bacteroides and Bifidobacterium species might play a crucial role in development of immune regulation.[102] Indeed, an absence of microbiota during this period of development leads to increases in the number of invariant

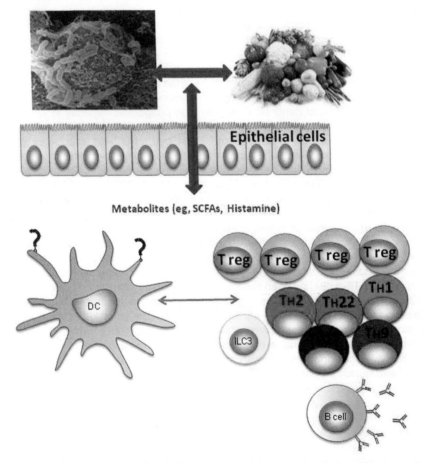

Fig. 2. Microbes and metabolites influence mucosal immune regulation. The type of microbes interacting with mucosal cells will influence host immune cell activity. Microbiome metabolism of dietary factors (eg, fiber) will also influence mucosal host cell activity, suggesting that microbiome-dietary interactions are important for immune homeostasis, resulting in balanced innate and adaptive responses.

natural killer T cells (iNKT) cells and in susceptibility to colitis and asthma in animal models. Early exposure to the gut microbiota suppresses the abundance of iNKT cells in the gut and lung, partly through the epigenetic suppression of the gene that encodes the chemokine chemokine (C-X-C motif) ligand 16.[67] Factors that can influence early life colonization include antibiotic treatment, method of delivery, maternal and infant diet, and biodiversity in the home, surrounding environment, and in family members. A delay in acquisition of a diverse microbiome or early life dysbiosis has been associated with an increased risk of later-life allergies and asthma. Children who developed asthma at school age had a lower gut microbiome diversity at 1 week or 1 month of age but not at 1 year of age compared with nonasthmatic children.[103] In another study, the early life relative abundance of the bacterial genera *Lachnospira*, *Veillonella*, *Faecalibacterium*, and *Rothia* was significantly decreased in children at risk of asthma. This dysbiosis was accompanied by reduced levels of fecal acetate and dysregulation of enterohepatic metabolites.[104] Colonization of mice with *Lachnospira*, *Veillonella*, *Faecalibacterium*, and *Rothia* mitigated airway inflammation in a model of allergic asthma, which raises the prospect that atopy or asthma could be averted by early therapy to correct dysbiosis.[104] In addition, decreased diversity of the Bacteroidetes phylum was reported in a separate study examining infants with atopic eczema.[105]

T_H2 cells dominate the immune system at birth. However, the human fetus has a functional immune system at a relative early status of development comprising $CD4^+$ and $CD8^+$ T cells but also FOXP3 T reg cells. One concept gaining support is that the developing fetus may become educated by whole bacteria or their genetic material that is provided via maternal serum. DNA from bifidobacteria and lactobacilli are found in the human placenta. In contrast, in utero exposure to potentially pathogenic bacteria, such us *Ureaplasma* species leads to immune dysregulation commonly ending in fatal complications.[106] Maternal consumption of probiotic-containing food components may reduce the risk for childhood allergic diseases, and mouse models demonstrate a reduced risk of inflammatory bowel diseases.[106] Epigenetic mechanisms may be critical as application of *Acinetobacter lwoffii* to pregnant mice reduced the airway hypersensitivity response of the offspring. The promoter region of interferon γ in $CD4^+$ T cells of the offspring had high levels of histone-4 acetylation, associated with enhanced transcription, whereas the IL-4 promoter region had lower levels of histone-4 acetylation. Moreover, exposure of pregnant mothers to the farm environment, which has high levels of *A lwoffii*, was associated with DNA demethylation of the FOXP3 locus and methylation of the T_H2-associated genes RAD50 and IL-13.[106]

Because the gut microbiota composition during the first months of life seems to be critical for the development of appropriate immune regulatory networks and thereby influence later-life disease risk, strategies to improve microbiome-immune response interactions (eg, using immunoregulatory probiotics) might be most effective at this age or even during pregnancy.

SUMMARY

Although it is clear that the microbiome significantly influences host immune maturation and immune activity, the molecular basis for these immunomodulatory mechanisms are only beginning to be elucidated. The presence of certain bacterial species or strains seems to be important, potentially because of the direct interactions with the host (eg, via PRR activation) or via their metabolic activity in vivo (eg, SCFAs generation). Diet is also important for the provision of the correct substrates for microbial metabolism. More accurate endotyping of patients with inflammatory disorders may be assisted by further analysis of the composition and metabolic activity of an individual's microbiome, and future clinical studies of new therapeutic agents should consider performing microbiome and metabolite analysis to determine if specific microbiome features correlate with responses to treatment. In addition, therapeutics directly targeting microbiome activities may be considered as complementary to existing drugs. Appropriately selected probiotics, prebiotics, or their combination may provide benefits for patients, particularly if administered early in life. A better description of the bacterial strains and metabolites, which influence immune function, will allow for improved design of future probiotic and prebiotic cocktails for prevention and treatment of immunologic disorders.

REFERENCES

1. Wang ZK, Yang YS, Chen Y, et al. Intestinal microbiota pathogenesis and fecal microbiota transplantation for inflammatory bowel disease. World J Gastroenterol 2014;20:14805–20.
2. Shanahan F, Quigley EM. Manipulation of the microbiota for treatment of IBS and IBD-challenges and controversies. Gastroenterology 2014;146:1554–63.
3. Frei R, Lauener RP, Crameri R, et al. Microbiota and dietary interactions: an update to the hygiene hypothesis? Allergy 2012;67:451–61.
4. Rodriguez B, Prioult G, Bibiloni R, et al. Germ-free status and altered caecal subdominant microbiota are associated with a high susceptibility to cow's milk allergy in mice. FEMS Microbiol Ecol 2011;76:133–44.
5. Frei R, Akdis M, O'Mahony L. Prebiotics, probiotics, synbiotics, and the immune system: experimental data and clinical evidence. Curr Opin Gastroenterol 2015; 31:153–8.
6. Schiavi E, Smolinska S, O'Mahony L. Intestinal dendritic cells. Curr Opin Gastroenterol 2015;31:98–103.
7. Konieczna P, Schiavi E, Ziegler M, et al. Human dendritic cell DC-SIGN and TLR-2 mediate complementary immune regulatory activities in response to Lactobacillus rhamnosus JB-1. PLoS One 2015;10:e0120261.
8. Bakdash G, Vogelpoel LT, van Capel TM, et al. Retinoic acid primes human dendritic cells to induce gut-homing, IL-10-producing regulatory T cells. Mucosal Immunol 2015;8:265–78.
9. Konieczna P, Ferstl R, Ziegler M, et al. Immunomodulation by Bifidobacterium infantis 35624 in the murine lamina propria requires retinoic acid-dependent and independent mechanisms. PLoS One 2013;8:e62617.
10. Konieczna P, Groeger D, Ziegler M, et al. Bifidobacterium infantis 35624 administration induces Foxp3 T regulatory cells in human peripheral blood: potential role for myeloid and plasmacytoid dendritic cells. Gut 2012;61:354–66.
11. Bimczok D, Kao JY, Zhang M, et al. Human gastric epithelial cells contribute to gastric immune regulation by providing retinoic acid to dendritic cells. Mucosal Immunol 2015;8:533–44.
12. Karimi K, Kandiah N, Chau J, et al. A Lactobacillus rhamnosus strain induces a heme oxygenase dependent increase in Foxp3+ regulatory T cells. PLoS One 2012;7:e47556.
13. Iida N, Dzutsev A, Stewart CA, et al. Commensal bacteria control cancer response to therapy by modulating the tumor microenvironment. Science 2013;342:967–70.
14. Sivan A, Corrales L, Hubert N, et al. Commensal Bifidobacterium promotes antitumor immunity and facilitates anti-PD-L1 efficacy. Science 2015;350:1084–9.

15. Vaishnava S, Yamamoto M, Severson KM, et al. The antibacterial lectin RegIIIγ promotes the spatial segregation of microbiota and host in the intestine. Science 2011;334:255–8.
16. Sonnenberg GF, Monticelli LA, Alenghat T, et al. Innate lymphoid cells promote anatomical containment of lymphoid-resident commensal bacteria. Science 2012;336:1321–5.
17. Zheng Y, Valdez PA, Danilenko DM, et al. Interleukin-22 mediates early host defense against attaching and effacing bacterial pathogens. Nat Med 2008;14: 282–9.
18. Ganal SC, Sanos SL, Kallfass C, et al. Priming of natural killer cells by nonmucosal mononuclear phagocytes requires instructive signals from commensal microbiota. Immunity 2012;37:171–86.
19. Kim YG, Udayanga KG, Totsuka N, et al. Gut dysbiosis promotes M2 macrophage polarization and allergic airway inflammation via fungi-induced PGE2. Cell Host Microbe 2014;15:95–102.
20. Hill DA, Siracusa MC, Abt MC, et al. Commensal bacteria-derived signals regulate basophil hematopoiesis and allergic inflammation. Nat Med 2012;18: 538–46.
21. Bain CC, Bravo-Blas A, Scott CL, et al. Constant replenishment from circulating monocytes maintains the macrophage pool in the intestine of adult mice. Nat Immunol 2014;15:929–37.
22. Franchi L, Kamada N, Nakamura Y, et al. NLRC4-driven production of IL-1β discriminates between pathogenic and commensal bacteria and promotes host intestinal defense. Nat Immunol 2012;13:449–56.
23. Sawa S, Cherrier M, Lochner M, et al. Lineage relationship analysis of RORγt+ innate lymphoid cells. Science 2010;330:665–9.
24. Sanos SL, Bui VL, Mortha A, et al. RORγt and commensal microflora are required for the differentiation of mucosal interleukin 22-producing NKp46+ cells. Nat Immunol 2009;10:83–91.
25. Satoh-Takayama N, Vosshenrich CA, Lesjean-Pottier S, et al. Microbial flora drives interleukin 22 production in intestinal NKp46+ cells that provide innate mucosal immune defense. Immunity 2008;29:958–70.
26. Sawa S, Lochner M, Satoh-Takayama N, et al. RORγt+ innate lymphoid cells regulate intestinal homeostasis by integrating negative signals from the symbiotic microbiota. Nat Immunol 2011;12:320–6.
27. Sonnenberg GF, Artis D. Innate lymphoid cell interactions with microbiota: implications for intestinal health and disease. Immunity 2012;37:601–10.
28. Kinnebrew MA, Buffie CG, Diehl GE, et al. Interleukin 23 production by intestinal CD103+CD11b+ dendritic cells in response to bacterial flagellin enhances mucosal innate immune defense. Immunity 2012;36:276–87.
29. Hepworth MR, Monticelli LA, Fung TC, et al. Innate lymphoid cells regulate CD4+ T-cell responses to intestinal commensal bacteria. Nature 2013;498: 113–7.
30. Hepworth MR, Fung TC, Masur SH, et al. Group 3 innate lymphoid cells mediate intestinal selection of commensal bacteria-specific CD4+ T cells. Science 2015; 348:1031–5.
31. Goto Y, Obata T, Kunisawa J, et al. Innate lymphoid cells regulate intestinal epithelial cell glycosylation. Science 2014;345:1254009.
32. Pickard JM, Maurice CF, Kinnebrew MA, et al. Rapid fucosylation of intestinal epithelium sustains host-commensal symbiosis in sickness. Nature 2014;514: 638–41.

33. von Moltke J, Ji M, Liang HE, et al. Tuft-cell-derived IL-25 regulates an intestinal ILC2-epithelial response circuit. Nature 2016;529:221–5.
34. Symonds EL, O'Mahony C, Lapthorne S, et al. Bifidobacterium infantis 35624 protects against salmonella-induced reductions in digestive enzyme activity in mice by attenuation of the host inflammatory response. Clin Transl Gastroenterol 2012;3:e15.
35. Scully P, Macsharry J, O'Mahony D, et al. Bifidobacterium infantis suppression of Peyer's patch MIP-1α and MIP-1β secretion during Salmonella infection correlates with increased local CD4+CD25+ T cell numbers. Cell Immunol 2013; 281:134–40.
36. Habil N, Abate W, Beal J, et al. Heat-killed probiotic bacteria differentially regulate colonic epithelial cell production of human β-defensin-2: dependence on inflammatory cytokines. Benef Microbes 2014;5:483–95.
37. Levy M, Thaiss CA, Zeevi D, et al. Microbiota-modulated metabolites shape the intestinal microenvironment by regulating NLRP6 inflammasome signaling. Cell 2015;163:1428–43.
38. Lin R, Jiang Y, Zhao X, et al. Four types of Bifidobacteria trigger autophagy response in intestinal epithelial cells. J Dig Dis 2014;15:597–605.
39. Wang L, Cao H, Liu L, et al. Activation of epidermal growth factor receptor mediates mucin production stimulated by p40, a Lactobacillus rhamnosus GG-derived protein. J Biol Chem 2014;289:20234–44.
40. Boonma P, Spinler JK, Venable SF, et al. Lactobacillus rhamnosus L34 and Lactobacillus casei L39 suppress Clostridium difficile-induced IL-8 production by colonic epithelial cells. BMC Microbiol 2014;14:177.
41. Ren DY, Li C, Qin YQ, et al. Lactobacilli reduce chemokine IL-8 production in response to TNF-α and Salmonella challenge of Caco-2 cells. Biomed Res Int 2013;2013:925219.
42. Sibartie S, O'Hara AM, Ryan J, et al. Modulation of pathogen-induced CCL20 secretion from HT-29 human intestinal epithelial cells by commensal bacteria. BMC Immunol 2009;10:54.
43. Turroni F, Taverniti V, Ruas-Madiedo P, et al. Bifidobacterium bifidum PRL2010 modulates the host innate immune response. Appl Environ Microbiol 2014;80: 730–40.
44. Couturier-Maillard A, Secher T, Rehman A, et al. NOD2-mediated dysbiosis predisposes mice to transmissible colitis and colorectal cancer. J Clin Invest 2013; 123:700–11.
45. Nigro G, Rossi R, Commere PH, et al. The cytosolic bacterial peptidoglycan sensor Nod2 affords stem cell protection and links microbes to gut epithelial regeneration. Cell Host Microbe 2014;15:792–8.
46. Ramanan D, Tang MS, Bowcutt R, et al. Bacterial sensor Nod2 prevents inflammation of the small intestine by restricting the expansion of the commensal Bacteroides vulgatus. Immunity 2014;41:311–24.
47. Bouskra D, Brézillon C, Bérard M, et al. Lymphoid tissue genesis induced by commensals through NOD1 regulates intestinal homeostasis. Nature 2008; 456:507–10.
48. Wlodarska M, Thaiss CA, Nowarski R, et al. NLRP6 inflammasome orchestrates the colonic host–microbial interface by regulating goblet cell mucus secretion. Cell. 2014;156:1045–59.
49. Kim HJ, Kim YJ, Lee SH, et al. Effects of Lactobacillus rhamnosus on allergic march model by suppressing Th2, Th17, and TSLP responses via CD4(+) CD25(+)Foxp3(+) Tregs. Clin Immunol 2014;153:178–86.

50. Liu Y, Fatheree NY, Mangalat N, et al. Human-derived probiotic Lactobacillus reuteri strains differentially reduce intestinal inflammation. Am J Physiol Gastrointest Liver Physiol 2010;299:1087–96.

51. Sakaguchi S, Wing K, Yamaguchi T. Dynamics of peripheral tolerance and immune regulation mediated by Treg. Eur J Immunol 2009;39:2331–6.

52. Atarashi K, Tanoue T, Oshima K, et al. Treg induction by a rationally selected mixture of Clostridia strains from the human microbiota. Nature 2013;500:232–6.

53. Atarashi K, Tanoue T, Shima T, et al. Induction of colonic regulatory T cells by indigenous Clostridium species. Science 2011;331:337–41.

54. Stefka AT, Feehley T, Tripathi P, et al. Commensal bacteria protect against food allergen sensitization. Proc Natl Acad Sci U S A 2014;111:13145–50.

55. Lyons A, O'Mahony D, O'Brien F, et al. Bacterial strain-specific induction of Foxp3+ T regulatory cells is protective in murine allergy models. Clin Exp Allergy 2010;40:811–9.

56. O'Mahony C, Scully P, O'Mahony D, et al. Commensal-induced regulatory T cells mediate protection against pathogen-stimulated NF-kappaB activation. PLoS Pathog 2008;4:e1000112.

57. Di Giacinto C, Marinaro M, Sanchez M, et al. Probiotics ameliorate recurrent Th1-mediated murine colitis by inducing IL-10 and IL-10- dependent TGF-β-bearing regulatory cells. J Immunol 2005;174:3237–46.

58. Karimi K, Inman MD, Bienenstock J, et al. Lactobacillus reuteri-induced regulatory T cells protect against an allergic airway response in mice. Am J Respir Crit Care Med 2009;179:186–93.

59. Tang C, Kamiya T, Liu Y, et al. Inhibition of Dectin-1 signaling ameliorates colitis by inducing Lactobacillus-mediated regulatory T cell expansion in the intestine. Cell Host Microbe 2015;18:183–97.

60. Groeger D, O'Mahony L, Murphy EF, et al. Bifidobacterium infantis 35624 modulates host inflammatory processes beyond the gut. Gut Microbes 2013;4:325–39.

61. Mortha A, Chudnovskiy A, Hashimoto D, et al. Microbiota-dependent crosstalk between macrophages and ILC3 promotes intestinal homeostasis. Science 2014;343:1249288.

62. Noval Rivas M, Burton OT, Wise P, et al. A microbiota signature associated with experimental food allergy promotes allergic sensitization and anaphylaxis. J Allergy Clin Immunol 2013;131:201–12.

63. Rosser EC, Oleinika K, Tonon S, et al. Regulatory B cells are induced by gut microbiota–driven interleukin-1β and interleukin-6 production. Nat Med 2014;20:1334–9.

64. Goto Y, Panea C, Nakato G, et al. Segmented filamentous bacteria antigens presented by intestinal dendritic cells drive mucosal Th17 cell differentiation. Immunity 2014;40:594–607.

65. Tanabe S. The effect of probiotics and gut microbiota on Th17 cells. Int Rev Immunol 2013;32:511–25.

66. Olszak T, Neves JF, Dowds CM, et al. Protective mucosal immunity mediated by epithelial CD1d and IL-10. Nature 2014;509:497–502.

67. Olszak T, An D, Zeissig S, et al. Microbial exposure during early life has persistent effects on natural killer T cell function. Science 2012;336:489–93.

68. Liang S, Webb T, Li Z. Probiotic antigens stimulate hepatic natural killer T cells. Immunology 2014;141:203–10.

69. Childs CE, Röytiö H, Alhoniemi E, et al. Xylo-oligosaccharides alone or in synbiotic combination with Bifidobacterium animalis subsp. lactis induce

bifidogenesis and modulate markers of immune function in healthy adults: a double-blind, placebo-controlled, randomised, factorial cross-over study. Br J Nutr 2014;111:1945–56.

70. Stanic B, van de Veen W, Wirz OF, et al. IL-10–overexpressing B cells regulate innate and adaptive immune responses. J Allergy Clin Immunol 2015;135: 771–80.

71. Mirpuri J, Raetz M, Sturge CR, et al. Proteobacteria-specific IgA regulates maturation of the intestinal microbiota. Gut Microbes 2014;5:28–39.

72. Lundell AC, Rabe H, Quiding-Järbrink M, et al. Development of gut-homing receptors on circulating B cells during infancy. Clin Immunol 2011;138:97–106.

73. Kawamoto S, Maruya M, Kato LM, et al. Foxp3+ T cells regulate immunoglobulin A selection and facilitate diversification of bacterial species responsible for immune homeostasis. Immunity 2014;41:152–65.

74. Kruglov AA, Grivennikov SI, Kuprash DV, et al. Nonredundant function of soluble LTα3 produced by innate lymphoid cells in intestinal homeostasis. Science 2013;342:1243–6.

75. Peterson DA, McNulty NP, Guruge JL, et al. IgA response to symbiotic bacteria as a mediator of gut homeostasis. Cell Host Microbe 2007;2:328–39.

76. Friman V, Nowrouzian F, Adlerberth I, et al. Increased frequency of intestinal Escherichia coli carrying genes for S fimbriae and haemolysin in IgA-deficient individuals. Microb Pathog 2002;32:35–42.

77. Bunker JJ, Flynn TM, Koval JC, et al. Innate and adaptive humoral responses coat distinct commensal bacteria with immunoglobulin A. Immunity 2015;43: 541–53.

78. Palm NW, de Zoete MR, Cullen TW, et al. Immunoglobulin A coating identifies colitogenic bacteria in inflammatory bowel disease. Cell. 2014;158:1000–10.

79. Sakai F, Hosoya T, Ono-Ohmachi A, et al. Lactobacillus gasseri SBT2055 induces TGF-b expression in dendritic cells and activates TLR2 signal to produce IgA in the small intestine. PLoS One 2014;9:e105370.

80. Dasgupta S, Erturk-Hasdemir D, Ochoa-Reparaz J, et al. Plasmacytoid dendritic cells mediate anti-inflammatory responses to a gut commensal molecule via both innate and adaptive mechanisms. Cell Host Microbe 2014;15:413–23.

81. Round JL, Mazmanian SK. Inducible Foxp3+ regulatory T-cell development by a commensal bacterium of the intestinal microbiota. Proc Natl Acad Sci U S A 2010;107:12204–9.

82. Jones SE, Paynich ML, Kearns DB, et al. Protection from intestinal inflammation by bacterial exopolysaccharides. J Immunol 2014;192:4813–20.

83. Tan J, McKenzie C, Potamitis M, et al. The role of short-chain fatty acids in health and disease. Adv Immunol 2014;121:91–119.

84. Thorburn AN, Macia L, Mackay CR. Diet, metabolites, and "western-lifestyle" inflammatory diseases. Immunity 2014;40:833–42.

85. Johnson-Henry KC, Pinnell LJ, Waskow AM, et al. Short-chain fructo-oligosaccharide and inulin modulate inflammatory responses and microbial communities in Caco2-bbe cells and in a mouse model of intestinal injury. J Nutr 2014;144:1725–33.

86. Jiang W, Sunkara LT, Zeng X, et al. Differential regulation of human cathelicidin LL-37 by free fatty acids and their analogs. Peptides 2013;50:129–38.

87. Arpaia N, Campbell C, Fan X, et al. Metabolites produced by commensal bacteria promote peripheral regulatory T-cell generation. Nature 2013;504:451–5.

88. Chang PV, Hao L, Offermanns S, et al. The microbial metabolite butyrate regulates intestinal macrophage function via histone deacetylase inhibition. Proc Natl Acad Sci U S A 2014;111:2247–52.

89. Singh N, Gurav A, Sivaprakasam S, et al. Activation of Gpr109a, receptor for niacin and the commensal metabolite butyrate, suppresses colonic inflammation and carcinogenesis. Immunity 2014;40:128–39.

90. Berndt BE, Zhang M, Owyang SY, et al. Butyrate increases IL-23 production by stimulated dendritic cells. Am J Physiol Gastrointest Liver Physiol 2012;303: 1384–92.

91. Arpaia N, Rudensky AY. Microbial metabolites control gut inflammatory responses. Proc Natl Acad Sci U S A 2014;111:2058–9.

92. Trompette A, Gollwitzer ES, Yadava K, et al. Gut microbiota metabolism of dietary fiber influences allergic airway disease and hematopoiesis. Nat Med 2014; 20:159–66.

93. Furusawa Y, Obata Y, Fukuda S, et al. Commensal microbe-derived butyrate induces the differentiation of colonic regulatory T cells. Nature 2013;504:446–50.

94. Zhang Z, Shi L, Pang W, et al. Dietary fiber intake regulates intestinal microflora and inhibits ovalbumin-induced allergic airway inflammation in a mouse model. PLoS One 2016;11:e0147778.

95. O'Mahony L, Akdis M, Akdis CA. Regulation of the immune response and inflammation by histamine and histamine receptors. J Allergy Clin Immunol 2011;128: 1153–62.

96. Frei R, Ferstl R, Konieczna P, et al. Histamine receptor 2 modifies dendritic cell responses to microbial ligands. J Allergy Clin Immunol 2013;132:194–204.

97. Smolinska S, Jutel M, Crameri R, et al. Histamine and gut mucosal immune regulation. Allergy 2014;69:273–81.

98. Smolinska S, Groeger D, Perez NR, et al. Histamine receptor 2 is required to suppress innate immune responses to bacterial ligands in patients with inflammatory bowel disease. Inflamm Bowel Dis 2016;22:1575–86.

99. Ferstl R, Frei R, Schiavi E, et al. Histamine receptor 2 is a key influence in immune responses to intestinal histamine-secreting microbes. J Allergy Clin Immunol 2014;134:744–6.

100. Gao C, Major A, Rendon D, et al. Histamine H2 receptor-mediated suppression of intestinal inflammation by probiotic Lactobacillus reuteri. MBio 2015;6: e01358–415.

101. Barcik W, Pugin B, Westermann P, et al. Histamine-secreting microbes are increased in the gut of adult asthma patients. J Allergy Clin Immunol 2016. [Epub ahead of print].

102. Abrahamsson TR, Wu RY, Jenmalm MC. Gut microbiota and allergy: the importance of the pregnancy period. Pediatr Res 2015;77:214–9.

103. Abrahamsson TR, Jakobsson HE, Andersson AF, et al. Low gut microbiota diversity in early infancy precedes asthma at school age. Clin Exp Allergy 2014;44: 842–50.

104. Arrieta MC, Stiemsma LT, Dimitriu PA, et al. Early infancy microbial and metabolic alterations affect risk of childhood asthma. Sci Transl Med 2015;7: 307ra152.

105. Abrahamsson TR, Jakobsson HE, Andersson AF, et al. Low diversity of the gut microbiota in infants with atopic eczema. J Allergy Clin Immunol 2012;129: 434–40.

106. Romano-Keeler J, Weitkamp JH. Maternal influences on fetal microbial colonization and immune development. Pediatr Res 2015;77:189–95.

Biology of the Microbiome 2: Metabolic Role

Jia V. Li, PhD[a,1], Jonathan Swann, PhD[a,1], Julian R. Marchesi, PhD[a,b,c,d,*]

KEYWORDS

- Metabonome • Microbiome • Mass spectrometry • NMR • Multi-variate data

KEY POINTS

- The human microbiome is a new frontier in biology and one that is helping to define what it is to be human.
- Recently, we have begun to understand that the "communication" between the host and its microbiome is via a metabolic superhighway.
- By interrogating and understanding the molecules involved, we may start to know who the main players are, and how to modulate them and the mechanisms of health and disease.

INTRODUCTION

Understanding mammalian biology has for the best part of 100 years been focused on trying to model how this system interacts with the environment. Since the discovery that DNA contains all the necessary information to recreate a new living organism and coupled with the revolution in gene sequencing, this focus turned to try to understand how host's genome interacts with its environment to influence the balance between health and disease. A significant component of this body of work has been focused on the role of microbial pathogens in driving disease phenotypes. However, there is a dearth of information that considers that the microbes colonizing the various niches of the human body may actually have coevolved with the host and provide essential functions not found in the host's genome. The role of mammalian microbiome is revealed, in extremis, when animals are reared in a sterile environment[1,2] and thus do not develop in the presence of a microbiota. The absence of the

[a] Section of Biomolecular Medicine, Division of Computational & Systems Medicine, Department of Surgery & Cancer, Faculty of Medicine, Imperial College London, Exhibition Road, South Kensington, London SW7 2AZ, UK; [b] Divison of Digestive Diseases, Department of Surgery & Cancer, Faculty of Medicine, Imperial College London, 10th Floor QEQM Building, St Mary's Hospital Campus, South Wharf Road, London W2 1NY, UK; [c] Department of Surgery & Cancer, Centre for Digestive and Gut Health, Imperial College London, Exhibition Road, South Kensington, London SW7 2AZ, UK; [d] School of Biosciences, Cardiff University, Museum Avenue, Cardiff CF10 3XQ, UK
[1] Both these authors contributed equally to this article.
* Corresponding author. School of Biosciences, Cardiff University, Museum Avenue, Cardiff, UK.
E-mail address: marchesijr@cardiff.ac.uk

Gastroenterol Clin N Am 46 (2017) 37–47
http://dx.doi.org/10.1016/j.gtc.2016.09.006
0889-8553/17/© 2016 Elsevier Inc. All rights reserved.

gastro.theclinics.com

microbiome has been shown to influence a very wide and disparate range of physiologic parameters, including cardiac size and output,[3] response to anesthesia,[4] and many other features of the mature mammalian system.[5] Although we can see a fundamental role for the microbiome in the development of a mature host, we are left with a dearth of mechanisms by which this process is driven.

WHY DO WE NEED TO KNOW WHAT METABOLITES ARE MADE?

The history of microbiology has been focused predominantly on understanding the role that pathogens play in disease, and this goes back to the time of Robert Koch and Louis Pasteur. However, in the last 15 years there has been a slow but inexorable move toward understanding how the commensal and mutualistic members of the human microbiome also contribute to host health and disease initiation. In the last 5 years, this interest in the microbiome has really expanded at an exponential rate. However, we cannot treat these organisms in a similar fashion to pathogenic microbes, because they have not evolved specific strategies to invade, colonize and reproduce in a hostile environment. Many of the functions and features that they possess, and on which we rely, do not conform to the virulence model that we have used to describe and understand pathogens. Many of the functions are actually part of that everyday metabolism of these organisms and as such cannot be considered as virulence factors. For example, for many anaerobic bacteria that colonize the large intestine the ability to ferment simple molecules, to extract energy from them, results in a wide range of metabolites that are bioactive and interact with a wide range of receptors within the host. Thus, the communication between this diverse set of organisms and its host is predominantly via a metabolite superhighway. Thus, to understand this communication we need to be able to characterize the wide array of metabolites that the bacteria produce in response to the environment in which they find themselves and understand how the host responds to these metabolites based on the genes that they have.

HOW DO ASSESS THEM AND WHAT CAN WE ASSESS: NUCLEAR MR AND MASS SPECTROMETRY, WHAT SAMPLES?

Microbial metabolites are typically present in feces, luminal contents and blood, particularly the hepatic portal vein blood, whereas host–microbial cometabolites are present more commonly in circulating blood and urine. Metabolic profiling approaches are increasingly used to study metabolic function of the gut microbiota. The practical implementation of metabolic profiling includes 5 steps: (1) sample collection and preparation, (2) biochemical composition analyses, (3) data analysis and integration (eg, statistically correlating metabolic and microbial data), (4) biomarker recovery and identification, and (5) validation and application.

Urine and blood plasma or serum collection is straightforward, whereas obtaining fecal samples is more challenging and rarely done at outpatient clinics. Moreover, fecal samples are complex in nature because they contain microbial and mammalian cells and food residues, in which the biological and chemical processes continue during postvoiding and sample handling. Hence, storing samples at a lower temperature and immediate sample processing reduce the variation induced by sample handling. Standard operating procedures for biofluid collection and the effects of various handling conditions on the biochemical composition have been reported previously.[6–8] Analytical platforms, including nuclear MR (NMR) spectroscopy and mass spectrometry (MS), are commonly used in metabolic profiling and can detect a wide range of microbial metabolites and host–microbial cometabolites. NMR spectroscopy is a robust analytical platform with high reproducibility and it generates the most easily accessible and comprehensive information on metabolite structures. Although the sensitivity of NMR spectroscopy is less than MS, it is nondestructive and requires minimum sample preparation. A single proton (^{1}H) NMR experiment using a 600 MHz NMR spectrometer takes about 5 to 10 minutes and can detect a wide range of metabolites including amino acids, fatty acids, phenols, indole, and other organic acids containing protons at low micromolar levels. Therefore, it serves as the first choice for global profiling. MS provide complementary molecular information (eg, molecular mass) and it is much more sensitive than NMR spectroscopy, but often requires preseparation techniques such as liquid chromatography (LC) and gas chromatography (GC). Depending on the metabolites of the interest, different methods can be used in LC to focus on subsets of molecules. For example, reversed phase chromatography is used to study nonpolar compounds, whereas hydrophilic interaction LC is used for detecting polar compounds. Both reversed phase LC-MS and hydrophilic interaction LC-MS are routinely used to analyze the same sample sets to achieve wider metabolite coverage. GC-MS is also a sensitive tool in metabolic profiling and commonly used to quantify short chain fatty acids. However, the drawback of GC-MS is that it requires derivatization of the samples, a long sample preparation procedure, and only volatile compounds or compounds that are volatile after derivatization can be detected. The main metabolic profiling platforms and their strengths and limitations have been summarized by Holmes and colleagues[9] in 2015. Detailed experimental protocols for global metabolic profiling[10–12] and bile acid profiling[13] have been published as well.

All of these analytical tools generate signal-rich data, which requires multivariate statistical analyses to extract useful information from the datasets. Multivariate data analysis methods, typically including principal component analysis, orthogonal projections to latent structures-discriminant analysis, and random forest, provide easy visualization of the metabolic similarities and differences between the samples or spectral data. Orthogonal projections to latent structures regression analysis is also used to statistically correlate metabolic data with other types of datasets, such as body weight, histologic scores, bacterial counts generated from 16S ribosomal RNA gene-based sequencing platform, cytokines, toxicity (**Fig 1** for an example). Such

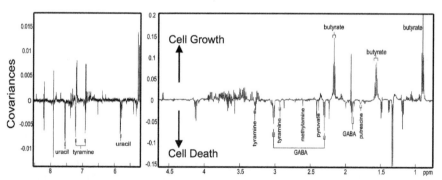

Fig. 1. Orthogonal projections to latent structures regression analyses of fecal water from a rat model of bariatric surgery against relative suspension growth values obtained from a 24-hour treatment of L5178Y cells. Peaks pointing upward in the loadings plots represent metabolites, which are positively correlated to the cell growth and vice versa. Red peaks reach a significance level of $P<.005$. GABA, gamma-aminobutyric acid; IS, indoxyl sulfate; PAG, phenylacetylglycine; p-cresyl sulf, p-cresyl sulfate; p-cresyl glu, p-cresyl glucuronide. (*Adapted from* Li JV, Reshat R, Wu Q, et al. Experimental bariatric surgery in rats generates a cytotoxic chemical environment in the gut contents. Front Microbiol 2011;2:183; with permission.)

correlation analysis between metabolic and microbial datasets allows further insight on metabolites that are likely to be associated with gut microbial composition. The statistical modeling results in a panel of spectral signals that are important for class discrimination (eg, treatment group vs control patients). Signal or feature identification can be challenging in global metabolic profiling. There are many publicly available databases such as human metabolome database[14] and METLIN,[15] software including Chenomx NMR Suite (Chenomx Inc, Edmonton, Ontario, Canada) and AMIX (Bruker, Billerica, MA) and published literature sources, that can assist in providing metabolite candidates for the selected features. Statistical total correlation spectroscopy analysis is a statistical tool to calculate correlation between the peaks from the same molecules or the same biological pathways.[16,17] Further analytical experiments should be carried out to confirm the metabolite identification. Various 2-dimensional NMR spectroscopic experiments can be used to elucidate the connectivity of protons and carbons of the metabolites. Tandem MS/MS can be used to obtain fragmentation patterns of the selected MS features to provide submolecular information for metabolite identification. In the case of targeted signals or metabolites at very low concentrations, solid phase extraction is often used to separate the signals of interest and concentrate it up for further 2-dimensional NMR experiments. In addition, metabolite candidates can be confirmed by spiking the standard compounds in the original biological samples and being tested by NMR spectroscopy or comparing the LC retention times and MS fragmentation patterns from the standards and the samples. Metabolite identification is a time-consuming step and is considered to be a bottle neck in the metabolic profiling approach. These metabolite identification methods are often combined to elucidate the structure of the targeted spectral signals. Approximate numbers of metabolites seen in different biofluids can be in the range of thousands for both urine[18] and serum.[19] Statistical validation can be carried out using methods such as *n*-fold cross-validation and permutation testing, whereas biological validation remains challenging owing to further requirement of knowledge of the target metabolic pathways, appropriate validation approaches and additional resources. Statistically and biologically validated output from metabolic profiling may eventually be applied to further mechanistic investigation, and clinical diagnosis and therapeutic decision making.

EXAMPLES OF USING METABOLIC PROFILING TO STUDY GUT MICROBIAL FUNCTIONALITY

The advancement of systems biology techniques, in particular metabolic profiling (metabolomics/metabonomics) and mathematical modeling approaches, has expanded the resolution at which we can study the metabolic contribution of the gut microbiota and their interaction with host biochemistry. A key strength of metabolic profiling is its holistic nature, simultaneously capturing vast amounts of metabolic information without bias, surpassing the need for a specific hypothesis allowing open questions to be asked. This property is ideal for studying the gut microbiota owing to its megavariate host-specific nature and our relatively limited understanding. Instead, metabolic profiling is a hypothesis-generating top-down approach that can illuminate linkages between the gut microbiota and host metabolic pathways for further evaluation.

Coupling these data-rich techniques with gnotobiotic (or germ-free or sterile) and antibiotic-treated animal models has allowed these biochemical associations to be elucidated and their relevance to health and disease to be studied. Pair-wise comparisons of the plasma metabolic phenotypes between gnotobiotic and conventionalized mice using an LC-MS and GC-MS–based approach highlighted the influential role of the gut microbiota on circulating amino acids and organic acids.[20] Differences were observed in the plasma levels of bioactive indole-containing metabolites derived from tryptophan such as indoxyl sulfate and indole-3-propionic acid. The absence of these metabolites in the gnotobiotic animals, coupled with their greater abundance of tryptophan, indicates that this tryptophan metabolism depends on the gut microbiota. Certain bacteria possess tryptophanase activity (a deamination of the amino acid) and can break down dietary tryptophan to indole. This molecule can be absorbed from the gut and metabolized in the liver to indoxyl before being sulphated to indoxyl-sulphate. Indole can also be further processed by a different set of intestinal bacteria to the antioxidant indole-3-propionic acid. The plasma of gnotobiotic animals also contained greater amounts of the amino acid tyrosine, whereas the conventional plasma contained greater amounts of the microbial-host cometabolite 4-cresyl-sulphate. Intestinal bacteria have been shown to metabolize dietary tyrosine to 4-cresol that, upon absorption from the gut, is sulphated in the liver to 4-cresyl sulfate (*p*-cresyl sulfate). These findings demonstrate the influence of the gut microbiota on the bioavailability of dietary amino acids, precursors for a range of essential bioactive metabolites.

Similarly, an ^{1}H NMR spectroscopy-based metabonomic approach was used to characterize the changes in the urinary metabolic profiles of gnotobiotic rats during 21 days of microbial colonization.[21] Here, the acquisition of the gut microbiota was accompanied by marked changes in the urinary biochemical profile. Elevations were noted in the excretion of hippurate, phenylacetylglycine, and 3- and 4-hydroxyphenyl-propionic acid. These are microbial-host cometabolites that result from the microbial metabolism of dietary components. Phenylacetylglycine arises from the bacterial metabolism of the amino acid phenylalanine to phenylacetate, which is conjugated with glycine in the rat liver to form phenylacetylglycine and with glutamine in the human liver to form phenylacetylglutamine. Hippurate is the glycine conjugate of benzoic acid that can be derived from the bacterial metabolism of phenylalanine, chlorogenic acid, and catechins. These molecules can be obtained from a range of polyphenolic compounds found in dietary components such as fruit, vegetables, tea, and coffee.[22] Interestingly, in a large-scale metabolic phenotyping study in humans from China, Japan, the United Kingdom, and the United States, hippurate excretion was found to be inversely associated with blood pressure, a major risk factor for cardiovascular disease.[23] Formate, a product of gut microbial fiber fermentation, was also inversely associated with blood pressure. Another metabonomic study characterized the systemic metabolic adaptation to gut colonization in gnotobiotic mice.[24] After 5 days of conventionalization, the metabolic strategy of the liver shifted from glycogenesis to lipogenesis. This observation was consistent with another study combining a transcriptomic and metabonomic approach to study metabolic response to colonization in the mouse jejunum. Here, 2 days of colonization resulted in the suppression of lipid catabolism (eg, β-oxidation) in the jejunum and activation of anabolic pathways (eg, lipogenesis, nucleotide synthesis, and amino acid synthesis).[25] Such biochemical reorientations occurred in parallel with a rapid increase in body weight. These observations indicate the intimate biochemical relationship between the gut microbiota and host and how the host metabolic phenotype is shaped with the development of the gut microbiota.

Antibiotic-treated animal models offer another tool for investigating microbial-host interactions. Gnotobiotic animals differ phenotypically from conventional animals raised in the presence of bacteria. Gnotobiotic animals have a reduced body weight, a lower metabolic rate, underdeveloped gut structure and absorptive capacity, and an immature immune system, and as such can obscure the interpretation of results.

Administering antibiotics to conventionally raised animals allows the influence of the gut microbiota on host biochemistry to be studied while preserving the conventional phenotype. This influence was demonstrated by administering the broad-spectrum antibiotics streptomycin and penicillin in the drinking water of rats for 8 days[26] and in an early study vancomycin to mice.[27] Swann and colleague used ^{1}H NMR spectroscopy to compare the urinary and fecal metabolic profiles of control, antibiotic suppressed and a group undergoing recolonization (4 days of antibiotics followed by 4 days of control treatment). In this study, antibiotic-induced suppression of the intestinal microbiota reduced the urinary excretion of hippurate, phenylpropionic acid, phenylacetylglycine, indoxyl-sulphate, trimethylamine-N-oxide (TMAO), and the short chain fatty acid, acetate. The excretion of the amino acids taurine and glycine, and the tricarboxylic acid cycle intermediates, citrate, 2-oxoglutarate, and fumarate was increased after microbial attenuation. In addition, all the short chain fatty acids (acetate, butyrate, propionate) were reduced in the feces of the antibiotic-treated rats. Short chain fatty acids arise from the bacterial fermentation of carbohydrates, including nondigestible polysaccharides. Because these products provide a significant energy source for the host, this represents a key function of the gut microbiota salvaging energy from the diet. A human study by Claesson and colleagues[28] correlated fecal metabolic and microbial profiles to highlight a putative statistical association between butyrate and the presence of *Ruminococcus* or *Butyricicoccus*. Microbial and metabolic profiling of the recolonizing animals revealed a cage-dependent bacterial recolonization. This difference was mirrored by cage-dependent differences in the metabolic signatures. This highlights the potential for environmental pressures to shape the gut bacterial reestablishment after antibiotic therapy, with downstream implications on the metabolic state of the host.

In addition to global profiling of low-molecular-weight metabolites, we can also target specific molecules or families of molecules, for example, bile acids and eicosanoids. Targeted profiling of the bile acid signature enables a detailed overview of the enterohepatic circulation to be gained and the influence of the gut microbiota to be studied.[13] The circulating and hepatic bile acid pool contains more than 30 known bile acids and the gut microbiota is responsible for driving the majority of this diversity.[29] Primary bile acids (cholic acid and chenodeoxycholic acid) are synthesized in the liver from cholesterol and are conjugated with either taurine or glycine before secretion into the bile. Upon ingestion of a meal, bile acids stored in the gallbladder are expelled from the gallbladder into the small intestine and although the majority are actively absorbed in the small intestine a minor amount (1%–5%; 200–800 mg/d in humans) reaches the colon. It is here that bile acids are modified by the resident microbiota. Many bacteria possess bile salt hydrolase enzymes that deconjugate the bile acid from its amino acid. Once deconjugated, further bacterial modifications can occur such as dehydroxylation giving rise to secondary bile acids such as deoxycholic acid and lithocholic acid. Modified bile acids can be absorbed and recycled to the liver, where they are reconjugated and secreted into the bile. This absorption forms the enterohepatic circulation whereby molecules are shuttled between the host liver and the microbiome. Although bile acids have a key role in lipid digestion and absorption, they are now also recognized as important signaling molecules serving as ligands for the nuclear receptor; farnesoid X receptor, and the plasma membrane–bound G-protein–coupled receptor, TGR5.[30,31] Through binding to these receptors bile acids can regulate genes involved in lipid[32–34] and glucose metabolism[35,36] and energy homeostasis.[37] Using a parallel transcriptomic and metabonomic approach the influence of the gut microbiota on the enterohepatic circulation and its signaling capacity was studied.[38] An LC-MS–based approach identified pronounced variation in the bile acid signatures of conventional and gnotobiotic rats with similar modulations induced by antibiotic treatment. The absence or attenuation of the gut microbiota shifted the bile acid signature to one dominated by taurine-conjugated bile acids and strikingly reduced the diversity of the bile acid pool. Such modulations impacted on the signaling function of the bile acid profile with significant alterations in the expression of genes and pathways regulated by bile acids. In addition to being measured in the blood and liver, bile acids were also measured in tissues outside of the enterohepatic circulation (kidney, heart), indicating a broader signaling role of these microbial–host cometabolites.

Metabolic profiling strategies applied to human studies have also expanded our understanding of the gut microbial contribution to host digestion and metabolism. This is well illustrated by the microbial metabolism of dietary choline to trimethylamine (TMA). Choline is predominantly derived from phosphatidylcholine found in animal sources in the diet. The microbial metabolism of choline involves the cleavage of the C–N bond to liberate TMA and acetaldehyde. Whereas acetaldehyde undergoes further microbial metabolism to ethanol, TMA is absorbed from the gut and oxidized in the liver to form TMAO by the flavin-containing monooxygenase 3 enzyme. TMA can also be demethylated to dimethylamine both endogenously and by the gut microbiota (PMID: 4091797). Microbial processing of choline is well established[39] and TMA and TMAO have been previously observed in biofluids from gnotobiotic and antibiotic-treated rodents.[21,26,40] However, recent work in humans has linked this activity to increased cardiovascular disease risk. In a global metabolic profiling study in humans, Wang and colleagues[41] found that 3 plasma metabolites were predictive of increased cardiovascular disease—namely, choline, its metabolite betaine, and TMAO. The role of these metabolites in increased cardiovascular disease risk was investigated by feeding them individually to mice. Both choline and TMAO were found to promote atherosclerosis and all 3 metabolites upregulated the expression of macrophage scavenger receptors known to contribute to the atherosclerotic process. The essential role of the gut microbiota in potentiating the bioactivity of choline through TMA production was confirmed using gnotobiotic mice. In a metabolic profiling study, microbial choline metabolism has also been shown to exacerbate nonalcoholic fatty liver disease, a condition caused by choline deficiency in mice.[42]

The potential for the gut microbiota to influence host drug metabolism has been demonstrated in a human study characterizing the metabolic fate of paracetamol/acetaminophen.[43] The metabolic output of the gut microbiota, specifically 4-cresol, was found to influence the phase II detoxification of this widely used analgesic; 4-cresol has toxic properties and requires detoxification by the host. The primary route of this detoxification is sulfation (both in the gastrointestinal tract and in the liver) before excretion in the urine. This is also the preferred route of detoxification for acetaminophen and both molecules are sulphated by the same human cytosolic sulfotransferase, SULT1A1. Because these 2 molecules compete for binding sites as well as for sulfate, the 4-cresol output of the gut microbiota can influence the ability of the host to sulfate acetaminophen. Alternative routes of detoxification including glucoronidation and phase I metabolism by the cytochrome P450 enzymes. Importantly, phase I metabolism results in the generation of the toxic intermediate, N-acetyl-p-benzoquinone imine. In this study, individuals excreting high amounts of 4-cresol before receiving a standard dose of acetaminophen were found to excrete lesser amounts of acetaminophen sulfate and greater amounts of acetaminophen glucuronide. Such an observation is not limited to acetaminophen and many xenobiotics are detoxified via sulfation. Interestingly, using a molecular epidemiology approach we have also observed 4-cresyl sulfate excretion to be positively correlated with age. This observation was found in both US and Taiwanese populations, suggesting that this age-associated change in the metabolic functionality of the gut microbiome is independent of diet and cultural influences. These data have particular relevance given the greater use of drug therapy with aging.[44]

The influence of the gut microbiota on idiosyncratic drug responses has also been demonstrated in a rodent study with the hepatotoxin, hydrazine.[40] In this metabolic profiling study, the protective effect of an established microbiome was demonstrated in rats with gnotobiotic animals showing a marked toxic response to a typically subtoxic dose. These studies demonstrate the potential of using a global metabolic profiling approach to characterize the metabolic functionality of the gut microbiota to predict the efficacy and safety of orally administered xenobiotics. This represents a step toward a precision medicine approach tailoring pharmacologic interventions to the metabolic status of the complete biological system including contributions from the host genome and the microbiome.

FUTURE DIRECTIONS

To maximize the potential of metabonomic approaches and using them for defining the role that microbes play in maintaining health and driving disease we predict that the follow areas of research will need to be developed.

- High throughput profiling of cellular responses to metabolites; currently, we do not have a platform that allow us to measure the responses of different cell types, for example, colonocytes or hepatocytes to doses or combinations of metabolites.
- A metabolic lexicon of bacteria—who makes what and from what substrate. The range of metabolites that different microbes make and from what, so we can predict how changes in the composition of the microbiota affects the metabonome is needed.
- The interactions between bacteria and their combined impact on the host. Many studies look at single organisms, but we are far from understanding how the microbes interact with each other and how this network affects the host via the metabolite axis.

SUMMARY

To understand how humans function now needs a systems based approach which incorporates the microbiome and its associated metabonome. The metabolic superhighway is the key avenue along which microbes influence the host's metabolism and physiology. To understand humans, we must start to understand and incorporate this knowledge into our model of the biology; otherwise, we will still be scrabbling around for explanations for disease for many years to come.

REFERENCES

1. Tlaskalova-Hogenova H, Vannucci L, Klimesova K, et al. Microbiome and colorectal carcinoma: insights from germ-free and conventional animal models. Cancer J 2014;20(3):217–24.
2. Marcobal A, Kashyap PC, Nelson TA, et al. A metabolomic view of how the human gut microbiota impacts the host metabolome using humanized and gnotobiotic mice. ISME J 2013;7(10):1933–43.
3. Gordon HA, Wostmann BS, Bruckner-Kardoss E. Effects of Microbial Flora on Cardiac Output and Other Elements of Blood Circulation. Proc Soc Exp Biol Med 1963;114:301–4.

4. Quevauviller A, Laroche MJ, Cottart A, et al. Anesthetic activity and comparative metabolism of hexobarbital in the germ-free and conventional mouse. Ann Pharm Fr 1964;22:339–44 [in French].

5. Smith K, McCoy KD, Macpherson AJ. Use of axenic animals in studying the adaptation of mammals to their commensal intestinal microbiota. Semin Immunol 2007;19(2):59–69.

6. Gratton J, Phetcharaburanin J, Mullish BH, et al. Optimized sample handling strategy for metabolic profiling of human feces. Anal Chem 2016;88(9):4661–8.

7. Siddiqui NY, DuBois LG, St John-Williams L, et al. Optimizing urine processing protocols for protein and metabolite detection. J Proteomics Bioinform 2015;2015(Suppl 14):003.

8. Teahan O, Gamble S, Holmes E, et al. Impact of analytical bias in metabonomic studies of human blood serum and plasma. Anal Chem 2006;78(13):4307–18.

9. Holmes E, Wijeyesekera A, Taylor-Robinson SD, et al. The promise of metabolic phenotyping in gastroenterology and hepatology. Nat Rev Gastroenterol Hepatol 2015;12(8):458–71.

10. Beckonert O, Keun HC, Ebbels TM, et al. Metabolic profiling, metabolomic and metabonomic procedures for NMR spectroscopy of urine, plasma, serum and tissue extracts. Nat Protoc 2007;2(11):2692–703.

11. Want EJ, Masson P, Michopoulos F, et al. Global metabolic profiling of animal and human tissues via UPLC-MS. Nat Protoc 2013;8(1):17–32.

12. Want EJ, Wilson ID, Gika H, et al. Global metabolic profiling procedures for urine using UPLC-MS. Nat Protoc 2010;5(6):1005–18.

13. Sarafian MH, Lewis MR, Pechlivanis A, et al. Bile acid profiling and quantification in biofluids using ultra-performance liquid chromatography tandem mass spectrometry. Anal Chem 2015;87(19):9662–70.

14. Wishart DS, Jewison T, Guo AC, et al. HMDB 3.0–the human metabolome database in 2013. Nucleic Acids Res 2013;41(Database issue):D801–7.

15. Smith CA, O'Maille G, Want EJ, et al. METLIN: a metabolite mass spectral database. Ther Drug Monit 2005;27(6):747–51.

16. Cloarec O, Dumas ME, Craig A, et al. Statistical total correlation spectroscopy: an exploratory approach for latent biomarker identification from metabolic 1H NMR data sets. Anal Chem 2005;77(5):1282–9.

17. Robinette SL, Lindon JC, Nicholson JK. Statistical spectroscopic tools for biomarker discovery and systems medicine. Anal Chem 2013;85(11):5297–303.

18. Bouatra S, Aziat F, Mandal R, et al. The human urine metabolome. PLoS One 2013;8(9):e73076.

19. Psychogios N, Hau DD, Peng J, et al. The human serum metabolome. PLoS One 2011;6(2):e16957.

20. Wikoff WR, Anfora AT, Liu J, et al. Metabolomics analysis reveals large effects of gut microflora on mammalian blood metabolites. Proc Natl Acad Sci U S A 2009;106(10):3698–703.

21. Nicholls AW, Mortishire-Smith RJ, Nicholson JK. NMR spectroscopic-based metabonomic studies of urinary metabolite variation in acclimatizing germ-free rats. Chem Res Toxicol 2003;16(11):1395–404.

22. Lees HJ, Swann JR, Wilson ID, et al. Hippurate: the natural history of a mammalian-microbial cometabolite. J Proteome Res 2013;12(4):1527–46.

23. Holmes E, Loo RL, Stamler J, et al. Human metabolic phenotype diversity and its association with diet and blood pressure. Nature 2008;453(7193):396–400.

24. Claus SP, Ellero SL, Berger B, et al. Colonization-induced host-gut microbial metabolic interaction. MBio 2011;2(2):e00271–310.

25. El Aidy S, Merrifield CA, Derrien M, et al. The gut microbiota elicits a profound metabolic reorientation in the mouse jejunal mucosa during conventionalisation. Gut 2013;62(9):1306–14.

26. Swann JR, Tuohy KM, Lindfors P, et al. Variation in antibiotic-induced microbial recolonization impacts on the host metabolic phenotypes of rats. J Proteome Res 2011;10(8):3590–603.

27. Yap IK, Li JV, Saric J, et al. Metabonomic and microbiological analysis of the dynamic effect of vancomycin-induced gut microbiota modification in the mouse. J Proteome Res 2008;7(9):3718–28.

28. Claesson MJ, Jeffery IB, Conde S, et al. Gut microbiota composition correlates with diet and health in the elderly. Nature 2012;488(7410):178–84.

29. Garcia-Canaveras JC, Donato MT, Castell JV, et al. Targeted profiling of circulating and hepatic bile acids in human, mouse, and rat using a UPLC-MRM-MS-validated method. J Lipid Res 2012;53(10):2231–41.

30. Houten SM, Watanabe M, Auwerx J. Endocrine functions of bile acids. EMBO J 2006;25(7):1419–25.

31. Eloranta JJ, Kullak-Ublick GA. The role of FXR in disorders of bile acid homeostasis. Physiology (Bethesda) 2008;23:286–95.

32. Hirokane H, Nakahara M, Tachibana S, et al. Bile acid reduces the secretion of very low density lipoprotein by repressing microsomal triglyceride transfer protein gene expression mediated by hepatocyte nuclear factor-4. J Biol Chem 2004; 279(44):45685–92.

33. Kast HR, Nguyen CM, Sinal CJ, et al. Farnesoid X-activated receptor induces apolipoprotein C-II transcription: a molecular mechanism linking plasma triglyceride levels to bile acids. Mol Endocrinol 2001;15(10):1720–8.

34. Watanabe M, Houten SM, Wang L, et al. Bile acids lower triglyceride levels via a pathway involving FXR, SHP, and SREBP-1c. J Clin Invest 2004;113(10):1408–18.

35. Katsuma S, Hirasawa A, Tsujimoto G. Bile acids promote glucagon-like peptide-1 secretion through TGR5 in a murine enteroendocrine cell line STC-1. Biochem Biophys Res Commun 2005;329(1):386–90.

36. Stayrook KR, Bramlett KS, Savkur RS, et al. Regulation of carbohydrate metabolism by the farnesoid X receptor. Endocrinology 2005;146(3):984–91.

37. Watanabe M, Houten SM, Mataki C, et al. Bile acids induce energy expenditure by promoting intracellular thyroid hormone activation. Nature 2006;439(7075): 484–9.

38. Swann JR, Want EJ, Geier FM, et al. Systemic gut microbial modulation of bile acid metabolism in host tissue compartments. Proc Natl Acad Sci U S A 2011; 108(Suppl 1):4523–30.

39. Asatoor AM, Simenhoff ML. The origin of urinary dimethylamine. Biochim Biophys Acta 1965;111(2):384–92.

40. Swann J, Wang Y, Abecia L, et al. Gut microbiome modulates the toxicity of hydrazine: a metabonomic study. Mol Biosyst 2009;5(4):351–5.

41. Wang Z, Klipfell E, Bennett BJ, et al. Gut flora metabolism of phosphatidylcholine promotes cardiovascular disease. Nature 2011;472(7341):57–63.

42. Dumas ME, Barton RH, Toye A, et al. Metabolic profiling reveals a contribution of gut microbiota to fatty liver phenotype in insulin-resistant mice. Proc Natl Acad Sci U S A 2006;103(33):12511–6.

43. Clayton TA, Baker D, Lindon JC, et al. Pharmacometabonomic identification of a significant host-microbiome metabolic interaction affecting human drug metabolism. Proc Natl Acad Sci U S A 2009;106(34):14728–33.
44. Swann JR, Spagou K, Lewis M, et al. Microbial-mammalian cometabolites dominate the age-associated urinary metabolic phenotype in Taiwanese and American populations. J Proteome Res 2013;12(7):3166–80.

Diet and the Microbiome

Nida Murtaza, MTech[1], Páraic Ó Cuív, PhD[1], Mark Morrison, PhD*

KEYWORDS

- Diet • Gut • Microbiota • Microbiome • Inflammatory bowel disease
- Irritable bowel syndrome

KEY POINTS

- Diet has a significant impact on the structure-function activities of the gut microbiota.
- Advances have been made in showing how host phenotype is shaped by the gut microbiota, and how diet may provide the selective pressure, in a positive or negative way, to sustain this relationship.
- Diet modification offers the opportunity in a clinical setting to reshape the gut microbiota for the relief of symptoms associated with functional disorders, and the therapeutic treatment of some gastrointestinal and extraintestinal diseases.
- However, studies need to continue to advance from microbiota profiling to function-based approaches and analyses, and more rigorous study designs also need to be used, to better differentiate between the cause and effect relationships of diet-microbiome interactions, and to translate microbiome research to medicine.

INTRODUCTION: WHAT IS THE MICROBIOME?

There are several extant definitions of the term "microbiome," a field of research that has become principally associated with the technological advances in DNA/RNA sequencing and computational biology. As such, the microbiome is still commonly defined as the collective genomic content of all microbes recovered from a habitat or ecosystem (eg, saliva and stool samples, skin swabs).[1] However, although such a definition captures the functional potential inherent to the microbiota (micro-), there

Disclosure Statement: The authors have no commercial or financial conflicts to disclose that are directly connected to the content of this publication. M. Morrison has been the recipient of speaker's honoraria, consulting fees, and participant support from several industry bodies including Janssen-Cilag (Australia), Danone-Murray Goulburn (Australia), and Yakult Honsha. The authors acknowledge research support provided by The University of Queensland, The Princess Alexandra Hospital Research Foundation, and the National Health and Medical Research Council of Australia. The Translational Research Institute is supported by a grant from the Australian Government.
The University of Queensland Diamantina Institute, The University of Queensland, Translational Research Institute, 37 Kent St, Brisbane, Queensland 4102, Australia
[1] Equal contribution.
* Corresponding author.
E-mail address: m.morrison1@uq.edu.au

is a need to place this knowledge in context with the interactions and processes contingent on the physicochemical attributes of their surrounding environment (-biome). This more holistic definition of the microbiome is applied throughout this article, in recognition of diet as a major influence on microbiome dynamics. By doing so, the concept of nutritional ecology is introduced: how the nutrient and its variations across temporal and spatial scales affect the gut microbiota. We contend that nutritional ecology will provide the mechanistic bases for understanding "diet and the microbiome," which will translate into improved diagnoses and treatments for functional and organic diseases.

GENERAL CONCEPTS AND APPROACHES OF MICROBIOME STUDIES

For the interested reader, Morgan and Huttenhower[2] present a well-structured and illustrated general overview of the techniques and approaches underpinning microbiome studies. Over the last two decades, microbiome studies have emphasized the use of polymerase chain reaction techniques targeting regions within the gene encoding 16S ribosomal RNA in prokaryotes (ie, bacteria principally, and archaea). When combined with the rapid advances in DNA sequencing technologies and a combination of ecologic, biostatistical, and computational methods, these 16S rRNA profiling methods have resulted in a taxonomy-based assessment of gut microbial communities resident in different regions of the gastrointestinal tract. Importantly, these approaches have afforded the differentiation of the microbiota to reveal specific microbes and microbial consortia indicative of alterations to gut homeostasis, which are generically referred to as "dysbiosis."[3,4] During the same period the National Institutes of Health Human Microbiome Project[5] has augmented these studies by producing the "reference genomes" of individual microbial species, which has supported the inference of the functional attributes inherent to the 16S rRNA profiles by such methods as PICRUSt.[6] However, and because of the continued advances in sequencing technologies, the time and cost constraints to "shotgun metagenome sequencing" are being relaxed, which affords a scale and depth of sequence coverage that provides an actual (rather than inferred) representation of the functional attributes inherent to the microbiota.[2]

These studies have also substantiated that the microbial communities of the gut are readily differentiated according to their microbial (and gene) density, diversity, and distribution; as affected by anatomic structure, host secretions, and digesta residence times at different sites. Although the esophageal, stomach, and small intestinal microbiota have now been characterised,[7] most studies that have advanced the mechanistic understanding of diet-microbiome interactions have been undertaken using stool/fecal samples and/or tissue samples collected from the large bowel. As such, the term "gut microbiome" has come to define this (terminal) region of the gastrointestinal tract. During the last 5 years in particular, shotgun metagenome sequencing of stool microbiota and the associated metagenome-wide association studies has revealed that the form and function of the stool microbiota is altered in patient cohorts with type-2 diabetes, cirrhosis, and colorectal cancer. These differences have not only provided insights of how microbial metabolism contributes to disease, but the identification of candidate gene and organismal biomarkers of health and disease.[8–11]

Critically, these methods have also shown the gut microbiota of humans (and other animals) is rapidly altered by changes in habitual or available diet, leading to the perception that diet may exert a stronger selective pressure on the gut microbiota than host genetics.[12,13] A particular focus in the last 10 years has related to obesity research, with Turnbaugh and colleagues[14] reporting an enrichment of microbial genes involved in carbohydrate, lipid, and amino acid metabolism in the obese adult gut. More recent studies have revealed that non-obese and obese individuals are characterized by variations in gene richness: subjects with a low gene count are characterized by increased adiposity, insulin resistance, and inflammation.[15,16] The difference in gene richness has been suggested to be predictive of previous weight gain and in mice, could be partially reversed following a dietary intervention for weight loss.[17] The links between diet and microbiome have also been further substantiated via fecal transplant studies in animal models. For instance, Turnbaugh and colleagues[18] were among the first to show how the transfer of an obese (or lean) phenotype to a naive host (ie, germ-free mice) can be effectively recapitulated using diet to exert the necessary selective pressure to sustain the microbiome. This type of an approach is being increasingly used to establish how either specific microbes or microbial consortia contribute to the onset of non-communicable metabolic and immune-mediated diseases.[19,20] Additionally, the benefits of existing and candidate next-generation probiotic strains, in terms of their capacity to attenuate inflammation and/or positively affect barrier function and host metabolism (eg, *Bifidobacterium* spp, *Faecalibacterium prausnitzii* and *Akkermansia muciniphila*), are being examined by their introduction to either germ-free or conventionally reared mice.[21–23]

Table 1 provides a summary of some recent advances in the understanding of how diet and the gut microbiome, from ecologic, metabolic and immunomodulatory contexts, can affect gut function and health. In addition to the other contributions provided in this issue, there are numerous books[38] and reviews of the topic, especially as it pertains to diet-microbiome (diet × microbiome) interactions during pregnancy and early life,[39,40] obesity and metabolic diseases,[41,42] and immune development and immune-mediated diseases.[3,4,24,26,43–45] Indeed, these interrelationships are now being defined from conception to grave: from their influences on fetal and infant developmental biology and homeostatic processes, to triggering a plethora of acute and chronic (extra) intestinal diseases, through to defining rules for microbiome restoration to better treat diseases and prevent relapse. Here, as a primer for gastroenterologists, we provide two examples of how diet has been used as a primary intervention that affects the microbiome: exclusive enteral nutrition (EEN) and diets with reduced fermentable oligo-, di-, monosaccharides and polyols (FODMAP) as induction therapies for Crohn's disease (CD) and irritable bowel syndrome (IBS), respectively. These two examples provide insights into how the microbiota is affected by these conditions, how diet can be managed to produce positive health outcomes, the consequences of these interventions on the microbiome, and why improved knowledge of diet × microbiome interactions is needed.

THE MICROBIOME AND INFLAMMATORY BOWEL DISEASE

The cause of inflammatory bowel disease (IBD) remains elusive because it is a multi-factorial disease influenced by the complex interplay between host genetic susceptibilities,[46] environmental, and lifestyle choices (eg, habitual diet, smoking).[47] With the global incidence and prevalence of IBD increasing, and reaching across to historically low-risk ethnic groups and countries,[48] the microbiome is widely perceived to represent the functional interface among these three components precipitating disease. Indeed, Sartor[49] proposed variations in the balance of the gut microbiota as a trigger for disease, and a large number of case-control and observational studies of the stool and mucosa-associated microbiota from patients with new-onset and chronic IBD now show an overall decrease in bacterial diversity of adult and pediatric patients with IBD during active disease, when compared with healthy control subjects. Reductions in bacterial lineages associated with the Gram-positive *Clostridium leptum* and

Table 1
Some recent examples of how diet and microbiome interact to affect gastrointestinal function and health

Diet	Ecological Effect	Microbiota Effect
Breastmilk	Provides human milk oligosaccharides	Promotes growth of Bifidobacteria and Lactobacillus[24]
Low FODMAP diet	Mitigates IBS symptoms	Alterations in bacterial taxa[25]
Exclusive enteral nutrition	Induces remission and promotes healing in CD	Alters structure-function activity of the microbiota[26,27]
Grains, resistant starches, "fibers"	Promotes SCFA production and reduced pH Anti-inflammatory effects	Suppresses growth of Gram-negative Enterobacteria Promotes growth of acetate and butyrate producers Stimulates Bifidobacteria and F. prausnitzii[28–30]

Dietary Metabolites	Metabolic and/or Immunomodulatory Effects	Microbiota Effect
SCFA	Metabolic effects via specific GPCR receptors Effects of butyrate on Treg cells	Variations in proportions and total SCFA produced[31] Loss of butyrate producing commensals with inflammation (eg, F. prausntizii)[32]
Trimethylamines	Risk factor for cardiovascular and renal disease	Microbial by-products of choline and creatinine[33]
Branched-chain amino acids	Promotes insulin resistance and diabetes	Enrichment of these pathways in microbiome of T2D[8]
Primary bile acid metabolites	Variations in host signaling via NR and GPCR	Gram-positive and sulfidogenic bacteria, Bacteroides[34]
Riboflavin precursors	Activation of MAIT cells	Produced mainly by Gram-negative enteric bacteria[35]
Anti-inflammatory peptides	Anti-inflammatory effects	Loss of F. prausnitzii associated with inflammation[36]
Polyphenols	Improve barrier function and proglucagon levels	Stimulation of A. muciniphila populations[37]

Abbreviations: CD, Crohn's disease; FODMAP, fermentable oligo-, di-, monosaccharides and polyols; GPCR, G protein-coupled receptors; IBS, irritable bowel syndrome; MAIT, mucosa associated invariant T cells; NR, nuclear receptors; SCFA, short chain fatty acids; T2D, type 2 diabetes.

Clostridium coccoides clusters are consistently reported in patients with IBD.[50,51] Members of these lineages are recognized to produce short chain fatty acids including butyrate during active growth in the large bowel, and at least some are implicated in driving the expansion of regulatory T-cell populations in the gut that suppress the inflammatory response.[52,53] Furthermore, reductions in the abundance of *F. prausnitzii*, which in healthy subjects may comprise approximately 5% of the total population, are frequently reported for patients with CD and ulcerative colitis (UC).[54–56] Longitudinal studies have also revealed that these changes are coincident with the onset of disease and that the restoration of these bacterial taxa is prognostic of better health outcomes.[55–58] Conversely, an increase in the relative abundance of pro-inflammatory Gram-negative bacteria principally affiliated with the Proteobacteria has been consistently identified in IBD,[50,51] and some *Bacteroides* spp have also been implicated in the onset of IBD and flares.[20] Much less is known about the diversity of the non bacterial members of the healthy gut microbiota. Our own studies revealed a strong signal for methane-producing archaea associated with colonic tissue,[59] although reductions in the absolute counts and taxonomic composition of archaea and fungi have been reported for patients with IBD compared with healthy subjects.[60–63] These findings strongly suggest that although the anti-inflammatory factors produced by such bacteria as *F. prausnitzii* are sustained and robust in healthy subjects, the growth, persistence and metabolic activity of these bacteria can be challenged by not-yet-identified factors that change within the gut milieu during active disease episodes. At the same time, pro-inflammatory bacteria seem to thrive in these same conditions but whether inflammation is the cause, or the consequence of these interrelationships still needs to be established.[64]

Starving the "Hungry Microbiome" as an Induction Therapy for Inflammatory Bowel Disease?

In some respects, the understanding of the contributions of diet to the cause and treatment of IBD has been historically marginalized, limited mainly to anecdotal observations, surveys, and reports rather than robust experimental designs.[26,43] However, and perhaps because of the rapid emergence of study of the gut microbiome, and the recognition of the dynamic relationships between diet and the microbiota, a more systematic assessment of these interrelationships has been forthcoming, offering new opportunities with real clinical impact. Currently, the most notable of these is the use of enteral feeding of a nutritionally replete liquid formula (EEN) in pediatric patients with CD, which can induce clinical remission and mucosal healing rates approaching 80% of newly diagnosed subjects.[65,66] Various types of EEN formulae exist and are classified as elemental (free amino acids), semi-elemental (peptides), or polymeric (proteins), with the polymeric formulae considered to be more palatable. The formulae do not vary in their ability to induce or maintain remission and moreover, they are superior to corticosteroids in their ability to induce mucosal healing in patients with CD, which is the greatest predictor of long-term health outcomes.[67,68] Although EEN is predominately used with pediatric patients it has also been shown to result in positive outcomes with adults, although it suffers from lower compliance.

Although the exact mechanisms of action remain unknown, EEN has been proposed to have positive impacts on the host and microbiota.[27,69] In general terms, studies of the stool microbiota have shown that EEN results in a further reduction in bacterial diversity, and in particular, reductions in those bacterial taxa assigned to the two most predominant phyla (ie, Firmicutes and Bacteroidetes).[70,71] In addition to EEN, recent systematic reviews have concluded that alternative dietary intervention strategies can modulate the symptoms of IBD.[72] In particular, the exclusion of foods that caused symptoms or that resulted in a blood serum IgG response to food antigens are associated with improved outcomes. Low residue or fiber diets do not exert a therapeutic effect, although there is limited evidence that a diet with reduced FODMAPs may also help control the functional symptoms associated with IBD.[73] Epidemiologic and animal studies have increasingly implicated high-fat diets and food additives, such as emulsifiers, as plausible triggers of IBD[74–76] and it remains to be determined whether these risks could be ameliorated by custom dietary interventions.

In summation, EEN either alone or in combination with exclusion diets, and in young patients with CD in particular, result in reductions in the bacterial diversity associated with stool and mucosal samples, and the period of "bowel rest" and mucosal healing afforded by EEN may result from limiting the growth of the hungry microbiome and minimizing their triggers of inflammation. In addition, as outlined in our recent review,[27] the process of mucosal healing that is characteristic of EEN treatments may also be partly supported by induction of the autophagy pathways to help repair damaged host cells. Surprisingly, however, current EEN formulations are considered to be ineffective for the treatment of UC, although it has been applied as an adjunct therapy; and exclusion diets specific for UC are in development (Levine and Lewindon, personal communication, 2016). However, randomized control trials have shown fecal microbiota transplants are a promising intervention for the treatment of UC, in addition to their use for the treatment of recalcitrant *Clostridium difficle* infections, although their impact in CD is more variable.[77] For these reasons, we believe that diet × microbiome interactions will soon be further understood and effectively managed, to provide synergistic interventions (eg, exclusion diets, partial enteral nutrition, and/or microbiota transplants) that will advance the treatment and clinical management of both major types of IBD.

THE CONUNDRUM OF DIET, MICROBIOME, AND IRRITABLE BOWEL SYNDROME

Thorough and excellent reviews of the diet × microbiome interactions affecting IBS treatment and symptom control have been recently published by Rajilić-Stovanović and colleagues[78] and Staudacher and Whelan.[25] In summary, there have been much fewer studies of diagnosed patients with IBS compared with patients with IBD, and most of these published studies have used 16S rRNA gene profiling studies as part of cross-sectional and observational studies. These studies have also principally used stool samples, often from cohorts representing more than one of the major subtypes of IBS: postinfectious IBS, constipation (IBS-C), diarrhea (IBS-D), and mixed. The findings of these profiling studies are best described as variable, with some genera assigned to the Firmicutes phylum, such as *Dorea, Roseburia, Ruminococcus* and *Blautia* spp.; along with members of the Gram-negative Proteobacteria being increased compared with healthy control subjects. Conversely, "good" bacteria, such as *Bifidobacterium, Collinsella* and *Faecalibacterium* spp, are often observed to be reduced in patients with IBS. Other bacterial taxa show mixed responses, either increased (or reduced) according to the IBS-C or IBS-D subtypes. Remarkable in this regard are the increase in methane-producing archaebacteria reported in patients with IBS-C, and the reductions in bacteria affiliated with the Bacteroidetes phylum in IBS subtypes other than IBS-D, where these groups have been reported to increase.[78] These variations are likely to be a consequence of how variations in gut transit time impose different selective pressures on the gut microbiota. For instance, bacteria with more rapid rates of growth are likely to be favored by the fast transit times associated with IBS-D, whereas microbes with slow growth rates and/or nutrient requirements including hydrogen and more reduced fermentation end-products (eg, formate, short chain alcohols and methylated amines) predominate in microbiomes with longer transit times (IBS-C).

The reviews noted previously also highlight the conundrum associated with the use of either probiotics or exclusion/reduction diets for treatment of IBS, because these interventions can result in somewhat contradictory effects on the gut microbiota. For instance, very low carbohydrate diets have been shown to improve the symptoms and quality of life in patients with IBS-D,[79] and a low FODMAP diet, compared with habitual diets in either the United Kingdom or Australia, has been shown via random-ized control and a randomized and blinded crossover trial, respectively, to be effective in controlling the symptoms of IBS.[80,81] Moreover, a study of patients with IBS who received either "standard" or "low FODMAP" diet advice concluded that patients who received the low FODMAP advice reported improvement in their IBS-associated symptoms, such as bloating and flatulence, than the patients who received standard dietary advice.[82] Importantly, the studies by Halmos and colleagues[83] also suggest that although diets low in FODMAPs reduce the symptoms of patients diag-nosed with IBS compared with when they consume a standard diet, no changes in the symptoms scores are observed in healthy controls subjects consuming either type of diet. In relative terms, there are scant reports of the microbiome changes associated with these diets, especially in terms of using the contemporary sequencing technolo-gies and approaches outlined previously. However, the quantification of key bacterial groups by species-specific polymerase chain reaction has been informative. In that context, Staudacher and colleagues[81] first reported a reduction in *Bifidobacterium* spp. (and IBS symptoms) in British subjects as a consequence of their intake of a low FODMAP diet, which seems contradictory to at least some of the findings linking Bifidogenic effects and IBS symptom improvement with probiotic use in IBS sufferers (see Staudacher and Whelan[25] for a detailed review). Halmos and colleagues[83] have since compared specific populations of bacteria in stool samples preserved from their previous study,[80] and the low FODMAP diet was linked with a reduction in the absolute abundance of total bacteria and specific taxa across healthy and IBS cohorts. These differences also translated into statistically significant reductions in the relative abun-dances of a major subdivision of the Gram-positive Firmicutes (Cluster XIVa) and *A. muciniphila*, widely considered to be a beneficial mucin-associated gut bacterium. Only one bacterium measured (*Ruminococcus torques*) showed a marginal increase in total abundance and a significant increase in relative abundance in response to the period of consuming a low FODMAP diet. Intriguingly, *R torques* is also known to be mucin-associated, and other bacteria taxonomically affiliated with this bacterium have been reported to be positively associated with IBS symptom severity, and capable of mixed acid fermentation and gas production from substrates, such as FODMAPs.[84,85]

Collectively, these findings demonstrate that much still needs to be defined in rela-tion to the diet × microbiome interactions for IBS symptom control and patient quality of life. In that context, Halmos and colleagues[83] recommend that until such knowledge is available, caution should be applied with long-term adherence to a low FODMAP diet, even in patients diagnosed with IBS, and its use by asymptomatic healthy per-sons should be avoided.

THE FUTURE: SHINING LIGHT ON MICROBIAL DARK MATTER

Here, we have presented an overview of the current evidence of the diet × microbiome interactions relevant to the use of exclusion diets, such as EEN and the low FODMAP diet, as induction therapies for the treatment of organic (CD) and functional gastrointes-tinal diseases (IBS), respectively. In summary, both dietary interventions result in an improvement in patient symptoms and in the case of CD, mucosal healing. Both inter-ventions also seem to starve specific members of the hungry microbiome in the large bowel and result in reductions in bacterial diversity. More specifically, and somewhat paradoxically, these interventions also tend to result in the reduction of key bacterial groups, such as *Bifidobacterium*, *Faecalibacterium* and *Akkermansia* spp., which are now widely recognized for their roles in providing anti-inflammatory effects and/or the promotion of barrier function. So what is missing? The available literature suggests the previously mentioned bacteria are among the first rate-limited in their growth and persistence with EEN and/or low FODMAP diets. As such, we are currently limited by a poor understanding of the substrate preferences, affinities, and maximal growth rates of these key bacterial groups. Are nutrients other than "functional fibers" and traditional prebiotic carbohydrates relevant to growth? Progress needs to be made in these areas if the nutritional ecology of the gut is to be managed and effectively targeted to promote the growth of these bacterial groups via the provision of niche-specific nutrients. Second, shotgun metagenomic sequencing has revealed that a substantial amount of the microbiota is comprised of "dark matter," either in the form of not-yet-cultured microbes and gene families that remain undefined in terms of the functionality[86] of their respective gene products.[87] Of further note is that a substantial amount of this microbial dark matter is specific to "healthy" control subjects, and not just the comparator case cohorts (eg, Qin and colleagues[8]). Knowledge also needs to extend beyond the bacterial world, to include lower eukaryotes and viruses. There is a growing need to bring (meta)genomes to life and illuminate the functional and ecologic contributions from all forms of microbial dark matter to gut function and health.

SUMMARY

Diet has a significant impact on the structure-function activity of the gut microbiota. Most of the research to date has focused on assessing the impact of diet on the fecal microbiota and less is known about the impact of diet on the mucosal associated microbiota and its relevance to gastrointestinal function, host health and well-being. Although much remains to be discovered, the development of therapeutic dietary interventions that support the rational modulation of the gut microbiota is now a much more realistic and attractive strategy to better support the clinical management of these chronic gut diseases.

ACKNOWLEDGMENTS

The authors are grateful for the helpful suggestions and discussions with Drs Daniel Burger, Jakob Begun, Peter Lewindon, Bradley Kendall, Rachelle Haikings and Gerald Holtmann during the preparation of this article.

REFERENCES

1. Human Microbiome Project Consortium. Structure, function and diversity of the healthy human microbiome. Nature 2012;486(7402):207–14.
2. Morgan XC, Huttenhower C. Chapter 12: Human microbiome analysis. PLoS Comput Biol 2012;8(12):e1002808.
3. Logan AC, Jacka FN, Prescott SL. Immune-microbiota interactions: dysbiosis as a global health issue. Curr Allergy Asthma Rep 2016;16(2):13.
4. Petersen C, Round JL. Defining dysbiosis and its influence on host immunity and disease. Cell Microbiol 2014;16(7):1024–33.
5. NIH HMP Working Group, Peterson J, Garges S, Giovanni M, et al. The NIH human microbiome project. Genome Res 2009;19(12):2317–23.
6. Langille MG, Zaneveld J, Caporaso JG, et al. Predictive functional profiling of microbial communities using 16S rRNA marker gene sequences. Nat Biotechnol 2013;31(9):814–21.
7. Stearns JC, Lynch MDJ, Senadheera DB, et al. Bacterial biogeography of the human digestive tract. Sci Rep 2011;1:170.

8. Qin J, Li Y, Cai Z, et al. A metagenome-wide association study of gut microbiota in type 2 diabetes. Nature 2012;490(7418):55–60.

9. Qin N, Yang F, Li A, et al. Alterations of the human gut microbiome in liver cirrhosis. Nature 2014;513(7516):59–64.

10. Wang T, Cai G, Qiu Y, et al. Structural segregation of gut microbiota between colorectal cancer patients and healthy volunteers. ISME J 2012;6(2):320–9.

11. Yu J, Feng Q, Wong SH, et al. Metagenomic analysis of faecal microbiome as a tool towards targeted non-invasive biomarkers for colorectal cancer. Gut 2015. [Epub ahead of print].

12. Carmody RN, Gerber GK, Luevano JM, et al. Diet dominates host genotype in shaping the murine gut microbiota. Cell Host Microbe 2015;17(1):72–84.

13. David LA, Maurice CF, Carmody RN, et al. Diet rapidly and reproducibly alters the human gut microbiome. Nature 2014;505(7484):559–63.

14. Turnbaugh PJ, Hamady M, Yatsunenko T, et al. A core gut microbiome in obese and lean twins. Nature 2009;457(7228):480–4.

15. Cotillard A, Kennedy SP, Kong LC, et al. Dietary intervention impact on gut microbial gene richness. Nature 2013;500(7464):585–8.

16. Le Chatelier E, Nielsen T, Qin J, et al. Richness of human gut microbiome correlates with metabolic markers. Nature 2013;500(7464):541–6.

17. Turnbaugh PJ, Bäckhed F, Fulton L, et al. Diet-induced obesity is linked to marked but reversible alterations in the mouse distal gut microbiome. Cell Host Microbe 2008;3(4):213–23.

18. Turnbaugh PJ, Ley RE, Mahowald MA, et al. An obesity-associated gut microbiome with increased capacity for energy harvest. Nature 2006;444(7122): 1027–31.

19. Cox LM, Yamanishi S, Sohn J, et al. Altering the intestinal microbiota during a critical developmental window has lasting metabolic consequences. Cell 2014; 158(4):705–21.

20. Palm NW, de Zoete MR, Cullen TW, et al. Immunoglobulin A coating identifies colitogenic bacteria in inflammatory bowel disease. Cell 2014;158(5):1000–10.

21. Martín R, Laval L, Chain F, et al. *Bifidobacterium animalis* ssp. lactis CNCM-I2494 restores gut barrier permeability in chronically low-grade inflamed mice. Front Microbiol 2016;7:608.

22. Miquel S, Leclerc M, Martin R, et al. Identification of metabolic signatures linked to anti-inflammatory effects of *Faecalibacterium prausnitzii*. MBio 2015;6(2).

23. Derrien M, Van Baarlen P, Hooiveld G, et al. Modulation of mucosal immune response, tolerance, and proliferation in mice colonized by the mucin-degrader akkermansia muciniphila. Front Microbiol 2011;2:166.

24. Doré J, Blottière H. The influence of diet on the gut microbiota and its consequences for health. Curr Opin Biotechnol 2015;32:195–9.

25. Staudacher HM, Whelan K. Altered gastrointestinal microbiota in irritable bowel syndrome and its modification by diet: probiotics, prebiotics and the low FODMAP diet. Proc Nutr Soc 2016;75(3):306–18.

26. Ruemmele FM. Role of diet in inflammatory bowel disease. Ann Nutr Metab 2016; 68(Suppl 1):33–41.

27. Ó Cuív P, Begun J, Keely S, et al. Towards an integrated understanding of the therapeutic utility of exclusive enteral nutrition in the treatment of Crohn's disease. Food Funct 2016;7(4):1741–51.

28. Filippo CD, Cavalieri D, Paola MD, et al. Impact of diet in shaping gut microbiota revealed by a comparative study in children from Europe and rural Africa. Proc Natl Acad Sci U S A 2010;107(33):14691–6.

29. Bindels LB, Walter J, Ramer-Tait AE. Resistant starches for the management of metabolic diseases. Curr Opin Clin Nutr Metab Care 2015;18(6):559–65.

30. Delcour JA, Aman P, Courtin CM, et al. Prebiotics, fermentable dietary fiber, and health claims. Adv Nutr 2016;7(1):1–4.

31. Morrison DJ, Preston T. Formation of short chain fatty acids by the gut microbiota and their impact on human metabolism. Gut Microbes 2016;7(3):189–200.

32. Kim CH, Park J, Kim M. Gut microbiota-derived short-chain fatty acids, T cells, and inflammation. Immune Netw 2014;14(6):277–88.

33. Aron-Wisnewsky J, Clément K. The gut microbiome, diet, and links to cardiometabolic and chronic disorders. Nat Rev Nephrol 2016;12(3):169–81.

34. Ridlon JM, Kang DJ, Hylemon PB, et al. Bile acids and the gut microbiome. Curr Opin Gastroenterol 2014;30(3):332–8.

35. Mondot S, Boudinot P, Lantz O. MAIT, MR1, microbes and riboflavin: a paradigm for the co-evolution of invariant TCRs and restricting MHCI-like molecules? Immunogenetics 2016;68(8):537–48.

36. Sokol H, Pigneur B, Watterlot L, et al. *Faecalibacterium prausnitzii* is an anti-inflammatory commensal bacterium identified by gut microbiota analysis of Crohn disease patients. Proc Natl Acad Sci U S A 2008;105(43):16731–6.

37. Roopchand DE, Carmody RN, Kuhn P, et al. Dietary polyphenols promote growth of the gut bacterium *Akkermansia muciniphila* and attenuate high-fat diet–induced metabolic syndrome. Diabetes 2015;64(8):2847–58.

38. Tuohy K, Rio DD. Diet-microbe interactions in the gut: effects on human health and disease. Academic Press; 2014.

39. Tamburini S, Shen N, Wu HC, et al. The microbiome in early life: implications for health outcomes. Nat Med 2016;22(7):713–22.

40. Ottman N, Smidt H, de Vos WM, et al. The function of our microbiota: who is out there and what do they do? Front Cell Infect Microbiol 2012;2:104.

41. Chilloux J, Neves AL, Boulangé CL, et al. The microbial-mammalian metabolic axis: a critical symbiotic relationship. Curr Opin Clin Nutr Metab Care 2016;19(4):250–6.

42. Karlsson F, Tremaroli V, Nielsen J, et al. Assessing the human gut microbiota in metabolic diseases. Diabetes 2013;62(10):3341–9.

43. Lee D, Albenberg L, Compher C, et al. Diet in the pathogenesis and treatment of inflammatory bowel diseases. Gastroenterology 2015;148(6):1087–106.

44. Gut microbiota–immune system crosstalk: implications for metabolic disease - diet-microbe interactions in the gut - Chapter 9. Available at: http://www.sciencedirect.com/science/article/pii/B9780124078253000095. Accessed September 12, 2016.

45. McCarville JL, Caminero A, Verdu EF. Novel perspectives on therapeutic modulation of the gut microbiota. Therap Adv Gastroenterol 2016;9(4):580–93.

46. Jostins L, Ripke S, Weersma RK, et al. Host-microbe interactions have shaped the genetic architecture of inflammatory bowel disease. Nature 2012;491(7422):119–24.

47. Ananthakrishnan AN. Epidemiology and risk factors for IBD. Nat Rev Gastroenterol Hepatol 2015;12(4):205–17.

48. Prideaux L, Kang S, Wagner J, et al. Impact of ethnicity, geography, and disease on the microbiota in health and inflammatory bowel disease. Inflamm Bowel Dis 2013;19(13):2906–18.

49. Sartor RB. Therapeutic manipulation of the enteric microflora in inflammatory bowel diseases: antibiotics, probiotics, and prebiotics. Gastroenterology 2004;126(6):1620–33.

50. Gevers D, Kugathasan S, Denson LA, et al. The treatment-naive microbiome in new-onset Crohn's disease. Cell Host Microbe 2014;15(3):382–92.

51. Kang S, Denman SE, Morrison M, et al. Dysbiosis of fecal microbiota in Crohn's disease patients as revealed by a custom phylogenetic microarray. Inflamm Bowel Dis 2010;16(12):2034–42.
52. Atarashi K, Tanoue T, Oshima K, et al. Treg induction by a rationally selected mixture of Clostridia strains from the human microbiota. Nature 2013; 500(7461):232–6.
53. Atarashi K, Tanoue T, Shima T, et al. Induction of colonic regulatory T cells by indigenous clostridium species. Science 2011;331(6015):337–41.
54. Sokol H, Seksik P, Furet JP, et al. Low counts of *Faecalibacterium prausnitzii* in colitis microbiota. Inflamm Bowel Dis 2009;15(8):1183–9.
55. De Cruz P, Kang S, Wagner J, et al. Association between specific mucosa-associated microbiota in Crohn's disease at the time of resection and subsequent disease recurrence: a pilot study. J Gastroenterol Hepatol 2015;30(2):268–78.
56. Mondot S, Lepage P, Seksik P, et al. Structural robustness of the gut mucosal microbiota is associated with Crohn's disease remission after surgery. Gut 2016; 65(6):954–62.
57. Shaw KA, Bertha M, Hofmekler T, et al. Dysbiosis, inflammation, and response to treatment: a longitudinal study of pediatric subjects with newly diagnosed inflammatory bowel disease. Genome Med 2016;8(1):75.
58. Nam Y-D, Chang H-W, Kim K-H, et al. Bacterial, archaeal, and eukaryal diversity in the intestines of Korean people. J Microbiol 2008;46(5):491–501.
59. Ó Cuív P, Aguirre de Cárcer D, Jones M, et al. The effects from DNA extraction methods on the evaluation of microbial diversity associated with human colonic tissue. Microb Ecol 2011;61(2):353–62.
60. Scanlan PD, Shanahan F, Marchesi JR. Human methanogen diversity and incidence in healthy and diseased colonic groups using mcrA gene analysis. BMC Microbiol 2008;8:79.
61. Blais Lecours P, Marsolais D, Cormier Y, et al. Increased prevalence of *Methanosphaera stadtmanae* in inflammatory bowel diseases. PLoS One 2014;9(2): e87734.
62. Sokol H, Leducq V, Aschard H, et al. Fungal microbiota dysbiosis in IBD. Gut 2016. [Epub ahead of print].
63. Liguori G, Lamas B, Richard ML, et al. Fungal dysbiosis in mucosa-associated microbiota of Crohn's disease patients. J Crohns Colitis 2016;10(3):296–305.
64. Burman S, Hoedt EC, Pottenger S, et al. An (Anti)-inflammatory microbiota: defining the role in inflammatory bowel disease? Dig Dis 2016;34(1–2):64–71.
65. Grover Z, Muir R, Lewindon P. Exclusive enteral nutrition induces early clinical, mucosal and transmural remission in paediatric Crohn's disease. J Gastroenterol 2014;49(4):638–45.
66. Soo J, Malik BA, Turner JM, et al. Use of exclusive enteral nutrition is just as effective as corticosteroids in newly diagnosed pediatric Crohn's disease. Dig Dis Sci 2013;58(12):3584–91.
67. Grover Z, Lewindon P. Two-year outcomes after exclusive enteral nutrition induction are superior to corticosteroids in pediatric Crohn's disease treated early with thiopurines. Dig Dis Sci 2015;60(10):3069–74.
68. Berni Canani R, Terrin G, Borrelli O, et al. Short- and long-term therapeutic efficacy of nutritional therapy and corticosteroids in paediatric Crohn's disease. Dig Liver Dis 2006;38(6):381–7.
69. Durchschein F, Petritsch W, Hammer HF. Diet therapy for inflammatory bowel diseases: the established and the new. World J Gastroenterol 2016;22(7):2179–94.

70. Quince C, Ijaz UZ, Loman N, et al. Extensive modulation of the fecal metagenome in children with Crohn's disease during exclusive enteral nutrition. Am J Gastroenterol 2015;110(12):1718–29 [quiz: 1730].

71. Kaakoush NO, Day AS, Leach ST, et al. Effect of exclusive enteral nutrition on the microbiota of children with newly diagnosed Crohn's disease. Clin Transl Gastroenterol 2015;6:e71.

72. Charlebois A, Rosenfeld G, Bressler B. The impact of dietary interventions on the symptoms of inflammatory bowel disease: a systematic review. Crit Rev Food Sci Nutr 2016;56(8):1370–8.

73. Gearry RB, Irving PM, Barrett JS, et al. Reduction of dietary poorly absorbed short-chain carbohydrates (FODMAPs) improves abdominal symptoms in patients with inflammatory bowel disease-a pilot study. J Crohns Colitis 2009;3(1):8–14.

74. Gulhane M, Murray L, Lourie R, et al. High fat diets induce colonic epithelial cell stress and inflammation that is reversed by IL-22. Sci Rep 2016;6:28990.

75. Chassaing B, Koren O, Goodrich JK, et al. Dietary emulsifiers impact the mouse gut microbiota promoting colitis and metabolic syndrome. Nature 2015; 519(7541):92–6.

76. Roberts CL, Rushworth SL, Richman E, et al. Hypothesis: increased consumption of emulsifiers as an explanation for the rising incidence of Crohn's disease. J Crohns Colitis 2013;7(4):338–41.

77. Rossen NG, MacDonald JK, de Vries EM, et al. Fecal microbiota transplantation as novel therapy in gastroenterology: a systematic review. World J Gastroenterol 2015;21(17):5359–71.

78. Rajilić-Stojanović M, Jonkers DM, Salonen A, et al. Intestinal microbiota and diet in IBS: causes, consequences, or epiphenomena? Am J Gastroenterol 2015; 110(2):278–87.

79. Austin GL, Dalton CB, Hu Y, et al. A very low-carbohydrate diet improves symptoms and quality of life in diarrhea-predominant irritable bowel syndrome. Clin Gastroenterol Hepatol 2009;7(6):706–8.e1.

80. Halmos EP, Power VA, Shepherd SJ, et al. A diet low in FODMAPs reduces symptoms of irritable bowel syndrome. Gastroenterology 2014;146(1):67–75.e5.

81. Staudacher HM, Lomer MCE, Anderson JL, et al. Fermentable carbohydrate restriction reduces luminal bifidobacteria and gastrointestinal symptoms in patients with irritable bowel syndrome. J Nutr 2012;142(8):1510–8.

82. Staudacher HM, Whelan K, Irving PM, et al. Comparison of symptom response following advice for a diet low in fermentable carbohydrates (FODMAPs) versus standard dietary advice in patients with irritable bowel syndrome: IBS symptom response to a low FODMAP diet. J Hum Nutr Diet 2011;24(5):487–95.

83. Halmos EP, Christophersen CT, Bird AR, et al. Diets that differ in their FODMAP content alter the colonic luminal microenvironment. Gut 2015;64(1):93–100.

84. Malinen E, Krogius-Kurikka L, Lyra A, et al. Association of symptoms with gastrointestinal microbiota in irritable bowel syndrome. World J Gastroenterol 2010; 16(36):4532–40.

85. Hynönen U, Rasinkangas P, Satokari R, et al. Isolation and whole genome sequencing of a Ruminococcus-like bacterium, associated with irritable bowel syndrome. Anaerobe 2016;39:60–7.

86. Cuív PÓ, Smith WJ, Pottenger S, et al. Isolation of genetically tractable most-wanted bacteria by metaparental mating. Sci Rep 2015;5:13282.

87. Qin J, Li R, Raes J, et al. A human gut microbial gene catalogue established by metagenomic sequencing. Nature 2010;464(7285):59–65.

Impact of Antibiotics on Necrotizing Enterocolitis and Antibiotic-Associated Diarrhea

Michael A. Silverman, MD, PhD[a],[*],[1], Liza Konnikova, MD, PhD[b],[c],[1], Jeffrey S. Gerber, MD, PhD[d]

KEYWORDS

- Antibiotics • Microbiome • Necrotizing enterocolitis • Antibiotic-associated diarrhea
- *Clostridium difficile* • Probiotics

KEY POINTS

- Antibiotics induce microbial dysbiosis.
- Neonatal intestinal dysbiosis may contribute to necrotizing enterocolitis (NEC).
- Microbiome information may help predict risk for antibiotic-associated diarrhea (AAD) and NEC.
- Microbiome modulation may help prevent disease.
- Antibiotics induce AAD by disrupting microbiota's metabolic functions.

INTRODUCTION

Antibiotics are commonly prescribed medications that have saved countless lives, yet their side effects pose significant health challenges. Antibiotics are the most frequently prescribed medications in children[1] and constitute a significant amount in adults.[2] Antibiotics function by either direct killing or inhibiting growth of bacteria. In either case, they work in conjunction with the host's immune system to resolve infections.

[a] Division of Infectious Diseases, Department of Pediatrics, The Children's Hospital of Philadelphia, Perelman School of Medicine, University of Pennsylvania, 3615 Civic Center Boulevard, Philadelphia, PA 19104, USA; [b] Department of Pediatric and Newborn Medicine, Brigham and Women's Hospital, 75 Francis Street, Boston, MA 02115, USA; [c] Department of Pediatrics, Harvard Medical School, Boston, MA 02115, USA; [d] Division of Infectious Diseases, Department of Pediatrics, The Children's Hospital of Philadelphia, University of Pennsylvania School of Medicine, 3535 Market Street, Philadelphia, PA 19104, USA
[1] Equal contributors.
* Corresponding author.
E-mail address: SILVERMAM1@EMAIL.CHOP.EDU

Gastroenterol Clin N Am 46 (2017) 61–76
http://dx.doi.org/10.1016/j.gtc.2016.09.010
0889-8553/17/© 2016 Elsevier Inc. All rights reserved.

gastro.theclinics.com

Antibiotics and the Microbiome

The intestinal microbiome is a complex ecosystem in which there is tremendous inter-dependence and crosstalk between microbial species, and between the microbes and their host. Although antibiotics target specific types of microbes (eg, vancomycin and gram-positive organisms), their effects on the microbiome go beyond just those clin-ically targeted microbes. For example, removing certain species of bacteria opens niches for other microbes to expand, which, in turn, can result in microbiome disrup-tions or microbial dysbiosis, such as when treatment with the gram-positive microbe-targeted antibiotic vancomycin leads to loss of some gram-negative taxa.[3] Not all antibiotics affect intestinal microbiota to the same degree. For example, vancomycin and metronidazole both drastically change the composition of the microbiota (in different ways) but the overall bacterial density is less following metronidazole treat-ment yet remains the same following vancomycin treatment.[3] The route of exposure also matters because parenteral antibiotic treatment can affect the intestinal micro-biome via biliary excretion of antibiotic into the intestinal lumen.[4] Thus, although anti-biotics are intended to target specific pathogenic microbes, their effects can be much more extensive, long-lasting, and unpredictable.[5] Antibiotic-induced dysbiosis con-tributes in the shorter term to antibiotic-associated diarrhea (AAD) and is epidemiolog-ically linked to a variety of longer-term health problems, including obesity, asthma, allergy, and inflammatory bowel disease.[5,6]

Microbiome of the Neonate

Neonates face enormous challenges at parturition, including developing tolerance to their new microbiota while maintaining immunity against infection. The initial coloniza-tion of the gastrointestinal (GI) tract is an intricate balance between the colonization of commensal bacteria that leads to the establishment of tolerance and the prevention of infections secondary to the selective recognition of pathogenic microbes by the host. These host-microbial interactions are critical for the development and function of both the GI tract and the immune system. For example, the microbiota of the GI tract reg-ulates angiogenesis,[7] enterocyte proliferation, and proper crypt formation,[8] along with development and function of gut-associated lymphoid tissue and the intestinal T cell populations that prevent intestinal inflammation.[9,10] In a healthy neonate, this early crosstalk between commensal bacteria and the host leads to pathogen recognition, epithelial barrier maturation, immune system development, and development of toler-ance to food antigens and commensal bacteria.[11]

Microbial exposures early in ontogeny are associated with a range of diseases from atopy and autoimmune disorders to obesity and cancer.[12] This process is thought to occur either through epigenetic epithelial and/or immune system changes or by providing a niche for specific microbial colonization that influences long-term health outcomes.[11] However, exactly how the microbiome is established, and the impact of prenatal and postnatal exposures on the development of the microbiome, is only starting to be elucidated but offers great promise in predicting, preventing, and treat-ing a variety of diseases.

The neonatal GI tract rapidly becomes colonized with microbiota. Newborn's initial microbiota is acquired by vertical transmission of the maternal microbiome during de-livery,[13–16] although there is evidence for[17–19] and against[20] low-level microbial colo-nization of the placenta in utero. The mode of delivery, either via vaginal or caesarian section, influences the acquisition of most of the initial microbes.[13,14,16] As such, pre-natal factors that affect the maternal microbiome also influence the newborn's microbiome.[6]

The neonatal microbiome follows a general developmental process although significant interindividual variation is prominent.[13,15,16] In the first month, facultative anaerobic microbes from the Enterobacteriaceae family, a large group of gram-negative bacteria that includes pathogens such as *Escherichia coli* along with nonpathogenic bacteria, dominates the neonatal microbiome. Over the next few months, the Enterobacteriaceae are succeeded by anaerobic bacteria, including the families Bifidobacteriaceae, Bacteroidaceae, Lachnospiraceae, and Ruminococcaceae.[13,15] Around the time of weaning, a varied mixture of bacterial families are present, including Clostridiaceae. One way to monitor the development of the microbiome is to use microbial ecology concepts, such as alpha diversity, that describe the number and distribution of species present in a given individual.[21] For example, alpha diversity is lower in infants than adults, reflecting the higher number of microbial species in the adult microbiome.[16] The microbiome of neonates and infants is rapidly changing but stabilizes into an adult-like microbiome by 3 years of age.[16,22] A multitude of factors, such as the maternal microbiome, mode of delivery, diet, and antibiotic exposure, influence this process.[6]

Moreover, murine models suggest that, not only is the fetus exposed to the maternal GI microbiome before delivery but that colonization of mice during gestation has direct effects on the development of the offspring's immune system.[23] These data raise the possibility that prenatal exposure to antibiotics or other means of altering maternal microbiomes can have profound implications for their offspring. In support of this, prenatal exposure to antibiotics has been associated with increased risk for obesity and asthma.[24,25]

Mode of delivery (cesarean section vs vaginal) also shapes the neonatal microbiome.[26] The microbiome of infants born vaginally is characterized by fecal resident microbes such as *Bifidobacterium longum* and *Bifidobacterium catenulatum*, whereas infants delivered by caesarian sections have environmental microbes as their predominant microbiota.[27] This difference is long-lasting and can be seen even in older infants[26] and children.[28] Moreover, studies have suggested a link between the caesarian-section–associated microbiome and long-term outcomes, such as asthma,[29] gastroenteritis, celiac disease,[30] and diabetes.[27,31]

Infant diet also contributes to the development and composition of the microbiome. The microbiomes of breastmilk-fed and formula-fed infants are quite distinct. Breastmilk is high in prebiotic compounds, such as human milk oligosaccharides, that enhance bacterial growth. It also contains live bacteria not found in formula that can influence the microbiome.[32] The microbiome of neonates fed a breastmilk diet is more abundant in *Bifidobacteria* and *Lactobacillus*.[26,33,34] Surprisingly, several studies have found that, although breastfed infants have higher bacterial counts, they have a lower species diversity than formula fed infants.[26,33,34]

Antibiotic Effects on the Microbiome

Postnatal exposure to antibiotics is another important factor that shapes the microbiome. Antibiotic treatment decreases alpha diversity of the individual's microbiome.[15,35] For example, a seminal study in 3 healthy adults showed that 5 days of standard dose (500 mg twice a day) antibiotic treatment with ciprofloxacin had a significant effect on roughly one-third of the bacterial taxa identified in the study. However, most of these disturbances only lasted approximately 4 weeks, although some taxa were still missing at 6 months after treatment.[35] Additional studies have corroborated these finding and demonstrated that some antibiotics have even more profound and long-lasting disruptions of the microbiome.[3,36] Further, antibiotic exposure in infants and young children may have significant impacts on the microbiota during critical periods of development. For example, the microbiomes of infants exposed to ampicillin and gentamicin perinatally showed a decrease in Actinobacteria, *Bifidobacterium* and *Lactobacillus* and an increase in Proteobacteria at 4 weeks of age, and continued to have a decrease in the alpha diversity of these species even by 8 weeks of age.[37] In a longer study that evaluated the microbiota of 43 infants form birth to age 2, Bokulich and colleagues[13] observed that early antibiotic exposure led to a decrease in the microbiome's alpha diversity and specific deficits in the *Clostridium* and *Ruminococcus* species. Moreover, they showed that early antibiotic exposure decreased stability and delayed the maturation of the intestinal microbiome.[13] Similarly, another longitudinal cohort of children from birth to age 3 also showed a decrease in the alpha diversity of the microbiota of children exposed to antibiotics.[15] Additionally, they showed that the species found in the microbiota of children exposed to antibiotics was dominated by a single strain rather than having multiple strains of the same species and, similarly to the previous study, had deficits in clostridium species. Finally, antibiotic-exposed microbiota had an expansion of antibiotics resistance genes[15] (**Fig. 1**).

Microbiome of the Preterm Infant

Preterm infants face a more difficult challenge to maintain homeostasis with their developing microbiomes. They have immature immune and GI systems, commonly receive multiple courses of antibiotics, and have abnormal feeding patterns. Not surprisingly, the colonization patterns of the GI tract differ in preterm and term infants.[38,39] The diversity of the premature infant's microbiota is even more limited than in full-term neonates, where many of the detectable species in premature infants' microbiomes are known neonatal pathogens.[38,39] Additional differences include fewer anaerobes, increased abundance of Firmicutes and Proteobacteria, and decreased abundance of Bacteroides, as well as a substantial delay in bifidobacterial colonization when compared with full-term neonates.[11,40,41]

NECROTIZING ENTEROCOLITIS

One of the most devastating emergencies of the premature infant is necrotizing enterocolitis (NEC), affecting up to 10% of all premature infants. Although the pathogenesis of NEC remains incompletely understood, there is growing appreciation that defects in the development of host-microbiome commensalism likely contributes. NEC is characterized by uncontrolled intestinal inflammation that can lead to tissue necrosis, perforation, and sepsis. It is associated with mortality rates as high as 30% and substantial short-term and long-term morbidity.[42] Prematurity is the predominant risk factor for NEC. Interestingly, most cases of NEC occur at 31 to 32 weeks

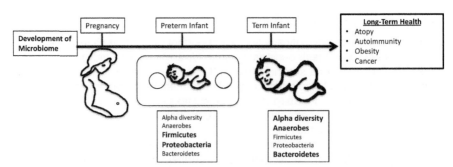

Fig. 1. Timeline of microbiome development in premature and term infants.

of corrected gestational age, independent of gestational age at birth, suggesting that host intrinsic developmental factors may affect the pathogenesis of NEC.[43]

Microbiome and Necrotizing Enterocolitis

Murine models of NEC have suggested that bacterial colonization of the intestine is essential to the development of NEC; however, no specific bacterial species has been identified as the causative agent for NEC.[44] Human cross-sectional studies have also failed to identify a causative bacterial agent for NEC.[41,45,46] Longitudinal analyses of fecal microbiomes from premature infants are beginning to shed some light on the differences in microbiome composition and colonization patterns between infants who develop NEC and those who do not. Several small, longitudinal studies have implicated a variety of bacterial species. For example, Torrazza and colleagues[47] showed that Proteobacteria and Actinobacteria were more abundant in stools of infants who later develop NEC, whereas Bifidobacteria and Bacteroidetes were less abundant in those infants. Fecal dysbiosis was also identified in a study by Morrow and colleagues[48] that similarly showed an increased abundance of microbes from the Proteobacteria and Firmicutes phyla preceding the development of NEC. Two separate small studies associated increased abundance of Clostridia species and Gammaproteobacteria with NEC.[49,50] In a cohort of 11 infants with NEC and 22 controls, Heida and colleagues[51] showed that the meconium of infants who subsequently developed NEC was enriched for *Clostridium perfringens* and *Bacteroides dorei* species when compared with control infants. Moreover, the abundance of staphylococci species was negatively associated with NEC development.[51] A recent large, multicenter study that analyzed stool samples from 166 infants of whom 46 developed NEC did not find any difference between the microbiome of the meconium in infants who developed NEC or controls. However, there were significant differences between groups by 1 month of age and, similarly to previous smaller studies, there was a higher abundance of Gammaproteobacteria before the diagnosis of NEC.[52] Additionally, there was a reduction in strict anaerobes and alpha diversity that preceded the development of NEC in infants born less than 27 weeks of age.[52] Taken together, these studies suggest that there is a clear dysbiosis with shifts toward increases in Gammaproteobacteria that precedes the development of NEC.

Antibiotics and Necrotizing Enterocolitis: Friend or Foe?

Although it remains controversial, prenatal and/or postnatal exposure to antibiotics might contribute to the dysbiosis preceding NEC. Several older randomized controlled trials (RCTs),[53] as well as animal studies, have shown that prophylactic administration of enteral antibiotics can prevent this disease.[49] Five RCTs have been conducted to evaluate the use of prophylactic enteral antibiotics (gentamicin, vancomycin, and kanamycin) for the prevention of NEC, all demonstrating significant reductions in rates of NEC,[53–57] with a subsequent meta-analysis showing an almost 50% reduction in the rates of NEC and a 70% reduction in NEC-related deaths.[58] However, these studies have limitations. The most recent study[53] was conducted in 1998 (and the others more than 30 years ago) and there was limited adjusting for confounding, accounting for diet and feeding schedules, or reporting of harmful side effects of the drugs. Further, the standard of care in the neonatal intensive care unit (NICU) has changed dramatically since then, with implementation of standardized feeding protocols, earlier introduction of enteral feeds, and use of donor human milk when maternal breast milk is not available, all of which have significantly reduced the rates of NEC.[59] As such, the applicability of these studies to the modern day NICU is uncertain. Additionally, there is concern that prolonged exposure to antibiotics will increase antibiotic resistance. Consistent with this, Boyle and colleagues[55] found that enteral kanamycin treatment was associated with an increase in antibiotic resistant bacteria. Interestingly, enteral vancomycin treatment was not associated with increased antibiotic resistance in this study but was associated with significant changes in the microbiota with predominance of gram-negative bacteria and yeasts, a milieu that could be harmful to the premature host.[53] Thus, before recommending empiric enteral antibiotic treatment of neonates at high risk for NEC, additional data are required to ensure that the potential benefits would outweigh the risks. Yet, these older RCTs, along with the new prospective characterization of the neonatal microbiome before the onset of disease, provide strong evidence for the importance of intestinal microbiota in the pathogenesis of NEC and raise enthusiasm for microbiota modulating therapy.

More recent studies have addressed whether parenteral antibiotics affect the risk for NEC. Premature neonates almost universally receive broad-spectrum antibiotics during their first 2 days of life and many receive more prolonged antibiotic courses for treatment of culture proven or culture-negative sepsis. Various retrospective studies have shown that prolonged antenatal[60] and postnatal antibiotic exposure is associated with an increased risk of developing NEC.[61–64] Specifically, a retrospective analysis of 97 matched pairs showed that prenatal exposure to ampicillin was significantly greater in infants with NEC.[60] Similarly, empirical (culture negative) antibiotics exposure for greater than 5 days has been associated with the development of NEC in numerous studies.[61–64]

This discordance in the effects of enteral versus parenteral administration of antibiotics on the effect of NEC suggests that it is not the use of the antibiotics per se that is detrimental but that alterations in the composition of the microbiome can either predispose to, or protect against, the development of NEC. Alternatively, residual confounding by indication might explain this association because patients who receive antibiotics may represent a sicker group with a higher risk for NEC that is independent of antibiotic exposure. Teasing this apart will require further study that explores NEC-associated pathogens such as Gammaproteobacteria in healthy and antibiotic-treated neonates.

Probiotics and Necrotizing Enterocolitis

Because intestinal dysbiosis is associated with the development of NEC, modulating the host's intestinal microbiome could be a way of preventing or ameliorating the disease. Probiotics have been extensively studied and, in general, seem to reduce the incidence of NEC. A recent meta-analysis of 20 RCTs[65] involving 5982 subjects, showed that the relative risk (RR) of NEC was reduced by almost 50% and overall mortality by 27% with the use of probiotics. However, these studies used various probiotics (*Lactobacillus*, *Bifidobacterium*, or *Saccharomyces* spp) and dosages. Subgroup analysis identified that *Lactobacillus* or a mixture of *Lactobacillus* and *Bifidobacterium* were most beneficial in reducing NEC. However, probiotics have not been used routinely to prevent NEC in the United States, owing to a lack of a product approved by the Food and Drug Administration (FDA) for this age group and little knowledge of potential adverse outcomes and long-term data. Additionally, a recent phase III trial failed to show a benefit to using *Bifidobacterium breve* BBG-001 in preventing NEC,[66] suggesting that this *Bifidobacterium* alone is not the optimal agent to use. Initially there was concern that the use of probiotics in premature infants would increase the risk of sepsis, which was extrapolated from case reports of probiotic-associated sepsis in immunocompromised and short bowel syndrome patients.[67] However, the meta-analysis did not show an increase in sepsis in infants

receiving probiotics.[65] Thus, probiotics
NEC, though the most effective and safe romising intervention for preventing
n has not been clearly identified.

ANTIBIOTIC-ASSOCIATED DIARRHEA

AAD, defined as diarrhea without a clear cause that is
ment, is among the most common medication side effec ted with antibiotic treat-
encounter.[68] Often, AAD is mild but can also be severe and patients and clinicians
in cases of *Clostridium difficile* infection (CDI).[68] Advances in reatening, especially
intestinal microbiome has set the foundation for microbiome-derstanding of the
prevent and treat AAD.   ed therapies to

Incidence of Antibiotic-Associated Diarrhea

Diarrhea occurs in up to 35% of patients who receive antibiotics.[68] AAD r ges in
severity from mild to life-threatening, and the incidence of diarrhea varies dep ding
on the antibiotic and the patient. Patients treated with amoxicillin-clavulanate nd
ampicillin have high rates of AAD (10%–25%), whereas fluoroquinolones, macrolides,
tetracyclines, and cephalosporins less often induce AAD.[68] A recent pediatric meta-
analysis reported AAD rates of 19.8%, 8.1%, and 1.2% for amoxicillin-clavulanate,
amoxicillin, and penicillin V, respectively.[69] Clindamycin was historically associated
with CDI in the original studies that linked CDI to pseudomembranous colitis[70,71]
and continues to cause a high rate of CDI.[72] However, almost any antibiotic can increase risk for CDI,[72] likely reflecting both the variation in the microbiota of patients
as well as the variable responses of different microbiota to different antibiotics.

Infectious Causes of Antibiotic-Associated Diarrhea

AAD has been recognized since the advent of antibiotics. More recently, CDI has
become a growing and significant problem. *Clostridium difficile* is a gram-positive,
spore forming, anaerobic, toxin-producing bacteria that lives in soil and the GI tract
of humans and animals. It is a significant cause of morbidity and mortality especially
in hospitalized patients. In 2011, there were an estimated half-million cases of CDI
and almost 30,000 deaths from this infection in the United States.[73] CDI is the leading
cause of death from gastroenteritis in the United States.[73] Patients may become colonized but remain asymptomatic or progress to symptomatic disease or CDI. The main
risk factors for CDI are antibiotic exposure along with advanced age, immune system
suppression, and prolonged hospital stay.[74]

Other pathogens beyond *Clostridium difficile* have been implicated as causing AAD
include *Klebsiella oxytoca*, *Staphylococcus aureus*, *Clostridium perfringens*, *Salmonella* spp, and *Candida* spp.[75] Most cases of AAD have not been linked to specific infectious agents, with only 10% to 20% due to CDI and a much smaller contribution
from the other known pathogens[75] (**Box 1**).

Mechanisms for Antibiotic-Associated Diarrhea

The most common mechanism is antibiotic-induced microbial dysbiosis, leading to
altered metabolism of key intestinal nutrients. Accumulation of certain metabolites
then induces an osmotic diarrhea. The second mechanism is loss of colonization
resistance and subsequent infection with pathogenic bacteria; for example, *Clostridium difficile*. A third is direct promotility action of specific antibiotics, such as erythromycin, which acts as a motilin agonist[68,76] (**Table 1**).

Box 1
Less-common infectious cause ...tic-associated diarrhea

Klebsiella oxytoca

Staphylococcus aureus

Clostridium perfringen'

Salmonella spp

Candida spp

Loss of Co~~l~~ **Metabolic Function**

The mec~~h~~ism for non-CDI AAD is thought to be due to altered microbial metabolism (see Ji~~a~~. Li and colleagues' article, "Biology of the Microbiome 2. Metabolic role," in this i~~ss~~ue). Normally, carbohydrates that were not absorbed in the small intestines wo~~ul~~d be fermented by colonic microbes to short-chain fatty acids (SCFAs), such as ~~b~~utyrate. It has been proposed that antibiotic-induced loss of colonic bacteria, such as clostridial species, leads to an increase in nonabsorbable carbohydrates in the large intestines. The excess carbohydrate load then induces an osmotic diarrhea.[77–79] Antibiotics clearly alter the intestinal metabolome,[80–82] yet there is little experimental evidence to directly connect these metabolic changes in the intestine to non-CDI AAD.[77,83] Additional study is needed to identify and test the causal relationship between specific antibiotic-induced metabolic perturbations and AAD (**Table 2**).

Loss of Colonization Resistance

Antibiotics decrease microbial community diversity and lead to decreased colonization resistance, which is the ability of the microbiota to prevent invasion of exogenous and potentially pathogenic microbes and to limit overgrowth of endogenous potentially pathogenic organisms—most notably Clostridium difficile. The mechanisms for colonization resistance are varied and include nutrient and physical niche competition between microbes, production of bacteriocins, and induction of a host response targeting specific microbes.[74] Although the association between antibiotic treatment and reduced colonization resistance has been observed for decades, the mechanisms have not been fully deciphered, yet recent discoveries offer some important hints. Studies involving the group of metabolites, or metabolome, of stool demonstrate that microbes regulate many metabolites and, not surprisingly, antibiotic treatment alters the metabolome with dramatic changes in bile acid, carbohydrate, and amino acid composition.[83]

Bile acids are important regulators of the Clostridium difficile lifecycle.[84,85] Primary bile acids induce germination of Clostridium difficile spores; however, secondary bile

Table 1
Mechanisms of antibiotic-associated diarrhea

Mechanisms of AAD	Consequence	Example
Loss of microbial metabolism	Increased metabolites lead to osmotic diarrhea	Amoxicillin-clavulanate
Loss of colonization resistance	Increased risk of infection by pathogen Clostridium difficile	Clindamycin
Direct promotility activity	Increased intestinal motility	Erythromycin

Table 2 Features of *Clostridium difficile* infection		
Features	***Clostridium difficile* Diarrhea**	**Non-CDI AAD**
Commonly implicated antibiotics	Clindamycin, cephalosporins, penicillins, fluoroquinolones	Clindamycin, cephalosporins, amoxicillin-clavulanate
Risk factors	Antibiotics, proton pump inhibitors, older age, hospital exposure, immune suppression, GI surgery	Previous AAD
History	Fevers, cramps	No fevers
Diarrhea	Mild to severe, fecal leukocytes positive	Usually mild, osmotic diarrhea
Mechanism	Loss of colonization resistance Altered bile acids	Loss of metabolic function Decreased fermentation of colonic carbohydrates to SCFAs
Treatment	Metronidazole or oral vancomycin, fecal microbial transplantation for recalcitrant cases, probiotics	Supportive, probiotics, antimotility agents

acids, generated by bacterial transformation of primary bile acids, inhibit *Clostridium difficile* growth and prevent its domination of the intestinal microbiome.[84] This is an elegant example of host–microbiota interactions generating colonization resistance from a pathogen that is mutually beneficial to the host and its microbiota. This balance is disrupted by antibiotic exposure that reduces bile acid–metabolizing bacteria, leading to lower secondary bile acids concentrations in the colon.[84] The loss of secondary bile acids relieves the inhibition on *Clostridium difficile* growth, allowing it to bloom to levels high enough to induce disease.[86] *Clostridium scindens*, a bile acid metabolizer, can prevent CDI in mice and, potentially, in humans.[86] This important finding lays the foundation for microbiome-targeted therapy to prevent CDI in humans.[74]

Competition of host-derived resources is another mechanism by which antibiotics predispose individuals to CDI. For example, antibiotics deplete microbes that use host-derived sialic acids. *Clostridium difficile* growth is enhanced in the presence of sialic acids. Therefore, antibiotic treatment predisposes the host to CDI by providing an overabundance of sialic acids that may promote CDI.[74,87]

Antibiotic-Associated Diarrhea Prevention

The cornerstone of AAD and CDI prevention is thoughtful and appropriate use of antibiotics along with proper precautions to prevent spread of *Clostridium difficile*.[88] Another more novel approach is to protect the intestinal microbiome from antibiotic effects by selectively inactivating antibiotics in the intestines. Concurrent administration of an intravenous beta lactam or cephalosporin antibiotic with an enteral beta lactamase that is not systemically absorbed prevents parenteral antibiotic from disrupting the intestinal microbiome.[89] This approach, which cleverly uses bacterial antibiotic resistance to benefit patients, is undergoing phase II clinical trials.[89]

CDI is associated with fecal microbiome changes that precede infection, including decreased alpha diversity, loss of SCFA-producing microbes, and elevated proportions of Proteobacteria.[90] The bile metabolizing microbe *Clostridium scindens* has been associated with protection from CDI in mice and humans.[86] Additional research is need to investigate whether this information could be help identify patients at high risk for developing CDI and perhaps offer novel microbiome-targeted therapies.

Antibiotic-Associated Diarrhea Treatment

AAD usually resolves with antibiotic cessation but this is not clinically feasible in patients with serious bacterial infection. Although antiperistaltic agents are not recommended for patients with CDI, they can provide symptom relief for patients with noninfectious AAD. Specific treatments for CDI AAD include antibiotic treatment, such as vancomycin or metronidazole[88]; fecal microbial transplantation (see Stephen M. Vindigni and Christina M. Surawicz's article, "Fecal Microbial Transplantation," in this issue); and probiotic therapy.

Probiotics for Antibiotic-Associated Diarrhea

Probiotics are formulations of live microorganisms intended to provide health benefits when administered into the body through alterations in the host microbiota, its metabolic function, or direct effects on the host. A multitude of organisms have been used as probiotics for the prevention or treatment of human disease. This point is worth emphasizing when considering the use of probiotics because the effectiveness and safety of various probiotics may differ based on both the properties of the specific probiotic and the characteristics of the recipient. The most commonly used probiotics include *Lactobacillus*, *Bifidobacterium*, and *Saccharomyces*, *Enterococcus*, and *Bacillus* spp, delivered either by pill or capsule, or through food.[91]

As previously outlined, the pathogenesis of AAD involves antibiotic-induced dysbiosis (resulting in an altered metabolic state) or diminished colonization resistance (providing a niche for infection with pathogenic bacteria). Therefore, supplementing the gut microbiota with bacteria that are robust to these disruptions by stabilizing it against the threat of dysbiosis from offending agents (eg, antibiotics), or creating a barrier to colonization with invading pathogens (eg, *Clostridium difficile*), or altering the microbiota's metabolic functions is an attractive preventive strategy.[92]

Probiotics for Antibiotic-Associated Diarrhea and Clostridium difficile Infection

Several studies examining the benefits of probiotics for AAD and/or CDI have been conducted, reflecting the diversity of microbial composition, host, and delivery vehicle. A recent systematic review and meta-analysis examined the impact of probiotics (*Lactobacillus*, *Bifidobacterium*, *Saccharomyces*, *Streptococcus*, *Enterococcus*, and/or *Bacillus*) on AAD in adults and children.[93] Of 63 RCTs (11,811 participants) that reported enough information for meta-analysis, probiotic use was associated with a lower rate of AAD compared with subjects who did not receive probiotics (RR 0.58), an effect that remained unchanged when stratified by age category. A Cochrane review assessed the efficacy of probiotics for the prevention of AAD in children, including 23 studies with nearly 4000 subjects receiving *Bacillus*, *Bifidobacterium*, *Clostridium*, *Lactobacilli*, *Lactococcus*, *Leuconostoc*, *Saccharomyces*, or *Streptococcus* spp, either alone or in combination.[94] Overall, 8% of children receiving probiotics experienced AAD versus 19% of those who did not (RR 0.46, number needed to treat 10). Adverse effects were rare and not associated with probiotic use.

Two large systematic reviews and meta-analyses examining the impact of probiotics on CDI in adults and children have also been conducted. Johnston and colleagues[95] analyzed data from 20 RCTs, including nearly 4000 subjects receiving *Bifidobacterium*, *Lactobacillus*, *Saccharomyces*, or *Streptococcus* spp, and found that probiotic use was associated with a 66% (RR 0.34) reduction in CDI rates compared with controls. This effect was similar for both adults and children, and probiotic use was not associated with adverse effects. A similar Cochrane review of 31 studies with nearly 4500 subjects found a similar (64%) reduction in CDI, which occurred in 2.0% of probiotic recipients and 5.5% of controls.[94]

Despite the consistency of findings across these systematic reviews and meta-analyses, 2 subsequently conducted multicenter RCTs highlight that some questions remain about the efficacy of probiotics for AAD and CDI. An RCT of nearly 3000 subjects greater than 65 years old found no benefit of Lactobacilli and Bifidobacterium use for the prevention of AAD (10.8% receiving probiotics vs 10.4% receiving placebo, RR 1.04, 95% CI 0.84–1.28) or CDI (0.8% vs 1.2%, RR 0.71, 95% CI 0.34–1.47).[96] Another multicenter RCT found no benefit of Saccharomyces boulardii for prevention of AAD in 477 adults from 15 hospitals using systemic antibiotics (HR 1.02, 95% CI .55–1.90).[97] Although the balance of evidence from systematic reviews and meta-analysis supports the use if pro-biotics for prevention of AAD and CDI, these large, multicenter trials highlight that the observed benefits likely do not apply to all probiotic formulations or patient populations.

Safety of Probiotics

To help inform the risk-benefit ratio of probiotic use for preventing AAD and CDI, examining probiotic safety is critical. Overall, probiotic administration seems to be safe with few if any side effects.[91] Several case reports document infections with organisms found in probiotics, typically occurring in hosts with immune-compromising conditions, such as prematurity, the presence of central venous access, or neutropenia.[98] However, these complications seem to be rare and generally treatable with antimicrobial therapy and/or removal of the infected device. Of note, because most probiotics are sold as dietary supplements, FDA scrutiny of probiotics is limited.[99] Thus, hospital formulary and drug-use and evaluation committees, and prescribing clinicians (in the ambulatory setting) should review any products considered for patient use and to verify responsible manufacturing practices.

The data previously summarized suggest that probiotics decrease the incidence of AAD and CDI in some populations of adults and children and that they are generally safe. However, several areas require further study, including the optimal microbial composition, dose, and timing of administration, as well as efficacy and safety in hosts with compromised immunity. Better defining the structure and function of the gut microbiome as it relates to the pathogenesis of AAD and CDI has the potential to generate customized probiotics for more effective prevention of these common and sometimes devastating conditions.[86]

REFERENCES

1. Chai G, Governale L, McMahon AW, et al. Trends of outpatient prescription drug utilization in US children, 2002-2010. Pediatrics 2012;130(1):23–31.

2. Hicks LA, Bartoces MG, Roberts RM, et al. US outpatient antibiotic prescribing variation according to geography, patient population, and provider specialty in 2011. Clin Infect Dis 2015;60(9):1308–16.

3. Robinson CJ, Young VB. Antibiotic administration alters the community structure of the gastrointestinal microbiota. Gut Microbes 2010;1(4):279–84.

4. Giuliano M, Barza M, Jacobus NV, et al. Effect of broad-spectrum parenteral antibiotics on composition of intestinal microflora of humans. Antimicrob Agents Chemother 1987;31(2):202–6.

5. Willing BP, Russell SL, Finlay BB. Shifting the balance: antibiotic effects on host-microbiota mutualism. Nat Rev Microbiol 2011;9(4):233–43.

6. Tamburini S, Shen N, Wu HC, et al. The microbiome in early life: implications for health outcomes. Nat Med 2016;22(7):713–22.

7. Stappenbeck TS, Hooper LV, Gordon JI. Developmental regulation of intestinal angiogenesis by indigenous microbes via Paneth cells. Proc Natl Acad Sci U S A 2002;99(24):15451–5.

8. Joly F, Mayeur C, Messing B, et al. Morphological adaptation with preserved proliferation/transporter content in the colon of patients with short bowel syndrome. Am J Physiol Gastrointest Liver Physiol 2009;297(1):G116–23.

9. Turnbaugh PJ, Ley RE, Hamady M, et al. The human microbiome project. Nature 2007;449(7164):804–10.

10. Uronis JM, Mühlbauer M, Herfarth HH, et al. Modulation of the intestinal microbiota alters colitis-associated colorectal cancer susceptibility. PLoS One 2009; 4(6):e6026.

11. Groer MW, Luciano AA, Dishaw LJ, et al. Development of the preterm infant gut microbiome: a research priority. Microbiome 2014;2:38.

12. Fujimura KE, Slusher NA, Cabana MD, et al. Role of the gut microbiota in defining human health. Expert Rev Anti Infect Ther 2010;8(4):435–54.

13. Bokulich NA, Chung J, Battaglia T, et al. Antibiotics, birth mode, and diet shape microbiome maturation during early life. Sci Transl Med 2016;8(343):343ra82.

14. Dominguez-Bello MG, Costello EK, Contreras M, et al. Delivery mode shapes the acquisition and structure of the initial microbiota across multiple body habitats in newborns. Proc Natl Acad Sci U S A 2010;107(26):11971–5.

15. Yassour M, Vatanen T, Siljander H, et al. Natural history of the infant gut microbiome and impact of antibiotic treatment on bacterial strain diversity and stability. Sci Transl Med 2016;8(343):343ra81.

16. Palmer C, Bik EM, DiGiulio DB, et al. Development of the human infant intestinal microbiota. PLoS Biol 2007;5(7):e177.

17. Stout MJ, Conlon B, Landeau M, et al. Identification of intracellular bacteria in the basal plate of the human placenta in term and preterm gestations. Am J Obstet Gynecol 2013;208(3):226.e1-7.

18. Aagaard K, Ma J, Antony KM, et al. The placenta harbors a unique microbiome. Sci Transl Med 2014;6(237):237ra65.

19. Satokari R, Grönroos T, Laitinen K, et al. Bifidobacterium and Lactobacillus DNA in the human placenta. Lett Appl Microbiol 2009;48(1):8–12.

20. Lauder AP, Roche AM, Sherrill-Mix S, et al. Comparison of placenta samples with contamination controls does not provide evidence for a distinct placenta microbiota. Microbiome 2016;4(1):29.

21. Costello EK, Stagaman K, Dethlefsen L, et al. The application of ecological theory toward an understanding of the human microbiome. Science 2012;336(6086): 1255–62.

22. Yatsunenko T, Rey FE, Manary MJ, et al. Human gut microbiome viewed across age and geography. Nature 2012;486(7402):222–7.

23. Gomez de Aguero M, Ganal-Vonarburg SC, Fuhrer T, et al. The maternal microbiota drives early postnatal innate immune development. Science 2016; 351(6279):1296–302.

24. Mueller NT, Whyatt R, Hoepner L, et al. Prenatal exposure to antibiotics, cesarean section and risk of childhood obesity. Int J Obes 2015;39(4):665–70.

25. Metsala J, Lundqvist A, Virta LJ, et al. Prenatal and post-natal exposure to antibiotics and risk of asthma in childhood. Clin Exp Allergy 2015;45(1):137–45.

26. Madan JC, Hoen AG, Lundgren SN, et al. Association of cesarean delivery and formula supplementation with the intestinal microbiome of 6-week-old infants. JAMA Pediatr 2016;170(3):212–9.

27. Neu J, Rushing J. Cesarean versus vaginal delivery: long-term infant outcomes and the hygiene hypothesis. Clin Perinatol 2011;38(2):321–31.

28. Salminen S, Gibson GR, McCartney AL, et al. Influence of mode of delivery on gut microbiota composition in seven year old children. Gut 2004;53(9):1388–9.

29. Renz-Polster H, David MR, Buist AS, et al. Caesarean section delivery and the risk of allergic disorders in childhood. Clin Exp Allergy 2005;35(11):1466–72.

30. Decker E, Engelmann G, Findeisen A, et al. Cesarean delivery is associated with celiac disease but not inflammatory bowel disease in children. Pediatrics 2010; 125(6):e1433–40.

31. Cardwell CR, Stene LC, Joner G, et al. Caesarean section is associated with an increased risk of childhood-onset type 1 diabetes mellitus: a meta-analysis of observational studies. Diabetologia 2008;51(5):726–35.

32. Fernandez L, Langa S, Martin V, et al. The human milk microbiota: origin and potential roles in health and disease. Pharmacol Res 2013;69(1):1–10.

33. Azad MB, Konya T, Maughan H, et al. Gut microbiota of healthy Canadian infants: profiles by mode of delivery and infant diet at 4 months. CMAJ 2013;185(5): 385–94.

34. Bezirtzoglou E, Tsiotsias A, Welling GW. Microbiota profile in feces of breast- and formula-fed newborns by using fluorescence in situ hybridization (FISH). Anaerobe 2011;17(6):478–82.

35. Dethlefsen L, Huse S, Sogin ML, et al. The pervasive effects of an antibiotic on the human gut microbiota, as revealed by deep 16S rRNA sequencing. PLoS Biol 2008;6(11):e280.

36. Pamer EG, Ubeda C, Buffie CG, et al. Profound alterations of intestinal microbiota following a single dose of clindamycin results in sustained susceptibility to *Clostridium difficile*-induced colitis. Infect Immun 2011;80(1):62–73.

37. Fouhy F, Guinane CM, Hussey S, et al. High-throughput sequencing reveals the incomplete, short-term recovery of infant gut microbiota following parenteral antibiotic treatment with ampicillin and gentamicin. Antimicrob Agents Chemother 2012;56(11):5811–20.

38. Mai V, Young CM, Ukhanova M, et al. Fecal microbiota in premature infants prior to necrotizing enterocolitis. PLoS One 2011;6(6):e20647.

39. Morowitz MJ, Denef VJ, Costello EK, et al. Strain-resolved community genomic analysis of gut microbial colonization in a premature infant. Proc Natl Acad Sci U S A 2011;108(3):1128–33.

40. Moles L, Gomez M, Heilig H, et al. Bacterial diversity in meconium of preterm neonates and evolution of their fecal microbiota during the first month of life. PLoS One 2013;8(6):e66986.

41. Claud EC, Keegan KP, Brulc JM, et al. Bacterial community structure and functional contributions to emergence of health or necrotizing enterocolitis in preterm infants. Microbiome 2013;1(1):20.

42. Walker WA, Neu J. Necrotizing enterocolitis. N Engl J Med 2011;364(3):255–64.

43. Yee WH, Soraisham AS, Shah VS, et al. Incidence and timing of presentation of necrotizing enterocolitis in preterm infants. Pediatrics 2012;129(2):e298–304.

44. Afrazi A, Sodhi CP, Richardson W, et al. New insights into the pathogenesis and treatment of necrotizing enterocolitis: toll-like receptors and beyond. Pediatr Res 2011;69(3):183–8.

45. Raveh-Sadka T, Thomas BC, Singh A, et al. Gut bacteria are rarely shared by co-hospitalized premature infants, regardless of necrotizing enterocolitis development. Elife 2015;4. http://dx.doi.org/10.7554/eLife.05477.

46. Normann E, Fahlén A, Engstrand L, et al. Intestinal microbial profiles in extremely preterm infants with and without necrotizing enterocolitis. Acta Paediatr 2013; 102(2):129–36.

47. Torrazza RM, Ukhanova M, Wang X, et al. Intestinal microbial ecology and environmental factors affecting necrotizing enterocolitis. PLoS One 2013;8(12): e83304.

48. Morrow AL, Lagomarcino AJ, Schibler KR, et al. Early microbial and metabolomic signatures predict later onset of necrotizing enterocolitis in preterm infants. Microbiome 2013;1(1):13.

49. Zhou Y, Shan G, Sodergren E, et al. Longitudinal analysis of the premature infant intestinal microbiome prior to necrotizing enterocolitis: a case-control study. PLoS One 2015;10(3):e0118632.

50. Sim K, Shaw AG, Randell P, et al. Dysbiosis anticipating necrotizing enterocolitis in very premature infants. Clin Infect Dis 2015;60(3):389–97.

51. Heida FH, van Zoonen AGJF, Hulscher JBF, et al. A necrotizing enterocolitis-associated gut microbiota is present in the meconium: results of a prospective study. Clin Infect Dis 2016;62(7):863–70.

52. Warner BB, Deych E, Zhou Y, et al. Gut bacteria dysbiosis and necrotising enterocolitis in very low birthweight infants: a prospective case-control study. Lancet 2016;387(10031):1928–36.

53. Siu YK, Ng PC, Fung SC, et al. Double blind, randomised, placebo controlled study of oral vancomycin in prevention of necrotising enterocolitis in preterm, very low birthweight infants. Arch Dis Child Fetal Neonatal Ed 1998;79(2):F105–9.

54. Grylack LJ, Scanlon JW. Oral gentamicin therapy in the prevention of neonatal necrotizing enterocolitis. A controlled double-blind trial. Am J Dis Child 1978; 132(12):1192–4.

55. Boyle R, Nelson JS, Stonestreet BS, et al. Alterations in stool flora resulting from oral kanamycin prophylaxis of necrotizing enterocolitis. J Pediatr 1978;93(5): 857–61.

56. Egan EA, Mantilla G, Nelson RM, et al. A prospective controlled trial of oral kanamycin in the prevention of neonatal necrotizing enterocolitis. J Pediatr 1976;89(3): 467–70.

57. Rowley MP, Dahlenburg GW. Gentamicin in prophylaxis of neonatal necrotising enterocolitis. Lancet 1978;2(8088):532.

58. Bury RG, Tudehope D. Enteral antibiotics for preventing necrotizing enterocolitis in low birthweight or preterm infants. Cochrane Database Syst Rev 2001;(1): CD000405.

59. Haque K. Necrotizing enterocolitis - some things old and some things new: a comprehensive review. J Clin Neonatol 2016;5(2). 79–12.

60. Weintraub AS, Ferrara L, Deluca L, et al. Antenatal antibiotic exposure in preterm infants with necrotizing enterocolitis. J Perinatol 2012;32(9):705–9.

61. Cotten CM, Taylor S, Stoll B, et al. Prolonged duration of initial empirical antibiotic treatment is associated with increased rates of necrotizing enterocolitis and death for extremely low birth weight infants. Pediatrics 2009;123(1):58–66.

62. Abdel Ghany EA, Ali AA. Empirical antibiotic treatment and the risk of necrotizing enterocolitis and death in very low birth weight neonates. Ann Saudi Med 2012; 32(5):521–6.

63. Kuppala VS, Meinzen-Derr J, Morrow AL, et al. Prolonged initial empirical antibiotic treatment is associated with adverse outcomes in premature infants. J Pediatr 2011;159(5):720–5.

64. Alexander VN, Northrup V, Bizzarro MJ. Antibiotic exposure in the newborn intensive care unit and the risk of necrotizing enterocolitis. J Pediatr 2011;159(3):392–7.

65. Lau CS, Chamberlain RS. Probiotic administration can prevent necrotizing enterocolitis in preterm infants: a meta-analysis. J Pediatr Surg 2015;50(8):1405–12.

66. Costeloe K, Hardy P, Juszczak E, et al. Probiotics in Preterm Infants Study Collaborative G. Bifidobacterium breve BBG-001 in very preterm infants: a randomised controlled phase 3 trial. Lancet 2016;387(10019):649–60.

67. Land MH, Rouster-Stevens K, Woods CR, et al. *Lactobacillus* sepsis associated with probiotic therapy. Pediatrics 2005;115(1):178–81.

68. Bartlett JG. Clinical practice. Antibiotic-associated diarrhea. N Engl J Med 2002;346(5):334–9.

69. Kuehn J, Ismael Z, Long PF, et al. Reported rates of diarrhea following oral penicillin therapy in pediatric clinical trials. J Pediatr Pharmacol Ther 2015;20(2):90–104.

70. Tedesco FJ, Barton RW, Alpers DH. Clindamycin-associated colitis. A prospective study. Ann Intern Med 1974;81(4):429–33.

71. Bartlett JG. *Clostridium difficile* infection: historic review. Anaerobe 2009;15(6):227–9.

72. Owens RC, Donskey CJ, Gaynes RP, et al. Antimicrobial-associated risk factors for *Clostridium difficile* infection. Clin Infect Dis 2008;46(Suppl 1):S19–31.

73. Lessa FC, Mu Y, Bamberg WM, et al. Burden of *Clostridium difficile* infection in the United States. N Engl J Med 2015;372(9):825–34.

74. Vincent C, Manges AR. Antimicrobial Use, Human Gut Microbiota and *Clostridium difficile* Colonization and Infection. Antibiotics (Basel) 2015;4(3):230–53.

75. Larcombe S, Hutton ML, Lyras D. Involvement of bacteria other than *Clostridium difficile* in antibiotic-associated diarrhoea. Trends Microbiol 2016;24(6):463–76.

76. Peeters T, Matthijs G, Depoortere I, et al. Erythromycin is a motilin receptor agonist. Am J Physiol 1989;257(3 Pt 1):G470–4.

77. Binder HJ. Role of colonic short-chain fatty acid transport in diarrhea. Annu Rev Physiol 2010;72(1):297–313.

78. Clausen MR, Bonnén H, Tvede M, et al. Colonic fermentation to short-chain fatty acids is decreased in antibiotic-associated diarrhea. Gastroenterology 1991;101(6):1497–504.

79. Young VB, Schmidt TM. Antibiotic-associated diarrhea accompanied by large-scale alterations in the composition of the fecal microbiota. J Clin Microbiol 2004;42(3):1203–6.

80. Antunes LCM, Han J, Ferreira RBR, et al. Effect of antibiotic treatment on the intestinal metabolome. Antimicrob Agents Chemother 2011;55(4):1494–503.

81. Vrieze A, Out C, Fuentes S, et al. Impact of oral vancomycin on gut microbiota, bile acid metabolism, and insulin sensitivity. J Hepatol 2014;60(4):824–31.

82. Mellon AF, Deshpande SA, Mathers JC, et al. Effect of oral antibiotics on intestinal production of propionic acid. Arch Dis Child 2000;82(2):169–72.

83. Theriot CM, Young VB. Interactions between the gastrointestinal microbiome and *Clostridium difficile*. Annu Rev Microbiol 2015;69:445–61.

84. Theriot CM, Bowman AA, Young VB. Antibiotic-induced alterations of the gut microbiota alter secondary bile acid production and allow for *Clostridium difficile*

spore germination and outgrowth in the large intestine. mSphere 2016;1(1): e00045–115.

85. Wilson KH. Efficiency of various bile salt preparations for stimulation of *Clostridium difficile* spore germination. J Clin Microbiol 1983;18(4):1017–9.

86. Buffie CG, Bucci V, Stein RR, et al. Precision microbiome reconstitution restores bile acid mediated resistance to *Clostridium difficile*. Nature 2015;517(7533): 205–8.

87. Ng KM, Ferreyra JA, Higginbottom SK, et al. Microbiota-liberated host sugars facilitate post-antibiotic expansion of enteric pathogens. Nature 2013; 502(7469):96–9.

88. Cohen SH, Gerding DN, Johnson S, et al. Clinical practice guidelines for *Clostridium difficile* infection in adults: 2010 update by the Society for Healthcare Epidemiology of America (SHEA) and the Infectious Diseases Society of America (IDSA). Infect Control Hosp Epidemiol 2010;31(5):431–55.

89. Kaleko M, Bristol JA, Hubert S, et al. Development of SYN-004, an oral beta-lactamase treatment to protect the gut microbiome from antibiotic-mediated damage and prevent *Clostridium difficile* infection. Anaerobe 2016;41:58–67.

90. Vincent C, Stephens DA, Loo VG, et al. Reductions in intestinal Clostridiales precede the development of nosocomial *Clostridium difficile* infection. Microbiome 2013;1(1):18.

91. Hempel S, Newberry S, Ruelaz A, et al. Safety of probiotics to reduce risk and prevent or treat disease. Evid Rep Technol Assess (Full Rep) 2011;(200):1–645.

92. Parkes GC, Sanderson JD, Whelan K. The mechanisms and efficacy of probiotics in the prevention of *Clostridium difficile*-associated diarrhoea. Lancet Infect Dis 2009;9(4):237–44.

93. Hempel S, Newberry SJ, Maher AR, et al. Probiotics for the prevention and treatment of antibiotic-associated diarrhea: a systematic review and meta-analysis. JAMA 2012;307(18):1959–69.

94. Goldenberg JZ, Lytvyn L, Steurich J, et al. Probiotics for the prevention of pediatric antibiotic-associated diarrhea. Cochrane Database Syst Rev 2015;(12):CD004827.

95. Johnston BC, Ma SSY, Goldenberg JZ, et al. Probiotics for the prevention of *Clostridium difficile*-associated diarrhea: a systematic review and meta-analysis. Ann Intern Med 2012;157(12):878–88.

96. Allen SJ, Wareham K, Wang D, et al. Lactobacilli and bifidobacteria in the prevention of antibiotic-associated diarrhoea and *Clostridium difficile* diarrhoea in older inpatients (PLACIDE): a randomised, double-blind, placebo-controlled, multi-centre trial. Lancet 2013;382(9900):1249–57.

97. Ehrhardt S, Guo N, Hinz R, et al. *Saccharomyces boulardii* to prevent antibiotic-associated diarrhea: a randomized, double-masked, placebo-controlled trial. Open Forum Infect Dis 2016;3(1):ofw011.

98. Borriello SP, Hammes WP, Holzapfel W, et al. Safety of probiotics that contain lactobacilli or bifidobacteria. Clin Infect Dis 2003;36(6):775–80.

99. Degnan FH. The US Food and Drug Administration and probiotics: regulatory categorization. Clin Infect Dis 2008;46(Suppl 2):S133–6 [discussion: S144–51].

The Microbiome-Gut-Brain Axis in Health and Disease

Timothy G. Dinan, MD, PhD[a,b,]*, John F. Cryan, PhD[a,c]

KEYWORDS

- Microbiota • Psychobiotics • Short-chain fatty acids • Vagus nerve • GABA
- Serotonin

KEY POINTS

- Gut microbes can communicate with the brain through a variety of routes, including the vagus nerve, short-chain fatty acids (SCFAs), cytokines, and tryptophan.
- Psychobiotics are bacteria that when ingested in adequate amounts produce a positive mental health benefit.
- The brain-gut-microbiota axis represents a paradigm shift in neuroscience and provides a novel target for treating not only irritable bowel syndrome (IBS) but also conditions, such as depression, autism, and Parkinson disease.

INTRODUCTION

The human adult gut contains more than 1 kg of bacteria, essentially the same weight as the human brain.[1] It is generally estimated that the gut is inhabited by 10^{13} to 10^{14} microorganisms, which is significantly more than the number of human cells in the body, and contains more than 100 times as many genes as in the genome.[2] Amazingly, the genomic and biochemical complexity of the microbiota exceeds that of the brain. Studies of the brain-gut-microbiota axis have been described as a paradigm shift in neuroscience.[3] Increasing evidence points to appropriate diversity in the gut microbiota that is essential not only for gut health but also for normal physiologic functioning in other organs, especially the brain. An altered gut microbiota in the form of dysbiosis at the extremes of life, both in the neonate and in the elderly, can have a profound impact on brain function. Such a dysbiosis might emerge for a variety of reasons, including the mode of birth delivery, diet, and antibiotic and other drug exposure. Given that the brain is dependent on gut microbes for essential metabolic products,

[a] APC Microbiome Institute, University College Cork, Cork, Ireland; [b] Department of Psychiatry and Neurobehavioural Science, University College Cork, Cork, Ireland; [c] Department of Anatomy and Neuroscience, University College Cork, Cork, Ireland
* Corresponding author. Department of Psychiatry and Neurobehavioural Science, University College Cork, Cork.
E-mail address: t.dinan@ucc.ie

Gastroenterol Clin N Am 46 (2017) 77–89
http://dx.doi.org/10.1016/j.gtc.2016.09.007
0889-8553/17/© 2016 Elsevier Inc. All rights reserved.

it is not surprising that a dysbiosis can have serious negative consequences for brain function both from neurologic and mental health perspectives. Although much of the early data emerged from animal studies, mainly rodent based, there are now an increasing number of human studies translating the animal findings.

This review focuses on the routes of communication between the gut and brain, examines a prototypic disorder of the brain gut axis, explores the ways in which gut dysbiosis may evolve, and provides an up-to-date account of behavioral and neurologic pathologies associated with dysbiosis.

BRAIN-GUT-MICROBIOTA COMMUNICATION

The brain-gut-microbiota axis is a bidirectional communication system enabling gut microbes to communicate with the brain and the brain with the gut.[4] Although brain-gut communication has been a subject of investigation for decades, an exploration of gut microbes within this context has only featured in recent years. The mechanisms of signal transmission are complex and not fully elucidated but include neural, endocrine, immune, and metabolic pathways.[5,6] Preclinical studies have implicated the vagus nerve as a key route of neural communication between microbes of the gut and centrally mediated behavioral effects, as demonstrated by the elimination of central *Lactobacillus rhamnosus* effects after vagotomy[7] and that humans who have underwent vagotomy at an early age have a decreased risk of certain neurologic disorders.[8] The gut microbiota also regulates key central neurotransmitters, such as serotonin, by altering levels of precursors; for example, *Bifidobacterium infantis* has been shown to elevate plasma tryptophan levels and thus influence central serotonin (5HT) transmission.[9] Intriguingly, synthesis and release of neurotransmitters from bacteria has been reported: *Lactobacillus* and *Bifidobacterium* spp can produce γ-aminobutyric acid (GABA); *Escherichia*, *Bacillus*, and *Saccharomyces* spp can produce noradrenaline; *Candida, Streptococcus, Escherichia*, and *Enterococcus* spp can produce serotonin; *Bacillus* can produce dopamine; and *Lactobacillus* can produce acetylcholine.[10,11] These microbially synthesized neurotransmitters can cross the mucosal layer of the intestines, although it is highly unlikely that they directly influence brain function. Even if they enter the blood stream, which is by no means certain, they are incapable of crossing the blood-brain barrier (BBB). Their impact on brain function is likely to be indirect, acting on the enteric nervous system. SCFAs, which include butyrate, propionate, and acetate, are essential metabolic products of gut microbial activity and may exert central effects either through G-protein–coupled receptors, although such receptors are sparsely concentrated in the brain. It is more likely that they act as epigenetic modulators through histone deacetylases.[2] SCFAs are also involved in energy balance and metabolism and can modulate adipose tissue, liver tissue, and skeletal muscle and function.[12] Immune signaling from gut to brain mediated by cytokine molecules is another documented route of communication.[13] Cytokines produced at the level of the gut can travel via the bloodstream to the brain. Under normal physiologic circumstances, it is unlikely that they cross the BBB, but increasing evidence indicates a capacity to signal across the BBB and to influence brain areas, such as the hypothalamus, where the BBB is deficient. It is through the latter mechanism the cytokines interleukin (IL)-1 and IL-6 activate the hypothalamic-pituitary-adrenal (HPA) axis, bringing about the release of cortisol. This is the most potent activator of the stress system.

The HPA axis, which provides the core regulation of the stress response, can have a significant impact on the brain-gut-microbiota axis.[14–20] It is increasingly clear and probably of relevance in several pathologic conditions that psychological or physical stress can significantly dysregulate the HPA axis and subsequently the brain-gut-microbiota axis, for example, in IBS[21] (**Fig. 1**).

Multiple lines of approach have been used to interrogate the brain-gut-microbiota axis, especially in animal model systems; these include the use of germ-free animals, potential probiotic agents, antibiotics, animals exposed to pathogens and the use of stress to determine the effects of dysregulating the axis. The largest naturalistic study of a gut pathogen and the impact on the brain-gut axis was as a result of the Walkerton catastrophe. The contamination of the Walkerton (Walkerton, Ontario, Canada) water supply occurred in 2000 claimed 7 lives and left more than 2000 people ill. The *E coli* outbreak was caused by farm runoff contaminating the town's water supply. Those infected had significant risk of developing postinfective IBS and many had comorbid depression/anxiety.[22] To a greater extent than any prior study, this natural disaster provided clear cut support for the notion of postinfective IBS.

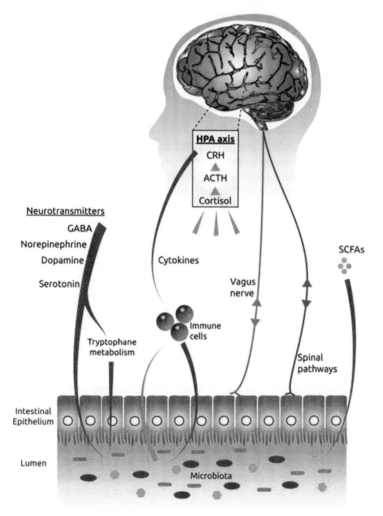

Fig. 1. Routes of communication between gut microbes and brain. These include the vagus nerve, SCFAs (butyrate, propionate, and acetate), cytokines, and tryptophan. ACTH, adreno-corticotropic hormone; CRH, corticotropin releasing hormone.

BRAIN-GUT-MICROBIOTA AXIS AND EXTREMES OF LIFE

The intestinal microbiota of newborn infants is characterized by low diversity and a relative dominance of the phyla Proteobacteria and Actinobacteria in the early post-natal period, a time at which there is enormous brain development. With the passage of time, the microbiota becomes more diverse, with the emergence and dominance of Firmicutes and Bacteroidetes.[23–25] Full-term, vaginally delivered babies born to healthy mothers who are breastfed and nonantibiotic treated have an optimal development of the neonatal microbiota.[26] The characteristic intestinal microbiota observed in healthy full-term infants is disturbed in preterm infants,[27] who are frequently delivered by caesarean section, receive antibiotics, and may have problems feeding.[28] Furthermore, preterm infants possess a functionally immature gut with low levels of acidity in the stomach, due to insufficient gastric acid secretion and their requirement for more frequent feeding.[28–30] These events lead to an increase in the prevalence of potentially pathogenic bacteria in the gastrointestinal (GI) tract and less microbial diversity than full term infants.[31–33] The extent to which these features play a role in the development of cerebral palsy and subsequent autism are the subject of research and ongoing debate.[34] What is clear is that complex brain maturation and the increasing sophistication of the gut microbiota are highly correlated. To date many assumptions are based on correlational data from which a causative impact cannot be conclusively concluded.

When the microbiota composition of elderly people in nursing homes are compared with those in the community, large-scale differences are detected. Those in nursing homes have a far less diverse microbiota and this has been attributed to a less varied diet.[35] It is possible, however, that pathologic factors that lead to admission into nursing homes, such as deteriorating cognitive function and less physical activity, might play an important role in the decreased microbial richness and not the less diverse diet. Ongoing studies should clarify this issue, and there is a challenge for the food industry to produce diets for the elderly that help to sustain microbial diversity.

What is abundantly clear is that a dysregulated gut microbiota either in early childhood or in an aging population significantly increases the likelihood of brain dysfunction. The precise relationship between these observations is far from understood. Determining the mechanisms and pathways underlying microbiota-brain interactions may yield novel insights into individual variations and perhaps enable the development of new treatments for a range of neurodevelopmental and neurodegenerative disorders, ranging from autism to Parkinson disease.

IRRITABLE BOWEL SYNDROME AS PROTOTYPE

IBS is the prototypic disorder of the brain-gut-microbiota axis, generally perceived as a having a biopsychosocial etiology[36] and frequently comorbid with depression or anxiety. The most important single risk factors are female gender, younger age, and preceding GI infections. Recent studies suggest that trauma in childhood, especially sexual abuse, may be an important risk factor.[37] The aspect of dysbiosis in IBS is important and is discussed elsewhere, but aspects of gut-to-brain communication are clearly altered. For example, elevated levels of plasma proinflammatory cytokines are found and there is an exaggerated pituitary-adrenal response to corticotropin-releasing hormone, together with augmented visceral pain responses. A recent study found that fasting serum levels of SCFAs did not differ between patients with IBS and controls.[38] The postprandial levels of total SCFAs, acetic acid, propionic acid, and butyric acid were found, however, significantly lower in patients with IBS compared with healthy controls. An epigenetic model of IBS has been proposed,[36] which is consistent with the potential epigenetic modulating effects of butyrate, the levels of which are altered substantially in the postprandial state.

Treatments of IBS that do not take into account this complex pathophysiology[37] are likely to be of limited benefit (**Fig. 2**).

DEPRESSION

IBS and depression are frequently comorbid and the latter is associated with the presence of biomarkers of inflammation, such as elevated IL-6, tumor necrosis factor (TNF)-α, and the acute-phase protein, C-reactive protein.[39] Similar elevated biomarkers of inflammation have been seen in anxiety states and are known to occur as a result of stress. The site at which these proinflammatory molecules is produced in depression is not known and it has yet to be determined whether the elevation is core to the pathophysiology or merely epiphenomenal. There is evidence from rodent studies to indicate that stress alters the gut barrier function, allowing lipopolysaccharide (LPS) and other molecules to gain access to the bloodstream, stimulating Toll-like receptor 4 and other Toll-like receptors, resulting in the production of inflammatory cytokines.[39] If this does occur in depression, which has yet to be definitively demonstrated, it would explain the proinflammatory phenotype observed.

Bercik and colleagues,[40] using germ-free and specific pathogen-free mice, demonstrated that the early life stress of maternal separation alters the HPA axis and colonic

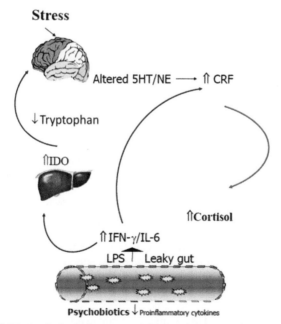

Fig. 2. Model of IBS. Psychological stress or infection leads to activation of the HPA axis, with elevation in cortisol and also changes in gut permeability. LPS enters the bloodstream, increasing proinflammatory cytokines and altering tryptophan metabolism. In turn this leads to alterations in serotonin (5HT) and glutamate neurotransmission. Psychobiotics may have an impact by decreasing gut permeability and signaling the brain via the vagus nerve and other routes. CRH, corticotropin releasing hormone; IDO, indoleamine 2,3-dioxygenase; IFN, interferon; NE, norepinephrine.

cholinergic neural regulation in a microbiota-independent fashion.[41] They showed, however, that the microbiota is required for the induction of anxiety-like behavior and behavioral despair. Colonization of adult germ-free maternally separated and control mice with the same microbiota produces distinct microbial profiles, which are associated with altered behavior in maternally separated mice but not in control mice. The results suggest that maternal separation–induced changes in host physiology lead to intestinal dysbiosis, which is a critical determinant of the abnormal behavior that characterizes this model of early-life stress. Prior studies in maternally separated rats demonstrated an altered behavioral phenotype when these animals reached maturity and also decreased diversity in the microbiota.[20] Does this decreased diversity translate to patients with major depression?

In a recent study the fecal microbiota was sequenced[41]; 46 patients with depression and 30 healthy controls were recruited. High-throughput pyrosequencing showed that, according to the Shannon index, increased fecal bacterial α-diversity was found in those currently depressed but not in a group who had responded to treatment. Bacteroidetes, Proteobacteria, and Actinobacteria were increased, whereas Firmicutes was significantly reduced. Despite the profound interindividual variability, levels of several predominant genera were significantly different between the depressives and controls. Notably, the depressives had increased levels of Enterobacteriaceae and Alistipes but reduced levels of Faecalibacterium. The investigators conclude that further studies are necessary to elucidate the temporal and causal relationships between gut microbiota and depression and to evaluate the suitability of the microbiome as a biomarker. When rats are given a humanized microbiota from depressed patients as opposed to healthy controls, they develop a depressive phenotype from a behavioral and immune perspective.[42]

AUTISM

Autism is a neurodevelopmental disorder whose prevalence is apparently on the increase. It is characterized by a failure of language acquisition and a lack of sociability. It is frequently associated with GI symptoms,[43] the relevance of which has been a longstanding source of controversy. Up to 70% of patients with the syndrome report abdominal symptoms and hence the view that it is a disorder of the brain-gut axis. The authors' group at the APC Microbiome Institute examined the behavior of mice raised in a germ-free environment.[44,45] The mice were tested in a 3-chamber apparatus, where a germ-free mouse was placed in the middle chamber with a familiar mouse in 1 chamber and a novel mouse in the third. The germ-free mouse spent as much time with the familiar as with the novel mouse; this is in contrast to the behavior of conventionally colonized mice who spend more time with the novel than the familiar mouse. Germ-free mice are also more likely to spend time with an empty chamber or an object than with another mouse, a decidedly abnormal behavior for a sociable animal. Colonization of the germ-free mice does partially normalize their behavior patterns. These behavioral changes are associated with significant alterations in underlying neurochemistry.

Work from the Patterson and Mazmanian[46] group in an animal model demonstrated that the microbiota modulates behavioral and physiologic abnormalities associated with neurodevelopmental disorders such as autism.[46] They used the maternal immune activation model induced by poly(I:C) injection during pregnancy and found altered GI barrier defects and microbiota alterations. Oral treatment with the human commensal *Bacteroides fragilis* was shown to correct gut permeability and interestingly stereotyped and other abnormal behaviors. Furthermore, a metabolite found in the abnormal animals was observed to transfer the phenotype to naïve animals and to be reduced by *B fragilis*.

Increasing attention is being paid to oxytocin the hypothalamic peptide, which has been shown to increase sociability. The oxytocin receptor knockout mouse shows considerable deficits in social behavior and some small-scale preliminary studies in humans indicate that intranasally administered oxytocin may positively alter social behavior patterns. A few large clinical trials are under way to test oxytocin and related therapies for autism spectrum disorder. There is still considerable debate as to whether or not the preclinical findings translate to the clinical setting and if they do which patients and which aspects of the syndrome are likely to benefit most. Intriguingly, a recent study indicates that probiotic bacteria can influence hypothalamic posterior pituitary activity and increase oxytocin levels, raising the possibility of influencing social behavior by targeting the gut microbiota.[47]

The fecal microbiota in patients with autism spectrum disorder has been sequenced.[48] In the most recently published study, Tomova and colleagues[48] examined the microbiota in Slovakian children. The fecal microbiota of autistic children showed a significant decrease of the Bacteroidetes/Firmicutes ratio and elevation of the amount of *Lactobacillus* spp. There was a modest elevation in *Desulfovibrio* spp and a correlation with the severity of autism. A probiotic diet normalized the Bacteroidetes/Firmicutes ratio and *Desulfovibrio* spp levels. As recently summarized by Mayer and colleagues,[3] there is a paucity of large comprehensive studies of the microbiome in autism. Again the 'chicken or egg' issue emerges: Are these changes induced by stereotyped diets seen in many individuals as a product of obsessional behavior patterns? Also the heterogeneous nature of the disease needs to be taken into account and much more effort is needed to tease out the exact role of the microbiome in both the etiology and treatment of the disorder.

PARKINSON DISEASE

In marked contrast to autism, Parkinson disease tends to be diagnosed generally in old age; it is the second most common neurodegenerative disorder and affects 1% to 2% of the population over 65 years of age. It is a movement disorder characterized by degeneration of the zona compacta neurons of the substantia nigra. The most common GI symptoms are constipation, appetite loss, weight loss, dysphagia, sialorrhea, and gastroesophageal reflux.[49] α-Synuclein aggregates, the major neuropathologic marker in Parkinson disease, are present in the submucosal and myenteric plexuses of the enteric nervous system, prior to their detection in the brain, which may indicate a gut to brain prion-like spread.[50]

The gut microbiota has been sequenced in patients with Parkinson disease.[51] On average, the abundance of Prevotellaceae in the feces of Parkinson disease patients was reduced by almost 80% compared with controls. A logistic regression analysis based on the abundance of 4 bacterial families and the severity of constipation identified Parkinson disease patients, with 66.7% sensitivity and 90.3% specificity. The relative abundance of Enterobacteriaceae was highly correlated with the severity of postural instability and gait difficulty. The findings suggest that the intestinal microbiome is altered in Parkinson disease and is related to motor phenotype. Large prospective studies beginning in the early stages of the disorder are required.

It has been suggested that microbiota transplantation might benefit patients with Parkinson disease but there is as yet no conclusive evidence.[52] Neither are there any reports of controlled trials of probiotics/psychotiotics.

PSYCHOBIOTICS

Psychobiotics were first defined as the family of probiotics that, ingested in appropriate quantities, had a positive mental health benefit.[53] Recently, the definition has been expanded to include prebiotics, which are dietary, soluble fibers for example, galactooligosaccharides (GOS) or fructooligosaccharides (FOS) that stimulate the growth of intrinsic commensal microbiota. There is now an enormous volume of preclinical data to support the concept of psychobiotics. Understandably, clinical data are less abundant but nonetheless emerging. Given the demonstrated efficacy of probiotics in IBS[54] and the high comorbidity between IBS and stress-related mental health issues, such as anxiety and depression, it is not surprising that certain probiotics might have a positive impact on mental health.

Tillisch and colleagues[55] administered healthy female participants either a placebo or a fermented dairy drink made from the probiotics (*Bifidobacterium animalis lactis*, *Streptococcus thermophiles*, *Lactobacillus bulgaricus*, and *Lactococcus lactis*), which were consumed over 4 weeks. Participants underwent functional MRI to determine how probiotic ingestion affected neuropsychological activity. During image acquisition, participants were shown emotional faces that are known to capture attention and cause brain activation. Relative to placebo, probiotic-treated participants showed decreased activity in a functional network associated with emotional, somatosensory, and interceptive processing, including the somatosensory cortex, the insula, and the periaqueductal gray. In marked contrast, placebo participants showed increased activity in these regions in response to emotional faces. This is interpreted as evidence of a probiotic-induced reduction in network-level neural reactivity to negative emotional information.

A recent prebiotic study carried out in Oxford University found a significant impact on stress responses.[56] Healthy male and female participants consumed either Bimuno-GOS (BGOS), FOS, or a placebo. In comparison to the other 2 groups, participants who consumed BGOS showed significantly reduced waking-cortisol responses, which are a robust marker of anxiety, stress, and depression risk.[57] Furthermore, participants completed an emotional dot-probe task measuring vigilance, or attention to negative stimuli, which is also a marker of anxiety and depression. Participants taking BGOS showed substantially attenuated vigilance on this task, suggesting reduced attention and reactivity to negative emotions. Overall, the data support the view that the specific prebiotic has anxiolytic activity.

Takada and colleagues[58] examined the effects of *Lactobacillus casei* strain Shirota (LcS) on gut-brain interactions under stressful conditions. Double-blind, placebo-controlled trials were conducted to examine the effects of LcS on psychological and physiologic stress responses in healthy medical students while undergoing examination stress. Subjects received LcS-fermented milk or placebo daily for 8 weeks prior to taking an examination. Subjective anxiety scores, salivary cortisol, and the presence of physical symptoms were analyzed. In a parallel animal study, rats were fed a diet with or without LcS for 2 weeks, then submitted to water avoidance stress (WAS). Plasma corticosterone concentration and the expression of cFos and corticotropin-releasing factor in the paraventricular nucleus were measured immediately after WAS. Academic stress resulted in increases in salivary cortisol and an increase in physical symptoms, both of which were significantly suppressed in the LcS group. In rats pretreated with LcS, WAS-induced increases in plasma corticosterone were significantly suppressed, and the number of corticotropin-releasing factor–expressing cells in the paraventricular nucleus was reduced. Intriguingly, intragastric administration of LcS was found to stimulate gastric vagal afferent activity in a dose-dependent manner. The results suggest that LcS may have a positive impact on stress responses by acting through the vagus nerve. In a study of university students, the authors have found that a *Bifidobacterium longum* decreased morning waking cortisol levels, reduced subjective levels of anxiety, and modestly improved aspects of cognitive functioning, an effect that was associated with altered encephalographic activity.

A large-scale cross-sectional study has examined the impact of probiotics on measures of social anxiety[59]; 710 young adults completed self-report measures of fermented food consumption, neuroticism, and social anxiety. An interaction model, controlling for demographics, general consumption of healthful foods, and exercise frequency, showed that exercise, neuroticism, and fermented food consumption significantly and independently predicted social anxiety. Furthermore, fermented food consumption also interacted with neuroticism in predicting social anxiety. For those with high neuroticism scores, a high frequency of fermented food consumption resulted in fewer symptoms of social anxiety. The data suggest that fermented foods containing probiotics may have a protective effect against social anxiety symptoms for those at higher genetic risk, as assayed by trait neuroticism.

Steenbergen and colleagues[60] tested a multispecies probiotic containing *Bifidobacterium bifidum*, *Bifidobacterium lactis*, *Lactobacillus acidophilus*, *Lactobacillus brevis*, *Lactobacillus casei*, *Lactobacillus salivarius*, and *Lactococcus lactis* in nondepressed individuals using a triple-blind, placebo-controlled, randomized, design; 20 healthy participants received a 4-week probiotic food-supplement intervention with the multispecies probiotics, whereas 20 control participants received an inert placebo for the same period. Subjects who received the 4-week multispecies probiotics intervention showed a significantly reduced overall cognitive reactivity to sad. The results provide evidence that probiotics may help reduce negative thoughts associated with sad mood.

Romijn and Rucklidge in their systematic review[61] add a note of caution to these optimistic findings, concluding that more trials are necessary before any definitive inferences can be made about the efficacy of probiotics in mental health applications. Further studies of a translational nature are required.

SUMMARY

The role of the microbiota-gut-brain access in the genesis of IBS symptoms is now largely accepted, although several questions remain unanswered. How does stress, especially early life stress, dysregulate the axis? Can IBS subtypes be delineated on the basis of the microbiota? If patients with IBS have comorbid psychiatric illness, does the latter resolve if the former is treated with probiotics?

There are an enormous number of preclinical studies implicating the gut microbiota in other stress-related conditions and in disorders at the extremes of life. Far more translational studies are required. The human studies to date support the view that the gut microbiota is altered in major depression and that psychobiotics, either in the form of prebiotics or probiotics, can have an impact on anxiety and depressive symptoms in healthy subjects. There is no clear indication of efficacy in diseased populations. In the neurodevelopmental disorder autism, which is usually diagnosed in early childhood, GI symptoms are common and an altered microbiota has been reported, whereas at the other end of the developmental spectrum, old age–related frailty correlates with decreased gut microbial diversity. Whether fecal microbiota transplantation is an appropriate therapeutic option in at least some brain-gut axis disorders remains to be determined.

ACKNOWLEDGMENTS

The authors are supported in part by Science Foundation Ireland in the form of a Centre grant (Alimentary Pharmabiotic Centre Grant Number SFI/12/RC/2273) and by the Health Research Board of Ireland (Grant Numbers HRA_POR/2011/23 and HRA_POR/2012/32) and received funding from the European Community's Seventh Framework Programme Grant MyNewGut under Grant Agreement No. FP7/2007-2013. The Centre has conducted studies in collaboration with several companies, including GSK, Pfizer, Cremo, Suntory, Wyeth, Nutricia, 4D Pharma, and Mead Johnson.

REFERENCES

1. Dinan TG, Stilling RM, Stanton C, et al. Collective unconscious: how gut microbes shape human behavior. J Psychiatr Res 2015;63:1–9.
2. Stilling RM, Dinan TG, Cryan JF. Microbial genes, brain & behaviour - epigenetic regulation of the gut-brain axis. Genes Brain Behav 2014;13(1):69–86.
3. Mayer EA, Knight R, Mazmanian SK, et al. Gut microbes and the brain: paradigm shift in neuroscience. J Neurosci 2014;34(46):15490–6.
4. Rhee SH, Pothoulakis C, Mayer EA. Principles and clinical implications of the brain-gut-enteric microbiota axis. Nat Rev Gastroenterol Hepatol 2009;6(5):306–14.
5. El Aidy S, Dinan TG, Cryan JF. Gut microbiota: the conductor in the orchestra of immune-neuroendocrine communication. Clin Ther 2015;37(5):954–67.
6. Grenham S, Clarke G, Cryan JF, et al. Brain-gut-microbe communication in health and disease. Front Physiol 2011;2:94.
7. Bravo JA, Forsythe P, Chew MV, et al. Ingestion of Lactobacillus strain regulates emotional behavior and central GABA receptor expression in a mouse via the vagus nerve. Proc Natl Acad Sci U S A 2011;108(38):16050–5.
8. Svensson E, Horvath-Puho E, Thomsen RW, et al. Vagotomy and subsequent risk of Parkinson's disease. Ann Neurol 2015;78(4):522–9.
9. Desbonnet L, Garrett L, Clarke G, et al. Effects of the probiotic Bifidobacterium infantis in the maternal separation model of depression. Neuroscience 2010;170(4):1179–88.
10. Lyte M. Microbial endocrinology in the microbiome-gut-brain axis: how bacterial production and utilization of neurochemicals influence behavior. PLoS Pathog 2013;9(11):e1003726.
11. Lyte M. Microbial endocrinology and the microbiota-gut-brain axis. Adv Exp Med Biol 2014;817:3–24.
12. Canfora EE, Jocken JW, Blaak EE. Short-chain fatty acids in control of body weight and insulin sensitivity. Nat Rev Endocrinol 2015;11(10):577–91.
13. El Aidy S, Dinan TG, Cryan JF. Immune modulation of the brain-gut-microbe axis. Front Microbiol 2014;5:146.
14. Wang Y, Kasper LH. The role of microbiome in central nervous system disorders. Brain Behav Immun 2014;38:1–12.
15. Tillisch K. The effects of gut microbiota on CNS function in humans. Gut microbes 2014;5(3):404–10.
16. Scott LV, Clarke G, Dinan TG. The brain-gut axis: a target for treating stress-related disorders. Mod Trends Pharmacopsychiatri 2013;28:90–9.
17. Moloney RD, Desbonnet L, Clarke G, et al. The microbiome: stress, health and disease. Mamm Genome 2014;25(1–2):49–74.

18. O'Mahony SM, Clarke G, Dinan TG, et al. Early-life adversity and brain development: Is the microbiome a missing piece of the puzzle? Neuroscience 2015. [Epub ahead of print].

19. O'Mahony SM, Hyland NP, Dinan TG, et al. Maternal separation as a model of brain-gut axis dysfunction. Psychopharmacology 2011;214(1):71–88.

20. O'Mahony SM, Marchesi JR, Scully P, et al. Early life stress alters behavior, immunity, and microbiota in rats: implications for irritable bowel syndrome and psychiatric illnesses. Biol Psychiatry 2009;65(3):263–7.

21. Dinan TG, Quigley EM, Ahmed SM, et al. Hypothalamic-pituitary-gut axis dysregulation in irritable bowel syndrome: plasma cytokines as a potential biomarker? Gastroenterology 2006;130(2):304–11.

22. Marshall JK, Thabane M, Garg AX, et al. Eight year prognosis of postinfectious irritable bowel syndrome following waterborne bacterial dysentery. Gut 2010; 59(5):605–11.

23. Backhed F. Programming of Host Metabolism by the Gut Microbiota. Ann Nutr Metab 2011;58:44–52.

24. Eckburg PB, Bik EM, Bernstein CN, et al. Diversity of the human intestinal microbial flora. Science 2005;308(5728):1635–8.

25. Qin J, Li R, Raes J, et al. A human gut microbial gene catalogue established by metagenomic sequencing. Nature 2010;464(7285):59–65.

26. Penders J, Thijs C, Vink C, et al. Factors influencing the composition of the intestinal microbiota in early infancy. Pediatrics 2006;118(2):511–21.

27. Dennison B. Definition of preterm delivery. Br Med J 1976;2(6049):1449.

28. Hoy CM, Wood CM, Hawkey PM, et al. Duodenal microflora in very-low-birthweight neonates and relation to necrotizing enterocolitis. J Clin Microbiol 2000; 38(12):4539–47.

29. Sondheimer JM, Clark DA. Gastric pH in healthy preterm infants - effect of age and feeding type. Gastroenterology 1985;88(5):1593.

30. Sondheimer JM, Clark DA, Gervaise EP. Continuous gastric pH measurement in young and older healthy preterm infants receiving formula and clear liquid feedings. J Pediatr Gastroenterol Nutr 1985;4(3):352–5.

31. Arboleya S, Binetti A, Salazar N, et al. Establishment and development of intestinal microbiota in preterm neonates. FEMS Microbiol Ecol 2012;79(3):763–72.

32. Chang JY, Shin SM, Chun J, et al. Pyrosequencing-based Molecular Monitoring of the Intestinal Bacterial Colonization in Preterm Infants. J Pediatr Gastroenterol Nutr 2011;53(5):512–9.

33. Jacquot A, Neveu D, Aujoulat F, et al. Dynamics and Clinical Evolution of Bacterial Gut Microflora in Extremely Premature Patients. J Pediatr 2011;158(3):390–6.

34. Mangiola F, Ianiro G, Franceschi F, et al. Gut microbiota in autism and mood disorders. World J Gastroenterol 2016;22(1):361–8.

35. Claesson MJ, Jeffery IB, Conde S, et al. Gut microbiota composition correlates with diet and health in the elderly. Nature 2012;488(7410):178–84.

36. Dinan TG, Cryan J, Shanahan F, et al. IBS: An epigenetic perspective. Nat Rev Gastroenterol Hepatol 2010;7(8):465–71.

37. Park SH, Videlock EJ, Shih W, et al. Adverse childhood experiences are associated with irritable bowel syndrome and gastrointestinal symptom severity. Neurogastroenterol Motil 2016;28(8):1252–60.

38. Undseth R, Jakobsdottir G, Nyman M, et al. Low serum levels of short-chain fatty acids after lactulose ingestion may indicate impaired colonic fermentation in patients with irritable bowel syndrome. Clin Exp Gastroenterol 2015;8:303–8.

39. Kelly JR, Kennedy PJ, Cryan JF, et al. Breaking down the barriers: the gut micro-biome, intestinal permeability and stress-related psychiatric disorders. Front Cell Neurosci 2015;9:392.
40. De Palma G, Blennerhassett P, Lu J, et al. Microbiota and host determinants of behavioural phenotype in maternally separated mice. Nat Commun 2015;6:7735.
41. Jiang H, Ling Z, Zhang Y, et al. Altered fecal microbiota composition in patients with major depressive disorder. Brain Behav Immun 2015;48:186–94.
42. Kelly JR, Borre Y, O'Brien C, et al. Transferring the blues: Depression-associated gut microbiota induces neurobehavioural changes in the rat. J Psychiatr Res 2016;82:109–18.
43. Li Q, Zhou JM. The microbiota-gut-brain axis and its potential therapeutic role in autism spectrum disorder. Neuroscience 2016;324:131–9.
44. Desbonnet L, Clarke G, Shanahan F, et al. Microbiota is essential for social devel-opment in the mouse. Mol Psychiatry 2014;19(2):146–8.
45. Borre YE, Moloney RD, Clarke G, et al. The impact of microbiota on brain and behavior: mechanisms & therapeutic potential. Adv Exp Med Biol 2014;817:373–403.
46. Hsiao EY, McBride SW, Hsien S, et al. Microbiota modulate behavioral and phys-iological abnormalities associated with neurodevelopmental disorders. Cell 2013;155(7):1451–63.
47. Erdman SE, Poutahidis T. Probiotic 'glow of health': it's more than skin deep. Benef Microbes 2014;5(2):109–19.
48. Tomova A, Husarova V, Lakatosova S, et al. Gastrointestinal microbiota in children with autism in Slovakia. Physiol Behav 2015;138:179–87.
49. Park H, Lee JY, Shin CM, et al. Characterization of gastrointestinal disorders in patients with parkinsonian syndromes. Parkinsonism Relat Disord 2015;21(5):455–60.
50. Felice VD, Quigley EM, Sullivan AM, et al. Microbiota-gut-brain signalling in Par-kinson's disease: Implications for non-motor symptoms. Parkinsonism Relat Dis-ord 2016;27:1–8.
51. Scheperjans F, Aho V, Pereira PA, et al. Gut microbiota are related to Parkinson's disease and clinical phenotype. Mov Disord 2015;30(3):350–8.
52. Dinan TG, Cryan JF. The impact of gut microbiota on brain and behaviour: impli-cations for psychiatry. Curr Opin Clin Nutr Metab Care 2015;18(6):552–8.
53. Dinan TG, Stanton C, Cryan JF. Psychobiotics: a novel class of psychotropic. Biol Psychiatry 2013;74(10):720–6.
54. Didari T, Mozaffari S, Nikfar S, et al. Effectiveness of probiotics in irritable bowel syndrome: Updated systematic review with meta-analysis. World J Gastroenterol 2015;21(10):3072–84.
55. Tillisch K, Labus J, Kilpatrick L, et al. Consumption of fermented milk product with probiotic modulates brain activity. Gastroenterology 2013;144(7):1394–401.
56. Schmidt K, Cowen PJ, Harmer CJ, et al. Prebiotic intake reduces the waking cortisol response and alters emotional bias in healthy volunteers. Psychopharma-cology 2015;232(10):1793–801.
57. Bhagwagar Z, Hafizi S, Cowen PJ. Increased salivary cortisol after waking in depression. Psychopharmacology 2005;182(1):54–7.
58. Takada M, Nishida K, Kataoka-Kato A, et al. Probiotic Lactobacillus casei strain Shirota relieves stress-associated symptoms by modulating the gut-brain interac-tion in human and animal models. Neurogastroenterol Motil 2016;28(7):1027–36.
59. Hilimire MR, DeVylder JE, Forestell CA. Fermented foods, neuroticism, and social anxiety: An interaction model. Psychiatry Res 2015;228(2):203–8.

60. Steenbergen L, Sellaro R, van Hemert S, et al. A randomized controlled trial to test the effect of multispecies probiotics on cognitive reactivity to sad mood. Brain Behav Immun 2015;48:258–64.

61. Romijn AR, Rucklidge JJ. Systematic review of evidence to support the theory of psychobiotics. Nutr Rev 2015;73(10):675–93.

The Gut Microbiome in Irritable Bowel Syndrome and Other Functional Bowel Disorders

Yehuda Ringel, MD, AGAF, FACG[a,b]

KEYWORDS

• Intestinal microbiota • Functional bowel disorders • Irritable bowel syndrome

KEY POINTS

- The emerging data from epidemiologic, microbiome, and physiology research in patients with functional bowel disorders (FBDs) provide evidence for a linkage between alterations in the intestinal microbiota and FBDs. However, currently most of the data is based on association studies, and the causality role of the microbiota in these disorders is not established.

- The growing evidence for compositional changes and the increasing recognition of the association between the intestinal microbiota and gut-brain functions that are relevant to the pathophysiology and/or clinical symptoms of FBDs have led to increased interest in manipulating the intestinal microbiota for the treatment of these disorders.

- Several therapeutic interventions targeting the intestinal microbiota have been suggested and are increasingly used in FBDs. These include dietary interventions aiming to modify the intestinal microbiota either directly by altering dietary substrate availability for intraluminal bacterial fermentation, prebiotics and probiotics or indirectly through effects on intestinal motility, transit and osmolarity. Nondietary interventions include antibiotics. Ongoing studies are currently exploring the potential role of fecal microbiota transplantation in patients with FBDs.

Conflict of Interest Statement: Consultant, advisory board, and/or research grants with Nestle, Procter & Gamble, Salix Pharmaceuticals, Danisco, Prometheus Therapeutics and Diagnostics, Ironwood, Takeda (Y. Ringel).

[a] Department of Gastroenterology, Beilinson Hospital, Petach Tikva 49100, Israel; [b] School of Medicine, University of North Carolina at Chapel Hill, 130 Mason Farm Rd, Chapel Hill, NC 27599, USA
E-mail address: ringel@med.unc.edu

IRRITABLE BOWEL SYNDROME AND FUNCTIONAL BOWEL DISORDERS

Functional bowel disorders (FBDs) are part of the larger group of functional gastrointestinal (GI) disorders characterized by symptoms attributed to the middle and lower GI tract that are not explained by structural or biochemical abnormalities. FBDs are subcategorized into several disorders, including irritable bowel syndrome (IBS), functional bloating, chronic idiopathic constipation, functional diarrhea, and unspecified functional bowel disorder. These disorders are distinguished by symptom-based diagnostic criteria and are traditionally diagnosed on the basis of characteristic GI symptoms and the absence of alarm features suggestive of organic disease.[1,2]

FBD are highly prevalent in Western countries, with IBS being the most prevalent (10%–20%) and best studied condition.[3] FBDs may have a considerable effect on patients' quality of life, daily functioning, and work productivity. The high prevalence of the disorders, their chronic nature, and the commonly associated non-GI comorbidities lead to significant utilization of health care services and socioeconomic burden.[4–6]

The pathogenesis of FBDs is multifactorial and not completely understood. Traditionally, the disorders have been thought to arise from abnormal function along the gut-brain axis with a variety of central and peripheral mechanisms that contribute to the initiation and perturbation of the GI motor and sensory functions leading to chronic, recurrent GI symptoms, including abdominal pain and discomfort, abdominal bloating, diarrhea, constipation, and alternating bowel movements.[7] The intensive research in this area over the past few years has implicated new theories and suggested additional new pathophysiologic mechanisms, including genetic predisposition,[8,9] peripheral GI factors,[10] extraintestinal neurohormonal and central factors.[11] Psychosocial aspects such as social learning, depression, anxiety, and somatization, are also recognized as important contributing factors, particularly to the clinical severity of the disorders.[12]

THE INTESTINAL MICROBIOTA

The microbiota comprising the human GI tract includes a complex community of microorganisms that are collectively referred to as the intestinal microbiota (the total community of organisms in the GI tract). In addition to bacteria, the intestinal microbiota includes archea, fungi, and viruses. Most of the bacteria in the GI tract are represented in 4 major bacterial phyla (divisions): Firmicutes (64%), Bacteroidetes (23%), Proteobacteria (8%) and Actinobacteria (3%).[13,14] The intestinal bacteria reside in an increasing density along the GI tract, with the highest density of about 10^{14} bacteria per gram of luminal content in the colon. There are more than 1000 different bacterial species; however, only about a third of them have been identified and characterized.

The intestinal microbiota is in close interaction with the human host and has a variety of physiologic effects, which are important for human health. At the peripheral level, intestinal commensal and pathogenic bacteria can affect the human host via multiple mechanisms, including by direct stimulation of enteric neurons and immune cells and indirectly via intraluminal metabolic effects. In addition, the intestinal microbiota can influence systemic physiologic processes through epithelial receptor-mediated signaling with effects beyond the GI tract.[15] For example, there is growing evidence for a bidirectional communication between the intestinal microbiota and the central (brain) nervous systems.[16] Indeed, studies in animal models have shown that products of microbiota have the potential to affect the excitability of enteric and vagal afferents neurons[17] as well as brain functions and behavior.[18] Conversely, the enteric mictobiota can be influenced through the brain effects on intestinal motility, secretion, and immune function,[19] thus creating the microbiota-gut-brain axis.[20]

THE INTESTINAL MICROBIOTA IN FUNCTIONAL BOWEL DISORDERS

Several lines of evidence support the relevance and importance of the intestinal microbiota in the pathogenesis and/or the clinical manifestation of FBDs. *The first line of evidence* comes from epidemiologic observations. Multiple epidemiologic studies have demonstrated that acute interruption of the intestinal microbiota is often associated with an increased risk for persistent functional GI symptoms. Several studies reported the development of persistent IBS symptoms following acute GI bacterial infection despite clearance of the initiating pathogen, a condition referred to as postinfectious IBS (PI-IBS). Indeed, acute gastroenteritis is currently recognized as the strongest identified predictor for the development of IBS with a 6- to 7-fold increased risk and average incidence of about 10%.[21,22] Although several predisposing factors for the development of persisting PI-IBS have been identified, including prior psychological morbidity, female gender, severity and duration of the initial infection, and the inflammatory/immune response to the infectious event,[22,23] the mechanisms underlying this disorder are still unclear. Nevertheless, a recent study comparing the intestinal microbiota between patients with or without IBS symptoms 6 months after gastroenteritis, patients with diarrhea-predominant IBS (IBS-D), and healthy controls has demonstrated that the microbiota of patients with PI-IBS is different from healthy controls but similar to the microbiota of patients with IBS-D, suggesting an ongoing postinfection alteration of the intestinal microbiota and possible shared pathophysiologic pathways with IBS-D.[24] Persistent increase in a range of mucosal inflammatory markers has also been reported in these patients.[25]

Another example for the development of persistent functional bowel symptoms following acute interruption of the intestinal microbiota is the use of antibiotics. The association between the use of antibiotics is less established because of relatively limited published data coming mainly from retrospective studies,[26] and the difficult interpretation of the data due to expected differences in the effect of the different types of antibiotics. For example, a large retrospective study of nearly 26,000 patients found that exposure to macrolides or tetracyclines was significantly associated with developing IBS, whereas treatment with cephalosporins or penicillins was not.[27] Nevertheless, a recent prospective case-control study has demonstrated that antibiotic therapy (all types) for extraintestinal infections was significantly associated with FBDs (odds ratio [OR] 1.90; 95% confidence interval [CI] 1.21–2.98) and even more so with IBS (OR 2.30; CI 1.22–4.33).[28]

The association between IBS and small-intestine bacterial overgrowth is commonly reported and has been suggested as a possible cause for IBS; however, the data on this association are nonconclusive, and the relationship is debatable.[29–31]

The second line of evidence comes from microbiology studies investigating the intestinal microbiota in patients with FBDs.[32–34] Most of the studies in this area have focused on characterizing the composition of the microbiota in patients with IBS and comparing it to the microbiota in healthy controls.[35] For convenience and practicality reasons, most of this research has been done on fecal samples as a representation of the overall bacterial makeup of the luminal intestinal microbiota. Only a few studies investigated the bacteria residing in the mucosal-associated microbiota, microorganisms in the thin layer of mucus adhering to the surface of the intestinal mucosa. In general, these studies have shown reduced microbial diversity and richness, and increased temporal instability in patients with IBS compared with healthy controls.[32,36–38] In addition, they provide evidence for compositional alterations at different levels of bacterial taxonomy. The most repeated observations in this area are increased levels of Firmicutes and decreased levels of Bacteroidetes[39] in patients with IBS compared with healthy controls. However, the differences in the abundance of specific species within these 2 microbial phyla are not consistent across studies.[24,38–40] Of interest are reports of decreased levels of bacteria with beneficial metabolic and anti-inflammatory properties, for example, Bifidobacteria, and *Faecalibacterium prausnitzii*,[41] and increased levels of potentially pathogenic bacteria, for example, *Streptococcus* spp (associated with increased interleukin-6 [IL-6] levels and stimulation of immune response) and mucin degraders bacteria, for example, members of the *Ruminococcus* spp in patients with IBS compared with healthy controls.[40]

Several studies investigated the intestinal microbiota in specific subtypes of IBS and attempted to compare the microbiota between clinically relevant IBS subgroups.[34,37–39] A recent study using high throughput pyrosequencing of the 16S rRNA gene on fresh fecal samples from a cohort of 60 patients with IBS and 20 healthy controls demonstrated significant differences in the microbiota between subgroups of patients with IBS that were categorized based on clinical symptoms of abdominal bloating and bowel characteristics (diarrhea predominant, constipation predominant, or mixed).[42]

Another recent study investigating both fecal and colonic mucosal microbiotas in patients with chronic constipation found that the colonic mucosal microbiota in constipated patients differ from that of controls with higher abundance of genera from Bacteroidetes in the constipation group. However, although the profile of the colonic mucosal microbiota discriminated between patients with constipation and controls with 94% accuracy, this association was independent of the physiologic measure of colonic transit. In contrast, the profile of the fecal microbiota was associated with colonic transit and methane production but not the clinical diagnosis of constipation.[43]

The latter 2 studies demonstrate 3 important points: (1) Alterations in the intestinal microbiota may have a role in the pathogenesis of specific symptoms (eg, abdominal bloating, constipation) associated with IBS and other FBDs; (2) The intestinal microbiota can affect relevant physiologic functions (eg, intestinal transit) as well as functional GI symptoms via different and independent mechanisms; (3) Both the intestinal luminal microbiota and the mucosa-associated microbiota are relevant and may have different effects on the human host.

The third line of evidence comes from physiologic studies that investigated the effects of the intestinal microbiota on gut-brain axis functions relevant to the pathophysiology of FBDs, including the following:

- GI sensory and motor functions,
- Intestinal barrier,
- Intestinal immune function,
- Intestinal neurohormonal function,
- Psychological factors.

Effects on gastrointestinal Sensorimotor Function

Most of the understanding of the effects of the intestinal microbiota on the GI sensory-motor function comes from animal studies. Early studies in germ-free rats (rats lacking microbiota) have demonstrated profound abnormalities in intestinal motor function including significantly delayed intestinal transit and a prolonged interdigestive migratory motor complex (MMC) period.[44] On the other hand, colonization of germ-free rats with either *Lactobacillus acidophilus* or *Bifidobacterium bifidum* partially increases interdigestive MMC activity and small-bowel transit time while colonization with *Escherichia coli* and *Micrococcus luteus* delays gut motility.[45] Thus, these studies demonstrate that the intestinal microbiota has an important role in maintaining normal intestinal motor function, and that different members of the intestinal microbiota can have different effects on intestinal motility.[45] Specifically relevant to FBD are more recent studies in which germ-free animals were colonized with fecal material from patients with IBS (ie, microbiota humanized mice). These studies have shown that the transfer of fecal material from patients with IBS to germ-free animals can induce alterations in intestinal transit[46] and greater pain responses to colonic balloon distension (ie, visceral hypersensitivity).[47,48] Taken together, these studies demonstrate that the 2 relevant physiologic functions of the disorder, abnormal motility and visceral hypersensitivity, are transferable via fecal material, thus supporting the possibility of a causal role for the intestinal microbiota in the pathophysiology of at least those 2 physiologic hallmarks of the disorder.

Effects on Intestinal Barrier

The GI barrier is composed of complex molecular tight junctions, intracellular and surface-membrane proteins that keep the enterocytes tightly sealed and regulate the passage of molecules across the epithelium. Loss of structural and functional integrity of the epithelial barrier could lead to exposure of the mucosa-associated immune system to luminal toxic and immunogenic particles and trigger immunologic responses that could eventually lead to a variety of GI disorders, including inflammatory bowel diseases and functional GI disorders.[49] Alterations in the integrity and function of the intestinal barrier have gained an increased interest as possible factors in the pathogenesis of IBS. Several studies in children and adult patients with IBS have demonstrated increased intestinal permeability in IBS compared with healthy controls.[50,51] The mechanisms related to the increased permeability in IBS are not clear. However, the observations that certain bacteria (*Vibrio cholera, Clostridium difficile,* and toxin-producing strains of *E coli*) can increase intestinal permeability, whereas certain probiotics can promote barrier integrity,[52] led to the suggestion that alterations in intestinal microbiota and mucosal immune functions could be important etiologic factors.[53]

The relevance of this hypothesis to FBDs is demonstrated by the following 3 studies. In the 2 studies, fecal supernatants from IBS patients were applied in vitro to colonic mucosa from mice[54] or to a model for intestinal barrier (Caco-2 cells system).[55] In both studies, the expression of a tight junction intracellular protein (zonula occludens; ZO-1) decreased and the permeability increased. In the third, more recent study, plasma from patients with IBS-D and healthy controls was applied to the Caco-2 model of intestinal barrier. Interestingly, exposure of plasma from the IBS-D patients to the basolateral cell led to an increase in permeability compared with exposure of plasma from healthy controls, thus suggesting also a possible systemic mechanism. Furthermore, the increased permeability effect in the latter study was attenuated by selective inhibition of mast cell tryptase, and gram-negative bacteria lipopolysaccharides (LPS) thus further support the idea that this effect is mediated by microbiota and immune factors.[56]

Effects on Intestinal Immune Function

Although IBS is not generally considered an inflammatory disease, there is growing evidence for the presence of dysregulated immune function and low-grade inflammation in some patients with IBS. Studies have demonstrated increased colonic infiltration of mucosal inflammatory and immune cells (most consistently reported are mast cells)[57] and increased levels of high-sensitivity C-reactive protein[58] and some inflammatory mediators (eg, IL-6 and IL-8) and inflammatory cytokines in patients with IBS compared with healthy individuals.[59,60] Abnormal polymorphisms in genes involved in immune and inflammatory responses have also been reported.[60] The interactions between the intestinal immune system and the intestinal microbiota are well documented,[61] and their relation to FBDs is reviewed in detail elsewhere. Important observations in this area are increased expression of Toll-like receptors (TLRs) specifically involved in activation of the innate immune response to enteric bacteria, including TLR4 (involved with recognition of bacterial LPS from gram-negative bacteria) and TLR5 (involved with recognition of flagellin, a common bacterial antigen present in most motile bacteria in the intestine). In line with these observations is the finding that TLR4-deficient mice have a significantly reduced number of enteric neurons and altered GI motility and that activation of TLR4 by enteric microbiota affects the enteric nervous system and intestinal motility.[62] Interestingly, a recent study has suggested that the microbiota effects on GI motility through TLRs could be mediated by affecting the expression of intestinal serotonin or 5-hydroxytryptamine (5-HT) receptors.[63] Also, in line with the observation of increased expression of TLR5 (involved with recognition of bacterial flagellin) is the finding of increased antiflagellin antibodies in IBS patients (mostly in PI-IBS, almost 30%) compared with healthy controls (only 7%).[64] These observations support the hypothesis that the intestinal luminal bacterial antigens could be the trigger of the immune activation that leads to alterations in intestinal physiology and functional bowel symptoms at least in a subset of patients.

Effects on Intestinal Neurohormonal Function

The role of the enteroendocrine system, and particularly the intestinal serotonin system, has been the focus of extensive research over the past decade. Serotonin or 5-HT is a monoamine neurotransmitter produced primarily (90%) by enterochromaffin cells in the GI tract. Indeed, 95% of this potent neurotransmitter is contained in the gut and only 5% in the central nervous system. The locally enteric release of 5-HT acts on specific intestinal receptors to affect multiple GI functions, including intestinal motility, sensation, and secretion.[65,66] The profound effects of serotonin on GI functions relevant to FBDs have led to the increased interest in targeting serotonin receptors (primarily 5-HT3 and 5-HT4 receptors) for development of pharmacologic interventions for these disorders.[67] An interesting association between the entering serotonergic system and the intestinal microbiota has been recently reported by an important study demonstrating that indigenous spore-forming microbes from mice and healthy human colons can produce specific metabolites that promote GI 5-HT biosynthesis by colonic enterochromaffin cells and that this microbiota-dependent 5-HT effect could have a significant impact on GI motility.[68]

Psychological Factors

Although most patients with FBDs do not meet criteria for diagnosis of psychiatric disorders, emotional distress and psychological difficulties are often clinically observed in these patients, and they are considered as contributing and risk factors for the onset, severity, duration, and response to treatment of the disorders.[69] Although it is not clear whether psychological and emotional distresses precede a diagnosis of FBDs or are consequences of them, they do have the capacity to affect physiologic functions relevant to the pathophysiology of the disorders. The effects of psychological disorders on motor, sensory, barrier, and immune functions are well documented and the relevance of these interactions to FBDs are usually discussed under the concept of gut-brain axis.[70] However, the increasing recognition of the regulatory effects of the intestinal microbiota on the bidirectional interactions between the central nervous system, the enteric nervous system, and the GI tract has broadened this concept, which is now referred to as "microbiota-gut-brain axis."[71]

The exact mechanisms of these interactions are not yet clear, but data from animal and a few human studies provide evidence for intestinal bacteria effect on pain experience and psychological, emotional, and behavioral disturbances that are often observed in association with FBDs.[71,72]

SUMMARY AND CLINICAL IMPLICATIONS

The emerging data from epidemiologic, microbiome, and physiology research in patients with FBDs provide evidence for a linkage between alterations in the intestinal microbiota and FBDs. However, currently most of the data is based on association studies, and the causality role of the microbiota in these disorders is not established. Furthermore, most of the research in this area had focused on differences in the composition of the microbiota (who is there?) and there is significantly less information on differences in the function of the microbiota (what are they doing?). The heterogeneity of the disorders and the inconsistent findings in the composition of the microbiota across studies do not enable using the microbiota as relevant markers for diagnosis, disease progression, and response to treatment. However, the growing evidence for compositional changes and the increasing recognition of the association between the intestinal microbiota and gut-brain functions that are relevant to the pathophysiology and/or clinical symptoms of FBDs have led to increased interest in manipulating the intestinal microbiota for the treatment of these disorders. Several therapeutic interventions targeting the intestinal microbiota have been suggested and are increasingly used in FBDs. These interventions include dietary interventions aiming to modify the intestinal microbiota either directly by altering dietary substrate availability for intraluminal bacterial fermentation or indirectly through effects on intestinal motility, transit, osmolality, pH, and so forth. The most popular and well-studied dietary interventions include avoidance of short highly fermentable carbohydrates; eg, low fermentable oligo-, di-, monosaccharides and polyols (FODMAP) diet[73] and supplementation of diet with prebiotics[74] and probiotics.[75] Nondietary interventions targeting the intestinal microbiota for the treatment of FBDs include antibiotics, particularly GI-directed, nonabsorbable antibiotics (eg, rifaximin).[76] Ongoing studies are currently exploring the potential role of fecal microbiota transplantation in patients with FBDs.[77]

REFERENCES

1. Longstreth GF, Thompson WG, Chey WD, et al. Functional bowel disorders. Gastroenterology 2006;130(5):1480–91.

2. Ringel Y, Drossman D. Irritable bowel syndrome. Philadelphia: Sanders Elsevier. Netter's textbook of internal medicine. 2nd edition. 2009. p. 419–25.

3. Saito YA, Schoenfeld P, Locke GR 3rd. The epidemiology of irritable bowel syndrome in North America: a systematic review. Am J Gastroenterol 2002;97(8):1910–5.

4. Chang JY, Locke GR 3rd, McNally MA, et al. Impact of functional gastrointestinal disorders on survival in the community. Am J Gastroenterol 2010;105(4):822–32.

5. Maxion-Bergemann S, Thielecke F, Abel F, et al. Costs of irritable bowel syndrome in the UK and US. Pharmacoeconomics 2006;24:21–37.

6. Peery AF, Crockett SD, Barritt AS, et al. Burden of gastrointestinal, liver, and pancreatic diseases in the United States. Gastroenterology 2015;149(7): 1731–41.e3.

7. Camilleri M, Di Lorenzo C. Brain-gut axis: from basic understanding to treatment of IBS and related disorders. J Pediatr Gastroenterol Nutr 2012;54:446–53.

8. Saito YA, Petersen GM, Locke GR 3rd, et al. The genetics of irritable bowel syndrome. Clin Gastroenterol Hepatol 2005;3(11):1057–65.

9. Levy RL, Jones KR, Whitehead WE, et al. Irritable bowel syndrome in twins: heredity and social learning both contribute to etiology. Gastroenterology 2001; 121:799–804.

10. Camilleri M. Peripheral mechanisms in irritable bowel syndrome. N Engl J Med 2012;367(17):1626–35.

11. Camilleri M. Physiological underpinnings of irritable bowel syndrome: neurohormonal mechanisms. J Physiol 2014;592(14):2967–80.

12. Drossman DA, Chang L, Bellamy N, et al. Severity in irritable bowel syndrome: a Rome Foundation Working Team report. Am J Gastroenterol 2011;106:1749–59.

13. Gill SR, Pop M, Deboy RT, et al. Metagenomic analysis of the human distal gut microbiome. Science 2006;312(5778):1355–9.

14. Backhed F, Fraser CM, Ringel Y, et al. Defining a healthy human gut microbiome: current concepts, future directions, and clinical applications. Cell Host Microbe 2012;12(5):611–22.

15. McClure R, Massari P. TLR-dependent human mucosal epithelial cell responses to microbial pathogens. Front Immunol 2014;5:386.

16. Cryan JF, Dinan TG. Mind-altering microorganisms: the impact of the gut microbiota on brain and behaviour. Nat Rev Neurosci 2012;13(10):701–12.

17. Bravo JA, Julio-Pieper M, Forsythe P, et al. Communication between gastrointestinal bacteria and the nervous system. Curr Opin Pharmacol 2012;12(6):667–72.

18. Yarandi SS, Peterson DA, Treisman GJ, et al. Modulatory effects of gut microbiota on the central nervous system: how gut could play a role in neuropsychiatric health and diseases. J Neurogastroenterol Motil 2016;22(2):201–12.

19. Kelly JR, Kennedy PJ, Cryan JF, et al. Breaking down the barriers: the gut microbiome, intestinal permeability and stress-related psychiatric disorders. Front Cell Neurosci 2015;9:392.

20. Moloney RD, Johnson AC, O'Mahony SM, et al. Stress and the microbiota-gut-brain axis in visceral pain: relevance to irritable bowel syndrome. CNS Neurosci Ther 2016;22(2):102–17.

21. Halvorson HA, Schlett CD, Riddle MS. Postinfectious irritable bowel syndrome—a meta-analysis. Am J Gastroenterol 2006;101(8):1894–9 [quiz: 1942].

22. Schwille-Kiuntke J, Enck P, Zendler C, et al. Postinfectious irritable bowel syndrome: follow-up of a patient cohort of confirmed cases of bacterial infection with Salmonella or Campylobacter. Neurogastroenterol Motil 2011;23(11): e479–88.

23. Marshall JK, Thabane M, Garg AX, et al. Eight year prognosis of postinfectious irritable bowel syndrome following waterborne bacterial dysentery. Gut 2010; 59:605–11.

24. Jalanka-Tuovinen J, Salojärvi J, Salonen A, et al. Faecal microbiota composition and host-microbe cross-talk following gastroenteritis and in postinfectious irritable bowel syndrome. Gut 2014;63(11):1737–45.

25. Sundin J, Rangel I, Kumawat AK, et al. Aberrant mucosal lymphocyte number and subsets in the colon of post-infectious irritable bowel syndrome patients. Scand J Gastroenterol 2014;49(9):1068–75.

26. Maxwell PR, Rink E, Kumar D, et al. Antibiotics increase functional abdominal symptoms. Am J Gastroenterol 2002;97(1):104–8.

27. Villarreal AA, Aberger FJ, Benrud R, et al. Use of broad-spectrum antibiotics and the development of irritable bowel syndrome. WMJ 2012;111:17–20.

28. Paula H, Grover M, Halder SL, et al. Non-enteric infections, antibiotic use, and risk of development of functional gastrointestinal disorders. Neurogastroenterol Motil 2015;27:1580–6.

29. Ford AC, Spiegel BM, Talley NJ, et al. Small intestinal bacterial overgrowth in irritable bowel syndrome: systematic review and meta-analysis. Clin Gastroenterol Hepatol 2009;7(12):1279–86.

30. Yu D, Cheeseman F, Vanner S. Combined oro-caecal scintigraphy and lactulose hydrogen breath testing demonstrate that breath testing detects oro-caecal transit, not small intestinal bacterial overgrowth in patients with IBS. Gut 2011; 60(3):334–40.

31. Posserud I, Stotzer PO, Bjornsson ES, et al. Small intestinal bacterial overgrowth in patients with irritable bowel syndrome. Gut 2007;56(6):802–8.

32. Rajilic-Stojanovic M, Jonkers DM, Salonen A, et al. Intestinal microbiota and diet in IBS: causes, consequences, or epiphenomena? Am J Gastroenterol 2015; 110(2):278–87.

33. Ringel Y, Carroll IM. Alterations in the intestinal microbiota and functional bowel symptoms. Gastrointest Endosc Clin N Am 2009;19(1):141–50.

34. Simren M, Barbara G, Flint HJ, et al. Intestinal microbiota in functional bowel disorders: a Rome foundation report. Gut 2013;62(1):159–76.

35. Ringel Y, Ringel-Kulka T. The intestinal microbiota and irritable bowel syndrome. J Clin Gastroenterol 2015;49(Suppl 1):S56–9.

36. Matto J, Maunuksela L, Kajander K, et al. Composition and temporal stability of gastrointestinal microbiota in irritable bowel syndrome–a longitudinal study in IBS and control subjects. FEMS Immunol Med Microbiol 2005;43:213–22.

37. Carroll IM, Ringel-Kulka T, Keku TO, et al. Molecular analysis of the luminal- and mucosal-associated intestinal microbiota in diarrhea-predominant irritable bowel syndrome. Am J Physiol Gastrointest Liver Physiol 2011;301(5):G799–807.

38. Carroll IM, Ringel-Kulka T, Siddle JP, et al. Alterations in composition and diversity of the intestinal microbiota in patients with diarrhea-predominant irritable bowel syndrome. Neurogastroenterol Motil 2012;24(6):521–30, e248.

39. Jeffery IB, O'Toole PW, Ohman L, et al. An irritable bowel syndrome subtype defined by species-specific alterations in faecal microbiota. Gut 2012;61(7): 997–1006.

40. Rajilic-Stojanovic M, Biagi E, Heilig HG, et al. Global and deep molecular analysis of microbiota signatures in fecal samples from patients with irritable bowel syndrome. Gastroenterology 2011;141(5):1792–801.

41. Machiels K, Joossens M, Sabino J, et al. A decrease of the butyrate-producing species Roseburia hominis and Faecalibacterium prausnitzii defines dysbiosis in patients with ulcerative colitis. Gut 2014;63(8):1275–83.

42. Ringel-Kulka T, Benson AK, Carroll IM, et al. Molecular characterization of the intestinal microbiota in patients with and without abdominal bloating. Am J Physiol Gastrointest Liver Physiol 2016;310(6):G417–26.

43. Parthasarathy G, Chen J, Chen X, et al. Relationship between microbiota of the colonic mucosa vs feces and symptoms, colonic transit, and methane production in female patients with chronic constipation. Gastroenterology 2016;150(2): 367–79.e1.

44. Caenepeel P, Janssens J, Vantrappen G, et al. Interdigestive myoelectric complex in germfree rats. Dig Dis Sci 1989;34(8):1180–4.

45. Husebye E, Hellström PM, Sundler F, et al. Influence of microbial species on small intestinal myoelectric activity and transit in germ-free rats. Am J Physiol Gastrointest Liver Physiol 2001;280(3):G368–80.

46. Kashyap PC, Marcobal A, Ursell LK, et al. Complex interactions among diet, gastrointestinal transit, and gut microbiota in humanized mice. Gastroenterology 2013;144:967–77.

47. Crouzet L, Gaultier E, Del'Homme C, et al. The hypersensitivity to colonic distension of IBS patients can be transferred to rats through their fecal microbiota. Neurogastroenterol Motil 2013;25:e272–82.

48. Crouzet L, Gaultier E, Del'Homme C, et al. The hypersensitivity to colonic distension of IBS patients can be transferred to rats through their fecal microbiota. Neurogastroenterol Motil 2013;25(4):e272–82.

49. Turner JR. Intestinal mucosal barrier function in health and disease. Nat Rev Immunol 2009;9:799–809.

50. Shulman RJ, Eakin MN, Czyzewski DI, et al. Increased gastrointestinal permeability and gut inflammation in children with functional abdominal pain and irritable bowel syndrome. J Pediatr 2008;153:646–50.

51. Dunlop SP, Hebden J, Campbell E, et al. Abnormal intestinal permeability in subgroups of diarrhea-predominant irritable bowel syndromes. Am J Gastroenterol 2006;101:1288–94.

52. Patel RM, Myers LS, Kurundkar AR, et al. Probiotic bacteria induce maturation of intestinal claudin 3 expression and barrier function. Am J Pathol 2012;180:626–35.

53. Camilleri M, Madsen K, Spiller R, et al. Intestinal barrier function in health and gastrointestinal disease. Neurogastroenterol Motil 2012;24:503–12.

54. Gecse K, Roka R, Ferrier L, et al. Increased faecal serine protease activity in diarrhoeic IBS patients: a colonic lumenal factor impairing colonic permeability and sensitivity. Gut 2008;57:591–9.

55. Piche T, Barbara G, Aubert P, et al. Impaired intestinal barrier integrity in the colon of patients with irritable bowel syndrome: involvement of soluble mediators. Gut 2009;58:196–201.

56. Ludidi S, Jonkers D, Elamin E, et al. The intestinal barrier in irritable bowel syndrome: subtype-specific effects of the systemic compartment in an in vitro model. PLoS One 2015;10(5):e0123498.

57. Barbara G, Stanghellini V, De Giorgio R, et al. Activated mast cells in proximity to colonic nerves correlate with abdominal pain in irritable bowel syndrome. Gastroenterology 2004;126:693–702.

58. Hod K, Ringel-Kulka T, Martin CF, et al. High-sensitive C-reactive protein as a marker for inflammation in irritable bowel syndrome. J Clin Gastroenterol 2016;50(3):227–32.

59. Matricon J, Meleine M, Gelot A, et al. Review article: associations between immune activation, intestinal permeability and the irritable bowel syndrome. Aliment Pharmacol Ther 2012;36:1009–31.

60. Ringel Y, Maharshak N. Bacteria, inflammation, and immune activation in the pathogenesis of irritable bowel syndrome. Am J Physiol Gastrointest Liver Physiol 2013;305(8):G529–41.

61. Hooper LV, Littman DR, Macpherson AJ. Interactions between the microbiota and the immune system. Science 2012;336:1268–73.

62. Anitha M, Vijay-Kumar M, Sitaraman SV, et al. Gut microbial products regulate murine gastrointestinal motility via Toll-like receptor 4 signaling. Gastroenterology 2012;143:1006–16.e4.

63. Forcén R, Latorre E, Pardo J, et al. Toll-like receptors 2 and 4 modulate the contractile response induced by serotonin in mouse ileum: analysis of the serotonin receptors involved. Neurogastroenterol Motil 2015;27(9):1258–66.

64. Schoepfer AM, Schaffer T, Seibold-Schmid B, et al. Antibodies to flagellin indicate reactivity to bacterial antigens in IBS patients. Neurogastroenterol Motil 2008;20:1110–8.

65. Gershon MD, Tack J. The serotonin signaling system: from basic understanding to drug development for functional GI disorders. Gastroenterology 2007;132:397–414.

66. Manocha M, Khan WI. Serotonin and GI disorders: an update on clinical and experimental studies. Clin Transl Gastroenterol 2012;3:e13.

67. Grover M, Camilleri M. Effects on gastrointestinal functions and symptoms of serotonergic psychoactive agents used in functional gastrointestinal diseases [review]. J Gastroenterol 2013;48(2):177–81.

68. Yano JM, Yu K, Donaldson GP, et al. Indigenous bacteria from the gut microbiota regulate host serotonin biosynthesis. Cell 2015;161(2):264–76.

69. van Tilburg MA, Palsson OS, Whitehead WE. Which psychological factors exacerbate irritable bowel syndrome? Development of a comprehensive model. J Psychosom Res 2013;74(6):486–92.

70. Al Omran Y, Aziz Q. The brain-gut axis in health and disease. Adv Exp Med Biol 2014;817:135–53.

71. Mayer EA, Savidge T, Shulman RJ. Brain gut microbiome interactions and functional bowel disorders. Gastroenterology 2014;146(6):1500–12.

72. Ringel-Kulka T, Goldsmith JR, Carroll IM, et al. Lactobacillus acidophilus NCFM affects colonic mucosal opioid receptor expression in patients with functional abdominal pain - a randomised clinical study. Aliment Pharmacol Ther 2014;40(2):200–7.

73. Staudacher HM, Irving PM, Lomer MC, et al. Mechanisms and efficacy of dietary FODMAP restriction in IBS. Nat Rev Gastroenterol Hepatol 2014;11(4):256–66.

74. Saulnier DM, Ringel Y, Heyman MB, et al. The intestinal microbiome, probiotics and prebiotics in neurogastroenterology. Gut Microbes 2013;4(1):17–27.

75. Floch MH, Walker WA, Sanders ME, et al. Recommendations for probiotic use—2015 update: proceedings and consensus opinion. J Clin Gastroenterol 2015;49(Suppl 1):S69–73.

76. Dupont HL. Review article: evidence for the role of gut microbiota in irritable bowel syndrome and its potential influence on therapeutic targets. Aliment Pharmacol Ther 2014;39(10):1033–42.

77. Pinn DM, Aroniadis OC, Brandt LJ. Is fecal microbiota transplantation (FMT) an effective treatment for patients with functional gastrointestinal disorders (FGID)? Neurogastroenterol Motil 2015;27(1):19–29.

Small Intestinal Bacterial Overgrowth and Other Intestinal Disorders

 CrossMark

Uday C. Ghoshal, MD, DNB, DM, FACG, RFF[a],*, Ujjala Ghoshal, MD[b]

KEYWORDS

- Gut microbiota • Malabsorption syndrome • Tropical sprue • Rifaximin
- Hydrogen breath tests

KEY POINTS

- The role of small intestinal bacterial overgrowth (SIBO) in various intestinal disorders, such as irritable bowel syndrome, celiac and Crohn disease, tropical sprue, gastrointestinal hypomotility states, hypochlorhydria, immunodeficiency states, and structural abnormalities, is increasingly understood.
- Though a bacterial count equal to or greater than 10^5 colony forming unit (CFU)/mL is considered diagnostic of SIBO, some experts suggest that a colony count equal to or greater than 10^3 CFU/mL should also be considered SIBO, particularly if coliforms are present in the upper gut.
- Hydrogen breath tests are popular noninvasive tests using different substrates such as glucose (though highly specific but quite insensitive) and lactulose (early-peak criteria is quite nonspecific and double-peak criteria is quite insensitive) to diagnose SIBO.
- The search for better diagnostic test for SIBO continues.
- Rifaximin is a quite safe and effective agent for treatment and retreatment of SIBO.

INTRODUCTION

The gastrointestinal (GI) tract harbors an enormous number of microbes, including bacteria, virus, fungus, and archaea.[1] Interestingly, the microbial cells in the gut (10^{14} cells) outnumber that in the human body (10^{13}).[2] Upper gut (stomach, duodenum, and jejunum) is relatively less populated with microbes ($0–10^3$ bacteria per mL of aspirate) due to the gastric acid barrier (**Fig. 1**).[1,3] The microbes in the upper gut are dominated by those that can resist gastric acid, such as *Helicobacter pylori* and lactobacilli. The distal small bowel and colon have more microbes (10^7 to 10^{12}).[1] Coliforms (Gram-negative nonspore-forming bacilli that ferment lactose) are

[a] Department of Gastroenterology, Sanjay Gandhi Postgraduate Institute of Medical Sciences, Lucknow 226014, India; [b] Department of Microbiology, Sanjay Gandhi Postgraduate Institute of Medical Sciences, Lucknow 226014, India
* Corresponding author.
E-mail address: udayghoshal@gmail.com

Gastroenterol Clin N Am 46 (2017) 103–120
http://dx.doi.org/10.1016/j.gtc.2016.09.008
gastro.theclinics.com

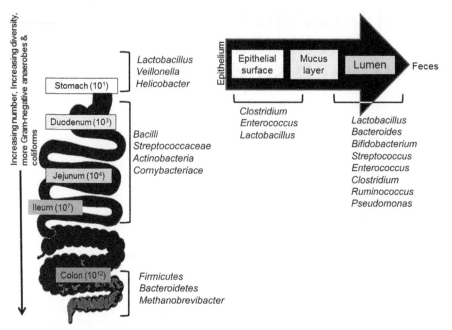

Fig. 1. Distribution of bacterial population in different parts of the human gastrointestinal (GI) tract from the luminal to epithelial surface.

present exclusively in the distal gut. Gut microbiota performs a variety of functions, such as barrier effect preventing invasion by the pathogenic organisms; regulation of immune function and motility; digestion of food; production of short-chain fatty acids, which regulate colonic water and electrolytes transport and are nutrient to the colonocytes; production of vitamins; metabolism of the drugs; detoxification of toxic compounds; and maintenance of overall homeostasis in the GI tract.[2,3] Hence, maintenance of normal gut flora (eubiosis) is essential for keeping an individual healthy. Abnormality in the gut flora (dysbiosis), including quantitative increase in small bowel bacteria (ie, small intestinal bacterial overgrowth [SIBO]), qualitative alteration in relative proportion of friendly bacteria and harmful ones, or change in location of bacteria (eg, colonic type bacteria in the small intestine), is known to be associated with several diseases.[2,4,5] Definition, etiologic factors, symptomatology, pathophysiology, diagnosis, and treatment of SIBO in relation to various intestinal disorders associated with it are reviewed in this article.

SIBO is defined as overgrowth of bacteria equal to or greater than 10^5 colony forming unit (CFU) per mL of jejunal aspirate.[3,4,6] Some authorities suggested that a colony count of equal to or greater than 10^3 CFU/mL of jejunal aspirate should also be considered SIBO, particularly if coliforms are found, especially in irritable bowel syndrome (IBS).[7,8] Understanding of the importance of SIBO in GI and hepatobiliary diseases is being increasingly recognized over time, as evidenced by publications on this issue (**Fig. 2**). **Table 1** lists the GI and hepatobiliary diseases associated with SIBO.[9,10]

ETIOLOGIC FACTORS AND PATHOGENESIS

Fig. 3 enumerates the various factors that predispose to SIBO, which shows that in addition to the structural causes, abnormalities in GI motility and gut defense are

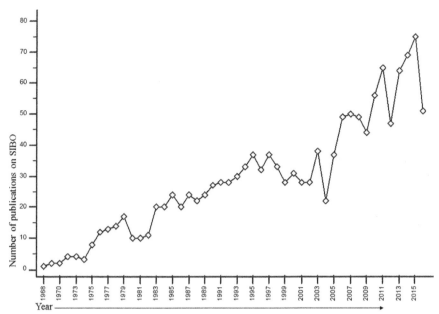

Fig. 2. Number of publications using search term "small intestinal bacterial overgrowth" in PubMed showing increasing recognition of this entity over time.

Table 1
Gastrointestinal and hepatobiliary diseases associated with small intestinal bacterial overgrowth

	Disease
GI diseases	IBS
	Tropical sprue
	Celiac disease
	Immunoproliferative small intestinal disease
	Inflammatory bowel disease, particularly Crohn disease
	Chronic intestinal pseudoobstruction
	Collagen diseases with small bowel involvement, such as progressive systemic sclerosis
	Gastric and enteric surgery
	Short bowel syndrome
	Visceral neuropathy (eg, diabetes mellitus, amyloidosis)
	Structural causes such as small intestinal diverticula, stricture, and fistula
	Lactose malabsorption
	Chronic proton pump inhibitor intake
	Immune deficiency states (combined variable immunodeficiency, hypogammaglobulinemia, T-cell deficiency)
Hepatic diseases	Cirrhosis of liver
	Spontaneous bacterial peritonitis
	Nonalcoholic fatty liver disease
Pancreatic disease	Chronic pancreatitis due to different causes

Abbreviations: GI, gastrointestinal; IBS, irritable bowel syndrome.

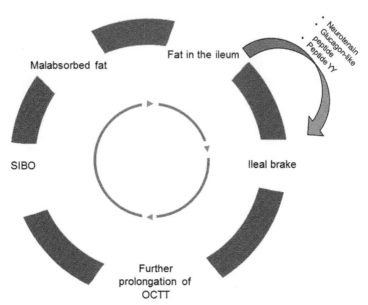

Fig. 3. How malabsorbed fat induces ileal brake while passing through the ileum, causing small bowel stasis and increasing bacterial overgrowth in the upper gut. OCTT, oro-cecal transit time; SIBO, small intestinal bacterial overgrowth.

risk factors for this condition.[10,11] Structural causes include intestinal stricture, enteroenteric fistula and anastomosis, diverticula, blind loop syndrome, incompetent ileocecal valve, and various GI surgical procedures, including those reducing gastric acid secretion.[10] Previously, recognition that SIBO can occur in absence of structural causes was somewhat less. However, it is being recognized more and more that a large proportion of patients diagnosed as having SIBO do not have any structural cause.[4,12–14]

Normal aboral motility of the gut pushes the intestinal content downward, preventing overgrowth of bacteria in upper gut.[15] In patients with abnormally slow motility, stagnation of intraluminal contents is associated with development of SIBO.[16] Mechanical factors due to previous GI surgery is an important cause of stasis.[17] However, functional stasis is being recognized increasingly as a cause for SIBO.[13,17] Phase III of fasting intestinal motility, called migratory motor complex (MMC), is an important mechanism to prevent SIBO and abnormal MMC has been shown to be associated with SIBO.[18,19] Treatment with some prokinetics, such as tegaserod, prevents recurrence of SIBO following its successful treatment.[20] Another mechanism of SIBO in patients with malabsorption syndromes, such as tropical sprue and celiac disease, is slowing of proximal gut motility by its inhibition caused by passage of unabsorbed fat through the ileum-liberating peptide YY, neurotensin, and glucagon-like peptide, a phenomenon called ileal brake (**Fig. 4**).[16,21,22] Hence, a vicious cycle sets in that is associated with slowing of small intestinal motility that leads to further small intestinal bacterial colonization (see **Fig. 4**).[22,23] Several systemic conditions may be associated with slowing of small intestinal motility, including hypothyroidism; diabetic autonomic neuropathy; other myoneuropathies affecting gut; and collagen diseases, such as progressive systemic sclerosis, systemic lupus erythematosus, and parkinsonism.[24–29]

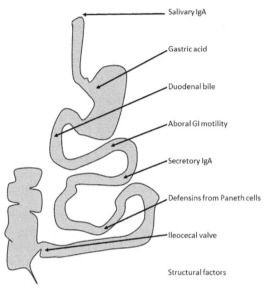

- Salivary IgA
- Gastric acid
- Duodenal bile
- Aboral GI motility
- Secretory IgA
- Defensins from Paneth cells
- Ileocecal valve
- Structural factors

Fig. 4. Major gut defense mechanisms preventing SIBO. GI, gastrointestinal; SIBO, small intestinal bacterial overgrowth.

The defense mechanisms of the gut, which prevent SIBO, include salivary immunoglobulin (Ig)-A, gastric acid, duodenal bile, pentavalent IgA in the intestinal secretion, and defensin (**Fig. 5**).[9,30] Defensins contribute to innate immunity of the gut. These are antimicrobial peptides secreted by Paneth cells located at the base of crypts of Lieberkuhn (see **Fig. 5**).[30,31] Density of Paneth cells is determined by the density of the bacteria in the gut and the need to keep the number of bacteria under check. For example, there are more Paneth cells in the ileum and right colon, where the numbers of bacteria are in excess, compared with the upper gut. In contrast, in the left colon

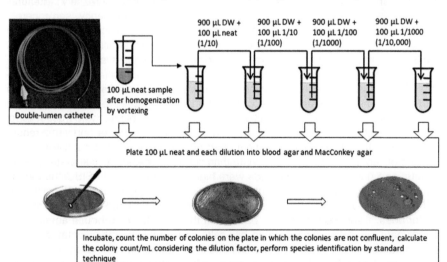

Fig. 5. Method of quantitative culture of upper gut aspirate for diagnosis of SIBO. DW, distilled water.

and rectum, though bacteria are more in number, there is no need to check their over-growth; therefore, the density of the Paneth cells is markedly less. Secreted defensins are sufficient to generate adequate microbicidal concentrations in the intestinal lumen maintaining eubiosis and inhibiting pathogenic microbes.[30,32] However, more data on the relationship between abnormality in this innate immune mechanism and SIBO are awaited.

Because mucosal immunity regulates gut microbiota and prevents SIBO, its defi-ciency is expected to cause bacterial overgrowth in the gut. However, data on this issue are limited to a few case reports and series on subjects with hypogammaglob-ulinemia or agammaglobulinemia, nodular lymphoid hyperplasia, or chronic lympho-cytic leukemia.[33–35] The bacteria overgrowing in the small bowel have been reported to translocate through the gut wall in subjects with hypogammaglobulinemia that is associated with strongyloidiasis, causing fatal septicemia.[36] More studies, however, are needed on this issue.

Hypochlorhydria caused by treatment with a proton pump inhibitor (PPI) is not an uncommon cause of SIBO as demonstrated by studies using quantitative small bowel aspirate culture and hydrogen breath tests (HBTs).[37,38] In an Italian study, subjects with gastroesophageal reflux disease (n = 450) treated with PPI more often had SIBO on glucose HBT (50%) compared with controls with IBS not receiving PPI (24.5%) and healthy subjects (6%).[37] In this study, use of PPI longer than 1 year was a risk factor for SIBO.[37] Similarly, higher frequency of SIBO with oral or fecal types of bacteria has been demonstrated by upper gut aspirate culture among subjects with different preparations and dosage of PPI compared with controls.[38] In a meta-analysis of 11 studies, an association between PPI use and SIBO was found when the gold standard method of duodenal or jejunal aspirate culture was used to diagnose it.[39]

HOW DOES SMALL INTESTINAL BACTERIAL OVERGROWTH CAUSE GUT DYSFUNCTIONS?

SIBO causes GI dysfunction and symptoms by several mechanisms, including pro-tracted inflammation, immune activation, alteration in motility, increase in intestinal permeability, deconjugation of bile salt, secondary lactase deficiency, serotonergic modulation, and water and nutrient malabsorption with increasing osmotic load and luminal contents.[4,11,40,41] In contrast to healthy subjects, the small bowel of subjects with SIBO contain colonic type bacteria, including Gram-negative aerobes and anaer-obes (eg, *Escherichia coli*, *Enterococcus* spp, *Klebsiella pneumonia*, and *Proteus mir-abilis*),[10,42,43] that ferment carbohydrates into gas,[44,45] causing symptoms such as bloating, distension, abdominal discomfort, and pain.[10] Moreover, the small bowel luminal content has a different metabolomic profile in subjects with than without SIBO.[46] In a study on 31 subjects with malabsorption syndrome and 10 disease-free controls, the malabsorption patients had higher quantities of total bile acids or cholesterol, lactate, acetate, and formate than controls. Quantities of acetate, lactate, formate, and unconjugated bile acids were higher in subjects with SIBO than those without. In subjects with malabsorption, the quantity of acetate positively correlated with the degree of SIBO, and unconjugated bile acids correlated with the degree of steatorrhoea,[46] suggesting that the bacteria in the small bowel produce acetate and deconjugate bile salts; deconjugated bile salts cause malabsorption of fat. Some of these metabolites are toxic to the small intestinal epithelium. For example, though these short-chain fatty acids are nutrients to colonocytes, these damage small intes-tinal epithelium and induce ileal brake, causing stasis and bacterial colonization.[4] Pa-tients with SIBO often have reduced villous height and inflammatory infiltrate in the epithelium.[22] SIBO is associated with increased intestinal permeability, which contributes to diarrhea and malabsorption[47]; moreover, the mucosal immune system is activated in patients with SIBO,[48,49] which may be related to passage of luminal antigens through leaky gut into the subepithelium.

SYMPTOMS OF SMALL INTESTINAL BACTERIAL OVERGROWTH

SIBO may contribute to a wide variety of symptoms, some of which are common to other GI diseases, posing considerable diagnostic challenge. Moreover, the symptoms may be incorrectly ascribed to primary disease causing SIBO and delaying its diagnosis. The symptoms of SIBO may be broadly divided into (1) those related to malabsorbed nutrients or metabolites in the GI tract and changes in intestinal permeability, (2) the nutritional consequences of malabsorption, and (3) systemic effects of gut inflammation and immune activation. The first group of symptoms includes bloating, flatulence, abdominal distension and discomfort, chronic diarrhea and steatorrhea (fat malabsorption), pale stool (due to dilution of bile pigment in a large volume of stool).[4,13] Abnormal small intestinal permeability may contribute to chronic diarrhea.[50] Some of the above symptoms mimic those of IBS. Hence, patients with SIBO may fulfill symptom-based criteria, such as that proposed by the Rome Foundation, for IBS.[4,51] The second group of symptoms are related to malabsorption of nutrients over a sufficiently long period of time, including weight loss, growth failure in children, and anemia.[3,13] Anemia in patients with SIBO may result from several mechanisms, such as iron and vitamin B12 deficiency resulting from malabsorption of these nutrients and poor intake due to associated anorexia.[52] Because B12 deficiency causes megaloblastic and iron deficiency microcytic anemia, a dimorphic blood picture may occur.[52] The associated diseases affecting proximal small bowel (site of iron absorption) and distal ileum (site of vitamin B12 absorption) may contribute to the deficiency of each of these nutrients. Because vegetarians may have a marginally lower B12 store, they are more prone to develop clinically obvious vitamin B12 deficiency. Interestingly, because bacteria synthesize folate, which is available to the host,[53] patients with SIBO are unlikely to have its deficiency. It is important to mention that by increasing the dietary intake the patients may compensate for the loss of nutrients and, hence, may not have features of deficiency; however, bowel symptoms are often present even in absence of nutritional deficiency. SIBO may be associated with systemic symptoms. Pimentel and colleagues[54] found that patients with fibromyalgia had higher frequency of SIBO than controls. Body ache and fatigue are reported by patients with SIBO. In advanced stages, patients may have neurologic manifestations of vitamin B12 deficiency, such as peripheral neuropathy and subacute combined degeneration of the spinal cord. The symptoms of SIBO tend to be chronic, existing for months to years, with fluctuation in intensity.

CLINICAL PREDICTORS OF SMALL INTESTINAL BACTERIAL OVERGROWTH

Because the presenting symptoms of SIBO are quite nonspecific and are reported in several other conditions affecting the GI tract and the diagnostic tests are neither very sensitive nor specific, a high degree of suspicion is required to diagnose SIBO. This highlights the importance of clinical predictors of SIBO. Chronic diarrhea and malabsorption syndrome predicts the presence of SIBO. In a study on 50 subjects with malabsorption syndrome due to various causes, such as tropical sprue, celiac disease, intestinal tuberculosis, panhypogammaglobulinemia, selective IgA deficiency, strongyloidiasis, acquired immunodeficiency syndrome, giardiasis, intestinal lymphangiectasia, structural lesions, and motility abnormality of gut, almost half had SIBO on jejunal aspirate culture.[14] Among subjects presenting as IBS, female gender, old age, marked bloating and flatulence, long-term treatment with PPI, narcotic intake, low hemoglobin, and diarrheal subtype of IBS were associated with SIBO.[3,55–57] In a recent study, higher small bowel bacterial colony count was associated with looser Bristol stool types.[6] Another study showed that *Ruminococcaceae-Bacteroides* enterotype growth potential positively correlated with Bristol stool scale scores.[58] Alcoholism, even in absence of chronic liver disease, is a predictor for occurrence of SIBO.[59] Although 1 study showed that prior cholecystectomy is associated with SIBO,[60] another study contradicted this observation.[59] Among subjects with celiac disease, nonresponse to gluten-free diet may be caused by SIBO and its treatment may lead to clinical remission.[61,62]

DIAGNOSIS OF SMALL INTESTINAL BACTERIAL OVERGROWTH

Table 2 enumerates the tests used to diagnose SIBO. Quantitative jejunal aspirate culture, which is performed by serial dilution technique (see **Fig. 5**), is currently considered the gold standard for diagnosis of SIBO.[16] A double-lumen catheter that avoids contamination by oropharyngeal flora is preferred to single-lumen cannula (see **Fig. 5**).[14] Bacterial colony counts in jejunal aspirate equal to or greater than 10^5 CFU/mL have conventionally been the defining cutoff for the diagnosis of SIBO.[16] However, recently, this has been challenged and a lower cutoff of equal to or greater than 10^3 CFU/mL has been suggested, particularly in presence of coliforms.[7] This is based on data suggesting that in several conditions, although bacterial colony counts are less than 10^5 CFU/mL, they are equal to or greater than 10^3 CFU/mL.[6,7] Moreover, jejunal aspirate in healthy subjects rarely grow bacteria equal to or greater than 10^3 CFU/mL on culture.[6,46] A recent randomized controlled trial among subjects with IBS also suggested that equal to or greater than 10^3 CFU/mL of jejunal aspirate should be the cutoff value for diagnosis of significant SIBO.[8] In this study, rates of symptomatic response among subjects with IBS with upper gut aspirate colony count of equal to or greater than 10^5 CFU, equal to or greater than 10^3 CFU, and less than 10^3 CFU/mL were 87.5%, 45.5%, and 14.2%, respectively.[8] One of the limitations of gut aspirate culture is that only 30% bacteria can be cultured.[4] Moreover, if air is used to inflate the gut during upper GI endoscopy, most of the anaerobes do not survive. In an earlier study using air during endoscopy, of 34 of 50 subjects with malabsorption syndrome in whom bacteria were cultured in jejunal aspirate, only 1 grew anaerobe.[14] Hence, either nitrogen or carbon dioxide gases should be used during

Table 2	
Tests used to diagnose small intestinal bacterial overgrowth	
Test Groups	**Diagnostic Tests**
Culture-based tests	Quantitative conventional culture of upper gut aspirate
	Quantitative culture of jejunal biopsy
	Culturomic method
HBT	Glucose HBT
	Lactulose HBT
	HBT combined with radionuclide gut transit tests
	D-xylose HBT
Carbon isotope breath test	^{14}C glycocholic acid breath test
Molecular methods	

insufflation. Due to the limitations previously mentioned, invasive nature of the procedure and need for good microbiological back up, upper gut aspirate culture is not used for diagnosis of SIBO in clinical practice.

HBTs are quite popular for the diagnosis of SIBO because they are noninvasive and inexpensive, in spite of the fact that they are neither highly sensitive nor specific.[3,63] The initial studies on SIBO in subjects with IBS were based on lactulose HBT.[4,51] A peak in hydrogen by 20 parts per million (ppm) above basal within 90 min was considered diagnostic of SIBO (**Fig. 6**). These studies presumed that orocecal transit time is always longer than 90 minutes.[54,64] Hence, a significant rise in hydrogen was expected to come from small bowel due to SIBO. However, several studies reported that orocecal transit time may be shorter than 90 minutes, even in healthy subjects (see **Fig. 6**).[51] In Indian and Taiwanese studies, orocecal transit time was often shorter (median: 65 min, range 40–110 min; mean 85 min, standard deviation 37 min, respectively).[22,65] While performing combined lactulose HBT and ^{99m}technetium (^{99m}Tc) scintigraphy, Yu and colleagues[66] demonstrated that the ^{99m}Tc reached the cecum before breath hydrogen increased in 88% of subjects (see **Fig. 6**). The conventional criterion for diagnosis of SIBO on lactulose HBT is based on occurrence of 2 peaks: 1 from small bowel due to SIBO and the other from colon (see **Fig. 6**). A few studies compared diagnostic performance of the early-peak and double-peak criteria for diagnosis of SIBO, considering quantitative jejunal aspirate culture as the gold standard. In an initial study on 83 subjects with malabsorption syndrome due to various causes, 32 (39.5%) had SIBO on aspirate culture.[16] The sensitivity and specificity of the double-peak criteria on lactulose HBT in this study were 31% and 86%, respectively.[16] In a recent study among 80 subjects with IBS, double-peak criteria on lactulose HBT had sensitivity and specificity of 0% and 98%, respectively; the corresponding values of early-peak criteria were 33% and 65%, respectively.[6] All these data suggest that the early-peak criteria on lactulose HBT are quite nonspecific and the double-peak criteria are insensitive to diagnose SIBO.[63] Hence, lactulose HBT cannot be recommended for the diagnosis of SIBO in clinical practice.

Diagnostic performance of glucose HBT has been evaluated considering the quantitative culture of upper gut aspirate culture in several studies. In a study on 83 subjects with malabsorption syndrome, sensitivity and specificity of glucose HBT were 44% and 80%, respectively.[16] In another study on 80 subjects with IBS, sensitivity of glucose HBT to diagnose SIBO was 27% and specificity was 100%.[6] In a recent study on 139 subjects with functional GI disorder, sensitivity and specificity of glucose HBT were 42% and 84%, respectively, considering jejunal aspirate culture as the gold standard.[67] These data suggest that, although specificity of glucose HBT is high, it misses the diagnosis of SIBO in three-fourths to two-thirds of subjects. Search for a noninvasive, sensitive, and specific diagnostic test for SIBO continues. In a recent retrospective study, lactulose HBT was combined with ^{99m}Tc-diethylene triamine pentaacetic acid to assess whether the rise in breath hydrogen is from small intestine due to SIBO or from cecum?[68] Because early-peak criterion on lactulose HBT is nonspecific due to the wide variation in orocecal transit time and double-peak criteria insensitive, a Chinese study evaluated a novel method of combined lactulose HBT and scintigraphic measurement of orocecal transit.[69] These investigators found that an equal to or greater than 5 ppm increase in breath H_2 before the arrival of radionuclide in the cecum identified SIBO with reasonable accuracy, which predicted response to treatment with rifaximin.[69] It seems that this method has great promise for diagnosis of SIBO in the future. However, more data are needed on this before its value in clinical practice can be decided.

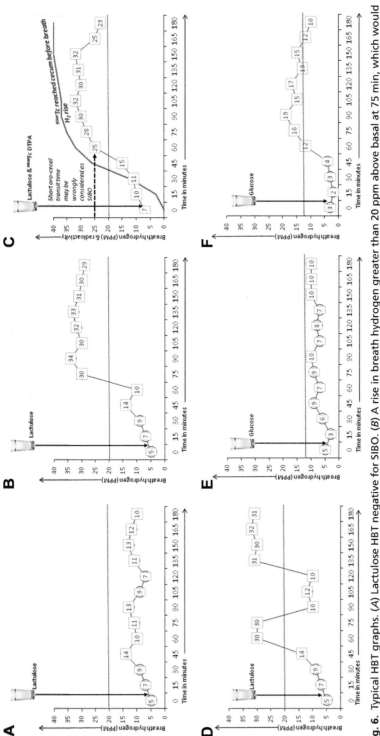

Fig. 6. Typical HBT graphs. (*A*) Lactulose HBT negative for SIBO. (*B*) A rise in breath hydrogen greater than 20 ppm above basal at 75 min, which would be fallaciously considered as SIBO according to the initial studies. (*C*) Although it reflects short orocecal transit time (*dotted line*), which is not unusual, such erroneous interpretation has been documented by combined lactulose HBT and radionuclide assessment of orocecal transit (*blue line*) using ^{99m}technetium-diethylene triamine pentaacetic acid (^{99m}Tc-DTPA), which showed ^{99m}Tc reached cecum before breath H2 increased. (*D*) Presence of SIBO on lactulose HBT shown by double-peak criterion. (*E*) Glucose HBT negative for SIBO. (*F*) Glucose HBT test positive for SIBO. Y axes denote breath hydrogen (parts per million) and X axes time in minutes in all the graphs. HBT, hydrogen breath test; PPM, parts per million; SIBO, small intestinal bacterial overgrowth.

D-xylose is a pentose sugar that is absorbed in the proximal small bowel and, hence, does not reach the colon. In patients with SIBO, D-xylose is metabolized by the bacteria in the small bowel, producing hydrogen that gets absorbed into the blood stream. The absorbed hydrogen is exhaled in the breath, which is estimated using a commercially available gas chromatograph. However, studies on diagnostic performance of this breath test are scanty. Hence, the D-xylose breath test is not popular in clinical practice. In the largest retrospective study on frequency of SIBO among 932 consecutive eligible subjects, 513 (55%) had SIBO.[70] This study, however, had limitation because the diagnosis of SIBO was not verified by any other method and the sensitivity and specificity of the D-xylose breath test to diagnose SIBO is not known.

Because bacteria in patients with SIBO deconjugate bile acids, the ^{13}C or ^{14}C glycocholic acid breath test has also been used for diagnosis of SIBO.[4] These tests involve oral administration of the bile acid ^{14}C or ^{13}C glycocholic acid, and detection of $^{14}CO_2$ or $^{13}CO_2$, which would be elevated in patients with SIBO.[4] However, data on the clinical utility of ^{13}C or ^{14}C glycocholic acid breath test are scanty. In an earlier study, the lactose-^{13}C ureide breath test was compared with glucose HBT, considering jejunal aspirate culture as the gold standard.[71] It had a sensitivity of 66.7% and a specificity of 100%, which were higher than glucose HBT.[71]

TREATMENT OF SMALL INTESTINAL BACTERIAL OVERGROWTH

The treatment in patients with SIBO is directed toward (1) altered gut microbiota, (2) nutritional deficiencies, (3) primary conditions predisposing to SIBO, and (4) prevention of recurrence. Altered microbiota is primarily treated by antibiotics (**Table 3**), although studies on probiotics and prebiotics are also reported. Various antibiotics that have been reported for treatment of SIBO include rifaximin; neomycin; tetracycline; doxycycline; fluoroquinolones, such as ciprofloxacin and norfloxacin; cotrimoxazole; and nitroimidazole.[11] An antibiotic used in treatment of SIBO should ideally be broad in its microbiological spectrum, targeting anaerobes, aerobes, Gram-positive as well as negative bacteria, poorly absorbed, selective in its action against overgrown small bowel bacteria but not the colonic microbes, and free from adverse effects. Rifaximin is the only agent that fulfills all these requirements.[72]

Rifaximin ($C_{43}H_{51}N_3O_{11}$), the structural analogue of rifampin, inhibits synthesis of bacterial RNA by binding to the β subunit of bacterial DNA-dependent RNA polymerase.[72] It is very poorly absorbed and is most active in presence of bile salt and, hence, on small bowel rather than colonic microbes.[72] Rifaximin has a very broad antimicrobial spectrum. In a study on 117 subjects with SIBO diagnosed on upper gut aspirate culture, rifaximin inhibited in vitro 85.4% of *Escherichia coli*, 43.6% of *Klebsiella* spp, 34.8% of *Enterobacter* spp, 54.5% of other *Enterobacteriaceae* spp, 82.6% of non-*Enterobacteriaceae* Gram-negative spp, 100% of *Enterococcus faecalis*, 100% of *Enterococcus faecium*, and 100% of *Staphylococcus aureus*.[73] In addition to modulation of microbiota, some evidence suggests that it may have additional mechanisms of action, including prevention of bacterial translocation across the gut mucosa, alteration in release and absorption of endotoxin and bacterial metabolites, antiinflammatory effect, and modulation of gut-immune signaling.[72,74] Hence, rifaximin has been considered as a gut microenvironment modulator,[72] abnormality in which is being understood to be an important mechanism of GI diseases, including functional bowel diseases.[75] In a dose-finding study on 90 subjects with SIBO diagnosed using glucose HBT, rifaximin 1200 mg per day was found superior to 800 and 600 mg per day.[76] However, in TARGET I and

Table 3
Studies on antibiotic treatment of small intestinal bacterial overgrowth

Antibiotics with Dosage	Duration	Subjects and Diagnostic Method	Outcome	Reference
Norfloxacin (800 mg/d), amoxicillin-clavulanic acid (1500 mg/d), Saccharomyces boulardii (1500 mg/d), placebo	7 d	10 subjects with SIBO (HBT, randomized crossover design)	Norfloxacin and amoxicillin-clavulanic acid effective compared with placebo or S boulardii	Attar et al,[82] 1999
Amoxicillin-clavulanic acid (500 mg 3 × d) and cefoxitin	7–10 d	55 subjects with diarrhea or malabsorption with SIBO (quantitative upper gut aspirate culture, uncontrolled design)	Eradicate more than 90% of species in subjects with SIBO	Bouhnik et al,[43] 1999
Rifaximin (1200 mg/d) or chlortetracycline (1 g/d)	7 d	21 subjects with SIBO (GHBT)	SIBO eradication higher with rifaximin (70%) than chlortetracycline (27%)	DiStefano et al,[79] 2000
Rifaximin (group 1: 600 mg/d; group 2: 800 mg/d; and group 3: 1200 mg/d)	7 d	90 subjects with SIBO (30 subjects in each group, GHBT)	Rate of normalization of GHBT was higher in group 3 (60% vs 17%, $P<.001$) than groups 1 and 2 (60% vs 27%, $P<.01$)	Lauritano et al,[76] 2005
Rifaximin (1600 mg/d) vs rifaximin (1200 mg/day)	7 d	80 subjects with SIBO (GHBT with methane measurement)	Rate of normalization of GHBT was greater with higher rather than lower dosage of rifaximin (80% vs 58%, $P<.05$)	Scarpellini et al,[85] 2007
Rifaximin (1200 mg/d) and metronidazole (750 mg/d)	7 d	142 subjects with SIBO (GHBT)	SIBO eradication higher with rifaximin (63.4% vs 43.7%, $P<.05$)	Lauritano et al,[78] 2009
Rifaximin (1200 mg/d) vs rifaximin with PHGG (1200 mg + 5 g/d)	10 d	77 subjects with SIBO (GHBT)	SIBO eradication: 62.1% in the rifaximin group and 85.0%, ($P = .036$) in the rifaximin with PHGG group	Furnari et al,[80] 2010
Norfloxacin (800 mg/d) or placebo	10 d	80 subjects with IBS (quantitative upper gut aspirate culture and GHBT)	Norfloxacin superior to placebo in symptom improvement and SIBO eradication. Higher bacterial colony count, greater response: $\geq 10^5$, 87.5%; $\geq 10^3$, 45.5%; and $<10^3$ CFU/mL, 14.2%	Ghoshal et al,[8] 2016

Abbreviations: d, day; GHBT, glucose hydrogen breath test; HBT, hydrogen breath test; PHGG, partially hydrolyzed guar gum; SIBO: small intestinal bacterial overgrowth.

II studies on a large cohort of subjects with IBS, 550 mg thrice daily dose was used.[77] Rifaximin has been found to be superior compared with chlortetracycline and metronidazole in the treatment of SIBO in 2 separate studies.[78,79] In a randomized controlled trial, rifaximin 1200 mg per day plus partially hydrolyzed guar gum 5 g per day for 10 days achieved higher rate of SIBO eradication (87%) and symptom improvement compared with an equivalent dose of rifaximin alone (62%).[80] A randomized trial of rifaximin followed by either probiotics or prebiotics did not show any difference in symptom improvement between the 2 groups.[81]

There are scanty data on other antibiotics for treatment of SIBO. In an in vitro study on antibiotic sensitivity pattern of bacteria cultured in 34 of 50 subjects with malabsorption syndrome, sensitivity to quinolones was more than that to tetracycline, ampicillin, erythromycin, and cotrimoxazole.[14] A recent randomized controlled trial found that presence of SIBO among subjects with IBS was a predictor for response to antibiotic treatment with norfloxacin.[8] In this study, 7 of 8 (87.5%) of 15 subjects with SIBO treated with norfloxacin became Rome III negative at 1 month compared with none of those treated with placebo. Interestingly, in this study, of 40 subjects treated with norfloxacin, 15 (37.5%) responded, showing that when not selected according to presence of SIBO, response rate was low.[8] In another study, subjects with SIBO diagnosed by combined lactulose HBT and scintigraphic measurement of orocecal transit, symptom resolution was more common among those with than those without SIBO.[69] In a randomized crossover trial on 10 subjects with SIBO, norfloxacin and amoxicillin-clavulanic acid were more effective in the treatment of bacterial overgrowth-related diarrhea than placebo or *Saccharomyces boulardii*.[82] The data on efficacy of probiotics and prebiotics in treatment of SIBO, however, are scanty.[11]

Because patients with SIBO often have nutritional deficiencies, corrective measures against these are of utmost importance. Secondary lactase deficiency resulting in lactose intolerance is common and avoidance of dietary lactose, at least for a short period of time, may reduce gas related symptoms, such as bloating, distension, flatulence, and osmotic diarrhea.[83] A low fermentable oligosaccharides, disaccharides, monosaccharides, and polyols (FODMAP) diet may also reduce these symptoms,[83] though a highly restrictive diet of this nature may also be counterproductive in relation of nutritional status. Because malabsorbed fat may increase abdominal bloating and small bowel bacterial colonization by causing stasis by ileal brake mechanism,[21,22] restricting fat during early course may be useful. Medium chain triglycerides may be useful in such patients. Deficiency of micronutrients, such as vitamin B12; calcium; fat-soluble vitamins, including vitamin D; and iron should be addressed. Because bacteria in patients with SIBO synthesize folate,[53] its supplementation is not needed except in patients with tropical sprue, who are deficient in it.[21]

Successful treatment of primary disease predisposing to SIBO is also useful in its treatment and in prevention of its recurrence. Recurrence of SIBO is not uncommon after successful treatment. During follow-up after successful eradication using rifaximin, 12.6%, 27.5%, and 43.7% had recurrence of SIBO on glucose HBT at 3, 6, and 9 months, respectively.[84] The TARGET I and II studies showed that 10-day treatment with rifaximin kept the symptom of IBS resolved for about 8 to 12 weeks.[77] In another recent study, symptom resolution persisted for 8 to 12 weeks after successful treatment with norfloxacin.[8] In a retrospective study, low-dose tegaserod was found to delay recurrence of SIBO after its successful treatment compared with no preventive measure or erythromycin treatment.[20] Recurrent symptoms can be successfully treated by retreatment with a microbiota-directed approach such as rifaximin.

SUMMARY

Gut microbiota, considered the largest organ of the human body, serve several important functions. Dysbiosis (abnormal gut microbiota) includes SIBO (quantitative increase in small bowel bacteria), qualitative alteration (ratio of friendly and harmful bacteria), or change in bacterial location (eg, colonic type bacteria in upper gut) and is increasingly realized to be associated with several diseases (eg, IBS, celiac disease, Crohn disease, tropical sprue, GI hypomotility states, hypochlorhydria, immunodeficiency states), in addition to the structural causes. Bacterial growth equal to or greater than 10^5 CFU/mL in culture of upper gut aspirate was conventionally considered as the gold standard for diagnosis of SIBO; however, recently, a cutoff equal to or greater than 10^3 CFU/mL is also being considered to suggest SIBO, particularly if colonic type bacteria are present in the upper gut. HBTs using different substrates (glucose, lactulose) are popularly used to diagnose SIBO, although these are neither very sensitive nor specific. Among currently available therapeutic options, rifaximin is the best treatment of SIBO due to its broad spectrum, lack of systemic absorption, and safety profile. Though recurrence of SIBO following successful treatment is common, it may be retreated with antibiotics such as rifaximin.

REFERENCES

1. Mackie RI, Sghir A, Gaskins HR. Developmental microbial ecology of the neonatal gastrointestinal tract. Am J Clin Nutr 1999;69:1035S–45S.
2. Prakash S, Rodes L, Coussa-Charley M, et al. Gut microbiota: next frontier in understanding human health and development of biotherapeutics. Biologics 2011;5:71–86.
3. Gabrielli M, D'Angelo G, Di Rienzo T, et al. Diagnosis of small intestinal bacterial overgrowth in the clinical practice. Eur Rev Med Pharmacol Sci 2013;17(Suppl 2):30–5.
4. Ghoshal UC, Srivastava D. Irritable bowel syndrome and small intestinal bacterial overgrowth: meaningful association or unnecessary hype. World J Gastroenterol 2014;20:2482–91.
5. Nagao-Kitamoto H, Kitamoto S, Kuffa P, et al. Pathogenic role of the gut microbiota in gastrointestinal diseases. Intest Res 2016;14:127–38.
6. Ghoshal UC, Srivastava D, Ghoshal U, et al. Breath tests in the diagnosis of small intestinal bacterial overgrowth in patients with irritable bowel syndrome in comparison with quantitative upper gut aspirate culture. Eur J Gastroenterol Hepatol 2014;26:753–60.
7. Khoshini R, Dai SC, Lezcano S, et al. A systematic review of diagnostic tests for small intestinal bacterial overgrowth. Dig Dis Sci 2008;53:1443–54.
8. Ghoshal UC, Srivastava D, Misra A, et al. A proof-of-concept study showing antibiotics to be more effective in irritable bowel syndrome with than without small-intestinal bacterial overgrowth: a randomized, double-blind, placebo-controlled trial. Eur J Gastroenterol Hepatol 2016;28:281–9.
9. Grace E, Shaw C, Whelan K, et al. Review article: small intestinal bacterial overgrowth–prevalence, clinical features, current and developing diagnostic tests, and treatment. Aliment Pharmacol Ther 2013;38:674–88.
10. Sachdev AH, Pimentel M. Gastrointestinal bacterial overgrowth: pathogenesis and clinical significance. Ther Adv Chronic Dis 2013;4:223–31.
11. Ghoshal UC, Shukla R, Ghoshal U, et al. The gut microbiota and irritable bowel syndrome: friend or foe? Int J Inflam 2012;2012:151085.
12. Ghoshal UC, Kumar S, Mehrotra M, et al. Frequency of small intestinal bacterial overgrowth in patients with irritable bowel syndrome and chronic non-specific diarrhea. J Neurogastroenterol Motil 2010;16:40–6.

13. Ghoshal UC, Mehrotra M, Kumar S, et al. Spectrum of malabsorption syndrome among adults & factors differentiating celiac disease & tropical malabsorption. Indian J Med Res 2012;136:451–9.
14. Ghoshal U, Ghoshal UC, Ranjan P, et al. Spectrum and antibiotic sensitivity of bacteria contaminating the upper gut in patients with malabsorption syndrome from the tropics. BMC Gastroenterol 2003;3:9.
15. Stotzer PO, Bjornsson ES, Abrahamsson H. Interdigestive and postprandial motility in small-intestinal bacterial overgrowth. Scand J Gastroenterol 1996;31:875–80.
16. Ghoshal UC, Ghoshal U, Das K, et al. Utility of hydrogen breath tests in diagnosis of small intestinal bacterial overgrowth in malabsorption syndrome and its relationship with oro-cecal transit time. Indian J Gastroenterol 2006;25:6–10.
17. Husebye E. The pathogenesis of gastrointestinal bacterial overgrowth. Chemotherapy 2005;51(Suppl 1):1–22.
18. Pimentel M, Soffer EE, Chow EJ, et al. Lower frequency of MMC is found in IBS subjects with abnormal lactulose breath test, suggesting bacterial overgrowth. Dig Dis Sci 2002;47:2639–43.
19. Vantrappen G, Janssens J, Hellemans J, et al. The interdigestive motor complex of normal subjects and patients with bacterial overgrowth of the small intestine. J Clin Invest 1977;59:1158–66.
20. Pimentel M, Morales W, Lezcano S, et al. Low-dose nocturnal tegaserod or erythromycin delays symptom recurrence after treatment of irritable bowel syndrome based on presumed bacterial overgrowth. Gastroenterol Hepatol (N Y) 2009;5:435–42.
21. Ghoshal UC, Kumar S, Misra A, et al. Pathogenesis of tropical sprue: a pilot study of antroduodenal manometry, duodenocaecal transit time & fat-induced ileal brake. Indian J Med Res 2013;137:63–72.
22. Ghoshal UC, Ghoshal U, Ayyagari A, et al. Tropical sprue is associated with contamination of small bowel with aerobic bacteria and reversible prolongation of orocecal transit time. J Gastroenterol Hepatol 2003;18:540–7.
23. Cook GC. Delayed small-intestinal transit in tropical malabsorption. Br Med J 1978;2:238–40.
24. Barboza JL, Okun MS, Moshiree B. The treatment of gastroparesis, constipation and small intestinal bacterial overgrowth syndrome in patients with Parkinson's disease. Expert Opin Pharmacother 2015;16:2449–64.
25. Akesson A, Akesson B, Gustafson T, et al. Gastrointestinal function in patients with progressive systemic sclerosis. Clin Rheumatol 1985;4:441–8.
26. Bharadwaj S, Tandon P, Gohel T, et al. Gastrointestinal manifestations, malnutrition, and role of enteral and parenteral nutrition in patients with scleroderma. J Clin Gastroenterol 2015;49:559–64.
27. Lyford G, Foxx-Orenstein A. Chronic Intestinal Pseudoobstruction. Curr Treat Options Gastroenterol 2004;7:317–25.
28. Marie I, Ducrotte P, Denis P, et al. Small intestinal bacterial overgrowth in systemic sclerosis. Rheumatology (Oxford) 2009;48:1314–9.
29. Miller LJ. Small intestinal manifestations of diabetes mellitus. Yale J Biol Med 1983;56:189–93.
30. Nakamura K, Sakuragi N, Takakuwa A, et al. Paneth cell alpha-defensins and enteric microbiota in health and disease. Biosci Microbiota Food Health 2016;35:57–67.
31. Ghosh D, Porter E, Shen B, et al. Paneth cell trypsin is the processing enzyme for human defensin-5. Nat Immunol 2002;3:583–90.
32. Salzman NH, Ghosh D, Huttner KM, et al. Protection against enteric salmonellosis in transgenic mice expressing a human intestinal defensin. Nature 2003;422:522–6.

33. Ghoshal UC, Goel A, Ghoshal U, et al. Chronic diarrhea and malabsorption due to hypogammaglobulinemia: a report on twelve patients. Indian J Gastroenterol 2011;30:170–4.

34. Rubio-Tapia A, Hernandez-Calleros J, Trinidad-Hernandez S, et al. Clinical characteristics of a group of adults with nodular lymphoid hyperplasia: a single center experience. World J Gastroenterol 2006;12:1945–8.

35. Smith GM, Chesner IM, Asquith P, et al. Small intestinal bacterial overgrowth in patients with chronic lymphocytic leukaemia. J Clin Pathol 1990;43:57–9.

36. Ghoshal UC, Ghoshal U, Jain M, et al. *Strongyloides stercoralis* infestation associated with septicemia due to intestinal transmural migration of bacteria. J Gastroenterol Hepatol 2002;17:1331–3.

37. Lombardo L, Foti M, Ruggia O, et al. Increased incidence of small intestinal bacterial overgrowth during proton pump inhibitor therapy. Clin Gastroenterol Hepatol 2010;8:504–8.

38. Fried M, Siegrist H, Frei R, et al. Duodenal bacterial overgrowth during treatment in outpatients with omeprazole. Gut 1994;35:23–6.

39. Lo WK, Chan WW. Proton pump inhibitor use and the risk of small intestinal bacterial overgrowth: a meta-analysis. Clin Gastroenterol Hepatol 2013;11:483–90.

40. Mathias JR, Clench MH. Review: pathophysiology of diarrhea caused by bacterial overgrowth of the small intestine. Am J Med Sci 1985;289:243–8.

41. Pimentel M, Kong Y, Park S. IBS subjects with methane on lactulose breath test have lower postprandial serotonin levels than subjects with hydrogen. Dig Dis Sci 2004;49:84–7.

42. Savage DC. Microbial ecology of the gastrointestinal tract. Annu Rev Microbiol 1977;31:107–33.

43. Bouhnik Y, Alain S, Attar A, et al. Bacterial populations contaminating the upper gut in patients with small intestinal bacterial overgrowth syndrome. Am J Gastroenterol 1999;94:1327–31.

44. Sachdev AH, Pimentel M. Antibiotics for irritable bowel syndrome: rationale and current evidence. Curr Gastroenterol Rep 2012;14:439–45.

45. Posserud I, Stotzer PO, Bjornsson ES, et al. Small intestinal bacterial overgrowth in patients with irritable bowel syndrome. Gut 2007;56:802–8.

46. Bala L, Ghoshal UC, Ghoshal U, et al. Malabsorption syndrome with and without small intestinal bacterial overgrowth: a study on upper-gut aspirate using 1H NMR spectroscopy. Magn Reson Med 2006;56:738–44.

47. Riordan SM, McIver CJ, Thomas DH, et al. Luminal bacteria and small-intestinal permeability. Scand J Gastroenterol 1997;32:556–63.

48. Srivastava D, Ghoshal U, Mittal RD, et al. Associations between IL-1RA polymorphisms and small intestinal bacterial overgrowth among patients with irritable bowel syndrome from India. Neurogastroenterol Motil 2014;26:1408–16.

49. Al-Khatib K, Lin HC. Immune activation and gut microbes in irritable bowel syndrome. Gut Liver 2009;3:14–9.

50. Kumar S, Ghoshal UC, Jayalakshmi K, et al. Abnormal small intestinal permeability in patients with idiopathic malabsorption in tropics (tropical sprue) does not change even after successful treatment. Dig Dis Sci 2011;56:161–9.

51. Ghoshal UC, Park H, Gwee KA. Bugs and irritable bowel syndrome: The good, the bad and the ugly. J Gastroenterol Hepatol 2007;25:244–51.

52. Lykova EA, Bondarenko VM, Parfenov AI, et al. Bacterial overgrowth syndrome in the small intestine: pathogenesis, clinical significance and therapy tactics. Eksp Klin Gastroenterol 2005;(6):51–7, 113. [in Russian].

53. Camilo E, Zimmerman J, Mason JB, et al. Folate synthesized by bacteria in the human upper small intestine is assimilated by the host. Gastroenterology 1996; 110:991–8.

54. Pimentel M, Wallace D, Hallegua D, et al. A link between irritable bowel syndrome and fibromyalgia may be related to findings on lactulose breath testing. Ann Rheum Dis 2004;63:450–2.

55. Choung RS, Ruff KC, Malhotra A, et al. Clinical predictors of small intestinal bacterial overgrowth by duodenal aspirate culture. Aliment Pharmacol Ther 2011;33: 1059–67.

56. Majewski M, McCallum RW. Results of small intestinal bacterial overgrowth testing in irritable bowel syndrome patients: clinical profiles and effects of antibiotic trial. Adv Med Sci 2007;52:139–42.

57. Reddymasu SC, Sostarich S, McCallum RW. Small intestinal bacterial overgrowth in irritable bowel syndrome: are there any predictors? BMC Gastroenterol 2010;10:23.

58. Vandeputte D, Falony G, Vieira-Silva S, et al. Stool consistency is strongly associated with gut microbiota richness and composition, enterotypes and bacterial growth rates. Gut 2016;65:57–62.

59. Gabbard SL, Lacy BE, Levine GM, et al. The impact of alcohol consumption and cholecystectomy on small intestinal bacterial overgrowth. Dig Dis Sci 2014;59: 638–44.

60. Sung HJ, Paik CN, Chung WC, et al. Small intestinal bacterial overgrowth diagnosed by glucose hydrogen breath test in post-cholecystectomy Patients. J Neurogastroenterol Motil 2015;21:545–51.

61. Tursi A, Brandimarte G, Giorgetti G. High prevalence of small intestinal bacterial overgrowth in celiac patients with persistence of gastrointestinal symptoms after gluten withdrawal. Am J Gastroenterol 2003;98:839–43.

62. Chang MS, Green PH. A review of rifaximin and bacterial overgrowth in poorly responsive celiac disease. Therap Adv Gastroenterol 2012;5:31–6.

63. Ghoshal UC. How to interpret hydrogen breath tests. J Neurogastroenterol Motil 2011;17:312–7.

64. Pimentel M, Chow EJ, Lin HC. Eradication of small intestinal bacterial overgrowth reduces symptoms of irritable bowel syndrome. Am J Gastroenterol 2000;95: 3503–6.

65. Lu CL, Chen CY, Chang FY, et al. Characteristics of small bowel motility in patients with irritable bowel syndrome and normal humans: an Oriental study. Clin Sci (lond) 1998;95:165–9.

66. Yu D, Cheeseman F, Vanner S. Combined oro-caecal scintigraphy and lactulose hydrogen breath testing demonstrate that breath testing detects oro-caecal transit, not small intestinal bacterial overgrowth in patients with IBS. Gut 2011; 60:334–40.

67. Erdogan A, Rao SS, Gulley D, et al. Small intestinal bacterial overgrowth: duodenal aspiration vs glucose breath test. Neurogastroenterol Motil 2015;27: 481–9.

68. Ning Y, Lou C, Huang Z, et al. Clinical value of radionuclide small intestine transit time measurement combined with lactulose hydrogen breath test for the diagnosis of bacterial overgrowth in irritable bowel syndrome. Hell J Nucl Med 2016;19(2):124–9.

69. Zhao J, Zheng X, Chu H, et al. A study of the methodological and clinical validity of the combined lactulose hydrogen breath test with scintigraphic oro-cecal transit test for diagnosing small intestinal bacterial overgrowth in IBS patients. Neurogastroenterol Motil 2014;26:794–802.

70. Schatz RA, Zhang Q, Lodhia N, et al. Predisposing factors for positive D-Xylose breath test for evaluation of small intestinal bacterial overgrowth: a retrospective study of 932 patients. World J Gastroenterol 2015;21:4574–82.
71. Berthold HK, Schober P, Scheurlen C, et al. Use of the lactose-[13C]ureide breath test for diagnosis of small bowel bacterial overgrowth: comparison to the glucose hydrogen breath test. J Gastroenterol 2009;44:944–51.
72. DuPont HL. Therapeutic effects and mechanisms of action of rifaximin in gastro-intestinal diseases. Mayo Clin Proc 2015;90:1116–24.
73. Pistiki A, Galani I, Pyleris E, et al. In vitro activity of rifaximin against isolates from patients with small intestinal bacterial overgrowth. Int J Antimicrob Agents 2014; 43:236–41.
74. Pimentel M. Review article: potential mechanisms of action of rifaximin in the management of irritable bowel syndrome with diarrhoea. Aliment Pharmacol Ther 2016;43(Suppl 1):37–49.
75. Barbara G, Feinle-Bisset C, Ghoshal UC, et al. The intestinal microenvironment and functional gastrointestinal disorders. Gastroenterology 2016;150:1305–18.
76. Lauritano EC, Gabrielli M, Lupascu A, et al. Rifaximin dose-finding study for the treatment of small intestinal bacterial overgrowth. Aliment Pharmacol Ther 2005; 22:31–5.
77. Pimentel M, Lembo A, Chey WD, et al. Rifaximin therapy for patients with irritable bowel syndrome without constipation. N Engl J Med 2011;364:22–32.
78. Lauritano EC, Gabrielli M, Scarpellini E, et al. Antibiotic therapy in small intestinal bacterial overgrowth: rifaximin versus metronidazole. Eur Rev Med Pharmacol Sci 2009;13:111–6.
79. Di Stefano M, Malservisi S, Veneto G, et al. Rifaximin versus chlortetracycline in the short-term treatment of small intestinal bacterial overgrowth. Aliment Pharma-col Ther 2000;14:551–6.
80. Furnari M, Parodi A, Gemignani L, et al. Clinical trial: the combination of rifaximin with partially hydrolysed guar gum is more effective than rifaximin alone in erad-icating small intestinal bacterial overgrowth. Aliment Pharmacol Ther 2010;32: 1000–6.
81. Rosania R, Giorgio F, Principi M, et al. Effect of probiotic or prebiotic supplemen-tation on antibiotic therapy in the small intestinal bacterial overgrowth: a compar-ative evaluation. Curr Clin Pharmacol 2013;8:169–72.
82. Attar A, Flourie B, Rambaud JC, et al. Antibiotic efficacy in small intestinal bacte-rial overgrowth-related chronic diarrhea: a crossover, randomized trial. Gastroen-terology 1999;117:794–7.
83. Deng Y, Misselwitz B, Dai N, et al. Lactose intolerance in adults: biological mech-anism and dietary management. Nutrients 2015;7:8020–35.
84. Lauritano EC, Gabrielli M, Scarpellini E, et al. Small intestinal bacterial overgrowth recurrence after antibiotic therapy. Am J Gastroenterol 2008;103:2031–5.
85. Scarpellini E, Gabrielli M, Lauritano CE, et al. High dosage rifaximin for the treat-ment of small intestinal bacterial overgrowth. Aliment Pharmacol Ther 2007;25: 781–6.

The Esophageal and Gastric Microbiome in Health and Disease

Richard H. Hunt, MB, FRCP, FRCP Ed, FRCPC*,
Mohammad Yaghoobi, MD, MSc (Epi), FRCPC

KEYWORDS

- Esophagus • Stomach • Microbiota • Gastric acidity • Health • Disease

KEY POINTS

- The esophagus and stomach are host to their own population of bacteria, which differs in health and disease.
- *Helicobacter pylori* uniquely colonizes only gastric mucosa, but an increasing number of bacteria is now isolated from the gastric juice and gastric mucosa, including *Lactobacillus*, which also colonizes gastric mucosa.
- The presence of *H pylori* alters the populations of other gastric bacteria with a marked reduction in diversity.
- Alterations in intragastric acidity may be the cause or the consequence of changes in the microbial populations of the stomach.
- Esophageal inflammation is associated with an altered microbiota in gastroesophageal reflux disease, Barrett's esophagus, eosinophilic esophagitis, and cancer.

INTRODUCTION

The microbiota of the esophagus and stomach have been the least systematically studied in the organs of the gastrointestinal tract and, until recently, most publications have reported phenomenological observations and associations rather than underlying physiologic or pathophysiologic mechanisms. The discovery of *Helicobacter pylori* by Marshall and Warren in 1982[1–3] has focused attention over the last 30 years on the unique characteristics of this bacterium to colonize and alter the immunologic and physiologic functions of the host.

The widely held view was that the gastric secretions of hydrochloric acid and the proteolytic enzyme pepsin ensured a sterile stomach despite numerous observations

Neither author has any conflicts to declare.
Division of Gastroenterology and Farncombe Family Digestive Health Research Institute, McMaster University, Hamilton, Ontario, Canada
* Corresponding author. Kilmartin, Pine Walk, Midhurst, West Sussex GU29 0AS, UK.
E-mail address: huntr@mcmaster.ca

by scientists from the late nineteenth century describing bacteria in the acidity of the stomach.[4] This may have influenced the commonly held view that *Helicobacter* species are the only organisms capable of colonizing the human stomach. *H pylori* research has increased the understanding of how it can modify its own microclimate, and it is now clear that other organisms also occupy the gastric mucosa and lumen.

Indeed, further investigations with modern techniques have shown that the microbiota of the stomach involves hundreds of phylotypes with a microbial density of between 10^1 and 10^3 colony-forming units (CFU)/g.[5-7] There are unique anatomic and physiologic features of the stomach that differentiate the microbiota here from that elsewhere in the gastrointestinal tract and especially the esophagus.

It is important to appreciate that the definitions and basic concepts and methodology for identifying bacteria and other microorganisms that constitute the microbiome and their interactions with the immune response, are covered earlier in this issue and also apply to the upper gastrointestinal microbiota. The terms microbiome and microbiota comprise the bacterial, fungal, viral, and potentially prion populations. However, this review addresses the bacterial components of the esophagus and stomach and the inherent differences that require consideration.

THE ESOPHAGEAL MICROBIOME IN HEALTH
Esophageal Microbial Flora

Under normal physiologic conditions, the esophagus acts as a conduit and does not retain food contents, which is in contrast to the oral cavity or the stomach and colon. Culture studies based on washings from the esophagus suggested that bacteria that were obtained from the esophagus were either swallowed from the oral cavity or reached the distal esophagus during reflux from the stomach.[8] A study of the bacterial flora of the oral cavity and the upper and lower esophagus, obtained by esophageal brushings and biopsy samples, revealed that *Streptococcus viridans* is the most common bacterium.[9] Methods of bacterial detection, which are independent of culture, are increasingly reported and characterize the diversity of the esophageal microbiota. In a group of healthy individuals, using broad-range 16S rDNA polymerase chain reaction (PCR) applied to esophageal biopsies, Pei and colleagues[10] found a range of microbial diversity with the most prevalent organisms being *Streptococcus*, *Prevotella*, and *Veillonella*. Fillon and colleagues[11] studied the esophageal microbiome by sampling with a new technique, the Enterotest capsule, an esophageal string test and an oral string and nasal swab. They found that the diversity at the phylum level was similar, and the most common genera were also *Streptococcus*, *Prevotella*, and *Veillonella*, similar to those found by Pei and colleagues.[10] In a study using PCR of biopsies from the distal esophagus in healthy volunteers, patients with either esophagitis or Barrett's esophagus (BE), Yang and colleagues[12] found that *Streptococcus* dominated in the healthy esophagus, whereas gram-negative anaerobes dominated in both esophagitis and BE. They further designated this division into 2 distinct types: type I and type II, respectively, for the 2 conditions.

THE ESOPHAGEAL MICROBIOME IN DISEASE

Several studies have reported changes in the microbiota of the lower esophagus in a variety of diseases, including reflux disease, BE, and esophageal carcinoma, in addition to eosinophilic esophagitis in a pediatric population.[13-15]

In patients with severe gastroesophageal reflux disease (GERD), Dunbar and colleagues[16] reported histologic changes characterized by T-lymphocyte predominant inflammation with papillary and basal cell hyperplasia with no loss of surface cells.

They suggest this inflammation may be cytokine mediated rather than the result of the usually attributed acid chemical injury. Another group suggests that pathogenesis might be driven by alterations of the esophageal microbiome with increasing gram-negative bacteria in esophagitis and BE.[12] With this increase in gram-negative bacteria, their lipopolysaccharide can upregulate gene expression and, through the TLR4 and NFKB pathway, proinflammatory cytokine production can also be increased.

As mentioned earlier, the microbiota in the healthy esophagus is dominated by *Streptococcus* species (type I) but gram-negative anaerobes predominate in the presence of inflammation and BE (type II).[14] In patients with BE,[17] the dynamic nature of the bacterial composition of the upper gastrointestinal tract was emphasized with some overlap between the esophageal and gastric microbiome, particularly of the antrum. *Streptococcus* and *Prevotella* spp dominated, and the ratio of these 2 species was associated with 2 known factors for esophageal adenocarcinoma in BE: the waist-to-hip ratio and the length of hiatal hernia.

Another report of Barrett's patients and controls[18] found 16 genera with 46 bacterial species, where 10 species were common to both Barrett's patients and controls. They found high levels of *Campylobacter* species (*Campylobacter concisus*, *Campylobacter rectus*) in 4 of 7 Barrett's patients (57%). These bacteria are more commonly linked to enteritis and periodontal infections, but these were not found in any of their controls. They suggested a possible link between nitrate-reducing species in BE and the potential for progression to adenocarcinoma. This group[19] also reported differences in the esophageal biofilm in disease, revealing *C concisus* dominance in reflux disease, with an increased expression of cytokines associated with carcinogenesis.

Esophageal Cancer

The rate of adenocarcinomas of the gastroesophageal junction and distal esophagus has been increasing over the past 3 decades, especially in white men in the developing world and is attributed to GERD, smoking, and alcohol consumption.[20] Conversely, *H pylori* infection has been proposed as protecting from distal esophageal cancer, likely through gastric atrophy leading to loss of acid secretion, cytokine or hormonal deregulation, and microbiome alteration.[14,21]

One study in healthy Chinese volunteers and patients using the Human Oral Microbe Identification Microarray, after adjusting for gender, smoking, age, antibiotic use, and a balloon sampling device, showed a significant positive association between microbial richness and pepsinogen I/II ratio and an inverse association with esophageal squamous dysplasia.[22] These findings suggested that individuals with lower microbial diversity were more likely to have chronic atrophic gastritis and squamous dysplasia in the esophagus. They also found a correlation between esophageal squamous dysplasia with the odds ratio (OR) being significantly decreased with increasing microbial richness.

Another study in Northern Iran, which is considered part of the "esophageal cancer belt," evaluated the gastric microbiota from the gastric fundic mucosa in patients with esophageal squamous cell carcinoma as compared with healthy controls.[23] They found higher numbers of *Clostridiales* and *Erysipelotrichales* species, belonging to the phylum Firmicutes, which were significantly associated with early squamous dysplasia and esophageal squamous cell cancer.

GASTRIC MICROBIOME IN HEALTH
Gastric Microbial Flora

Microbes in the human body interact not only with their host but also with each other, which can lead to a significant microbial imbalance or dysbiosis.[24] When considering bacteria, dysbiosis usually refers to increased levels of potentially harmful or harmful bacteria. Conversely, reduced levels of bacteria are considered to be beneficial. Historically, the stomach has been considered a germ-free environment due to the acidic milieu. However, observations reported by several scientists over the years, including Bottcher and Letulle (1875), Klebs (1881), Bizzozero (1893), Salomon (1896), Krienitz (1906), Edkins (1921), Doenges (1938), Freedberg and Barron (1940), Gorham (1940), and Steer and Colin-Jones (1975) all described finding bacteria in the stomach.[4] One of the most important contributions came from the Polish scientist, Walery Jaworski, in 1899, who was studying gastric juice from the human stomach. He reported spiral-shaped bacteria and, importantly, rod-shaped bacilli, which he isolated and cultured and demonstrated that they produced lactic acid.[25] Thus, he confirmed that more than one bacterial species could colonize the stomach simultaneously, and he speculated that spiral-shaped bacteria might be involved in the pathogenesis of stomach ulcer, stomach cancer, and achylia.

Marshall and Warren[3] described *Campylobacter pyloridis* in 1982 (renamed *H pylori* in 1989), and this dramatically refocused the concepts of bacteria and the stomach.[5-7] Studies to define the unique mechanisms by which *H pylori* successfully survives and replicates within the hostile, acidic milieu of the stomach suggest that this is likely to be a unique attribute. However, although pH values <4 largely prevent bacterial overgrowth, the acidic milieu is not capable of sterilizing the stomach.[7,26] Although *H pylori* is the best known and studied of the gastric bacteria, it is not the only microbial inhabitant of the gastric mucosa. As mentioned earlier, *Lactobacillus* species convert lactose to lactic acid acidifying the surface of the gastric mucous layer,[27] which explains its adaptation to the acidic environment and colonization of the stomach.[28-30] There are also other species that survive gastric acidity, including *Yersinia enterocolitica,* with an acid-activated urease mechanism, and *Vibrio cholera*, which expresses an acid tolerance mechanism that maintains the cytoplasm at pH of 4 to 5, although growth does not occur.[27,31]

The microbial density of the stomach is considered to be between 10^2 and 10^4 CFU/g.[6,7,32] However, like the rest of the intestinal microbiome, this is a dynamic situation with considerable fluctuations in microbial density changing with pH, whereby both the quantity and the proportion of genera also fluctuate.[33,34] Gastric juice is mainly composed of proteolytic enzymes and hydrochloric acid, which restricts the quantity of microorganisms entering the small intestine and reduces the risk of infection by pathogens.[35,36] Human gastric juice has an interprandial pH of between pH 1 and 2 in the gastric lumen, and this is also influenced by food ingestion and fluctuates to $\geq$pH 5. The pH within the stomach varies between the most acidic, parietal cell containing fundus, and the antrum. There is also a pH gradient from the gastric juice in the lumen to the surface of the cells of the gastric epithelium. The mucus layer consists of an inner mucus layer that is firmly attached to the epithelium and a variable mucus layer interfacing with the lumen.[37,38] Thus, across the relatively stable mucus layer overlying the gastric epithelium, the pH ranges from about 5.5 to 6.8 or even 7 at the surface of the gastric epithelial cells.[39,40]

To understand the dynamics of the gastric microbiota, it is necessary to consider the site of their isolation. Bacteria, and bacterial DNA, which are isolated from gastric juice, differ from bacterial isolates adhering to the mucosa, which is a more hospitable environment for colonization. During abnormal conditions, this balance may be different. Reduction of gastric acid secretion increases the risk of bacterial overgrowth and also influences the composition of intestinal or oral microorganisms, including pathogenic organisms[36] and those which can nitrosate dietary nitrate and nitrite, which are not normally cultured from a healthy stomach.[41] In this section, we review current knowledge concerning the gastric microbiota with a brief introduction on the role of *H pylori* and its relationship with other microorganisms associated with the gastric mucosa.

Helicobacter pylori

H pylori infection is the most common worldwide human infection and is associated with several important upper gastrointestinal conditions, including chronic gastritis, peptic ulcer disease, and gastric malignancy. It is the dominant gastric organism in *H pylori*–positive individuals when detected by conventional methods.[42–44] *H pylori* has specific characteristics allowing it to survive in low pH environment in the stomach by producing urease and ammonia.[45,46] Alkalinization enables the bacteria to survive through the variable acidity of the gastric juice and reach the higher pH of the mucous layer in close apposition to the surface epithelial cells. The acute inflammatory response to *H pylori* infection initiates the release of interleukin-8 and the recruitment of inflammatory cells, leading to a chronic active gastritis.[47,48] The production of catalase and superoxide by *H pylori* protect it from reactive oxygen and nitrogen species.[48] The immunology of the stomach and host response involved in the persistence of *H pylori* infection and the role of other organisms are an important new focus for current research into the gastric microbiome.[5]

Gastric Microbiota in Healthy Individuals

Soon after the discovery of *H pylori*, other bacteria such as *Veillonella*, *Lactobacillus*, and *Clostridium* were identified in the stomach.[49] The gastric microbiota differs from the oral cavity or pharynx,[32] which argues for the stomach comprising resident microbes rather than those that have relocated from the oropharynx or esophagus.

The presence of non–*H pylori* microorganisms in human gastric tissue has been documented by conventional methods, including histology[50] and the culture of gastric juice and mucosal biopsies.[51–53] *Clostridium* spp, *Lactobacillus* spp, and *Veillonella* sp are the most reported bacteria of the healthy human stomach based on culture studies.[49] Most of the bacteria are not easily cultured,[54] but the development of culture-independent molecular techniques based on 16S rRNA has revealed several other genera in the stomach, including *Neisseria*, *Haemophilus*, *Prevotella*, *Streptococcus*, and *Porphyromonas*.[32,42,55,56] In healthy individuals, the predominant bacteria are *Actinobacteria* (*Rothia*, *Actinomyces*, and *Micrococcus*), *Bacteroidetes* (*Prevotella* species), *Firmicutes* (*Streptococcus* and *Bacillus*), and *Proteobacteria* (which include *H pylori* as well as *Haemophilus*, *Actinobacillus*, and *Neisseria*), and the predominant genus is *Streptococcus*, which may originate from the oral or nasal cavities.[42,56–58] Interestingly, the presence of *Streptococci* was recently associated with peptic ulcer disease in one study from Malaysia.[59]

The reported variability in the gastric microbiota is in part due to geographic and cultural variations, but also due to the different methods of investigation used. Moreover, several studies show that the gastric microbiota in patients infected with *H pylori* is different from uninfected individuals.[58,60] For example, a Swedish study showed the gastric microbiota from *H pylori*–negative subjects displays a greater diversity than the microbiota of *H pylori*–positive patients.[58] However, in contrast, a study in 215 healthy Malaysians showed that the microbial diversity was not influenced by the presence of *H pylori*.[59] Thus, there might be geographic differences in the diversity of the human gastric microbiota, which result in variations in the interactions between *H pylori* and other gastric bacteria residing in the gastric mucosa. The human gastric microbiota was surveyed in 8 studies using 4 molecular methods: next-generation sequencing technologies,[32,58,61] Sanger sequencing of 16S rDNA,[62,63] a community fingerprinting method to define a library for Sanger sequencing,[44,64] and the PhyloChip.[60] Although there is considerable variation in the gastric microbiome between individuals at the genus level, the most frequently detected phyla detected in the stomach were *Proteobacteria, Firmicutes, Bacteroidetes, Actinobacteria,* and *Fusobacteria*. The most abundant phyla in the stomachs of *H pylori*–infected subjects were *Proteobacteria, Firmicutes,* and *Actinobacteria*. In the absence of *H pylori* infection, the most abundant phyla were the *Firmicutes, Bacteroidetes,* and *Actinobacteria*. Overall, *H pylori* is the most dominant species in the human stomach, comprising 72% to 99% of sequencing readouts with *Proteobacteria* the dominant phylum in those infected with *H pylori*.[42,58] In the absence of *H pylori* infection, analysis consistently reports the presence of *Streptococcus* spp.

These findings have been further tested in several in vitro and animal studies. The prolonged exposure to *H pylori* infection alters the composition of the microbiota in rodent stomachs.[65] In an animal model of *H pylori* infection, *Lactobacillus johnsonii, Lactobacillus murinus,* and *Lactobacillus reuteri* inhibited the growth of *H pylori* organisms in vitro.[66] In the same model, some *Lactobacillus, Bifidobacteria,* and *Saccharomyces* also prevented adhesion and colonization of *H pylori*.[66] *Streptococcus mitis*, which is a commensal microorganism of the human stomach, also inhibited the growth of *H pylori* and its conversion from a spiral to a coccoid form.[67] In another study, 2 *L reuteri* strains, isolated from gastric juice and biopsies, showed resistance to acid and a strong antimicrobial effect against *H pylori*.[68] The mechanism of altering the gastric microbiota by *H pylori* is unclear; however, one theory is direct killing of bacteria by the induction of host antimicrobial peptides, such as β-defensin 2[69] or cecropinlike peptide.[70] *H pylori* infection also induces an inflammatory cascade that may end in reduced gastric secretion from parietal cells and elevation of intragastric pH. The higher pH will eventually result in colonization by other microorganisms in the stomach,[71–74] and existing evidence also suggests that alteration of the gastric microbiota may predispose to the development of gastric cancer.[75]

Interaction Between H pylori and Other Microbiota

In the absence of *H pylori* infection, the structure and composition of the gastric microbiota most resemble that reported for the distal esophagus with unique differences due to *Proteobacteria*.[58,76] However, the effects of *H pylori* infection on the gastric microbiota are not fully understood. *H pylori* density increases with the onset of gastritis,[64] which may allow *H pylori* to outcompete other bacteria.[42] In one study, *H pylori* accounted for 93% to 97% of all reads in the infected stomach and also substantially decreased diversity because only 33 phylotypes were observed in *H pylori*–positive individuals compared with 262 phylotypes observed in *H pylori*–negative subjects.[58] However, several studies have reported the ability to detect *H pylori* sequences at extremely low levels in subjects who were *H pylori* negative by other diagnostic methods.[32,42,60,64] These results may reflect the host response, leading to reduction of *H pylori* or the presence of non–*H pylori Helicobacters*.[48] Regarding the uniformity of the microbiota within the stomach, several studies have found no differences in the microbiota of the antrum and corpus in their populations, with the exception of decreased *Prevotella* reported in the antrum of patients with gastritis.[42,56] In contrast, others have noted bacterial differences between subjects and between the antrum and corpus.[61] Thus, *H pylori* infection and the associated changes in the stomach alter the ecological niche of the gastric microbiota. However, the gastric microbiota also competes with *H pylori* for a gastric niche and may play an important role in the progression of disease. More studies involving the microbiota-host-environment interactions, including the effect of diet, geography, culture, and gender, are needed to fully understand the role of gastric bacteria in human health and disease.

Lactobacillus

Lactobacillus species are found in the stomachs of all mammals, and several studies have reported *Lactobacillus* species colonizing the human gastric mucosa.[32,52,53,77–80] *Lactobacilli* are rod-shaped, gram-positive, micro-aerophilic bacteria with some similarities to *H pylori*. The distinguishing feature of *Lactobacillus* metabolism is the conversion of lactose to lactic acid, and this leads to acidification of the bacterial microenvironment, resulting in acidification of the gastric mucous layer.[27] Acidophilic gastric *Lactobacilli* are able to adapt sufficiently to the acid environment and colonize the stomach due to these acidophilic properties.[28–30] Moreover, some *Lactobacilli* have a urease enzyme with an optimum activity at pH 3 to 4, which is similar to that of *H pylori*.[81,82]

Acidification of the gastric antral mucosa causes rapid inhibition of gastrin and a reduction in gastric acid secretion.[83–87] Thus, acid-generating *Lactobacilli* close to the surface of the antral gastric epithelium may decrease gastric acid secretion (**Fig. 1**). In contrast, *H pylori* alkalinizes the gastric antral mucosa, increasing gastrin and consequently also acid secretion.[88] Lactic acid produced by *Lactobacilli* neutralizes ammonia produced by *H pylori*, which would result in a null net effect on pH at the surface of the gastric epithelium when both *H pylori* and *Lactobacilli* are colonizing the stomach together[88] (see **Fig. 1**). The impact of *Lactobacilli* colonizing the gastric mucosa may be different in the antrum and body of the stomach; however, it can only result in acidification and thus trends to a lower mucosal surface pH, leading to subsequent inhibition of gastrin secretion. In support of this observation, a study in Finland found in *H pylori*–infected patients that taking a probiotic, which included *Lactobacillus rhamnosus*, significantly decreased serum gastrin-17.[89] Some *Lactobacilli* have an inhibitory effect on *H pylori*,[90,91] and probiotics isolated from dairy products or human feces have been shown to have suppressive effects on *H pylori*

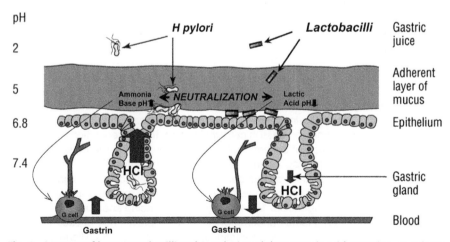

Fig. 1. Concept of how *Lactobacilli* and *H pylori* modulate gastric acid secretion. In culture, *Lactobacilli* can produce lactic acid (0.25 M–0.50 M), which can modulate gastric physiology by acidifying the mucus of the gastric antrum, thus lowering gastrin. In contrast, *H pylori* produces ammonia, which alkalinizes the antral mucus leading to gastrin secretion. Lactic acid at this concentration also modulates *H pylori* bacteria (George Sachs, personal communication, 2009). (*From* Padol IT, Hunt RH. The evolutionary impact of Lactobacilli on *H. pylori* and gastric acid secretion: did a century of dietary change alter the gastric microbiota? Helicobacter 2011;16(Suppl 1, P11.12):141; with permission.)

infection.[90,92] In a clinical trial on 40 *H pylori*–infected mice randomized to 4 groups undergoing triple therapy together with *Lactobacillus fermenti, Lactobacillus acidophilus*, and normal saline confirmed that *Lactobacillus* strains had a significant activity against *H pylori*.[93] Another study of 147 *H pylori*–infected patients showed that Will yogurt (a Korean brand of *L acidophilus* HY2177, *Lactobacillus casei* HY2743, *Bifidobacterium longum* HY8001, and *Streptococcus thermophilus* B-1) added to triple therapy increased the *H pylori* eradication rate, although adverse effects were unaltered.[94] Other studies also suggest that *Lactobacillus* preparations may increase eradication rates of *H pylori* infection or even limit related manifestations of disease or symptoms.[95–97] Lactic acid produced by *Lactobacilli* inhibits the growth of *H pylori* at concentrations of 1% and 3%.[98,99]

Further mechanisms by which *Lactobacillus* species may influence *H pylori* infection are by direct effects. *L reuteri* DSM17648 was found to act as a highly specific binding antagonist to *H pylori*.[100] In a single-blinded, randomized, placebo-controlled pilot study, this strain coaggregated the pathogen in vitro and in vivo and significantly reduced the load of *H pylori* in healthy, yet infected adults. The investigators then showed a rapid and efficient coaggregation of *H pylori* by a specific *Lactobacillus* strain under gastric conditions. Reducing the amount of *H pylori* in the stomach by selective bacteria-bacteria cell interaction might be a new way for treating *H pylori*, given that the eradication is associated with potential side effects or antibiotic resistance.[101] These investigators suggested that *Lactobacillus* interferes with *H pylori* motility and the organisms' adherence to the gastric mucosa by aggregating them and masking *H pylori* surface sites that are ordinarily available for binding to human epithelial cells.

Interestingly, a new strain of *L johnsonii* No. 1088 was isolated from the juice of a healthy Japanese male volunteer. *L johnsonii* has shown the best acid resistance among several *Lactobacilli* examined with greater than 10% of organisms surviving at pH of 1 after 2 hours. *L johnsonii* also inhibited the growth of *H pylori, Escherichia coli* O-157, *Salmonella typhimurium*, and *Clostridium difficile* in vitro and suppressed gastric acid secretion in mice. Although further studies are required, there might be a role for this microorganism in cotherapy for resistant *H pylori* infections.[102]

GASTRIC MICROBIOTA IN DISEASE
Gastric Cancer

There is increasing evidence on the potential role of the gastric microbiota in the development of gastric cancer by inducing and maintaining the carcinogenic pathways by stimulation of inflammation, increase in cell proliferation, the dysregulation of stem cell physiology, and production of several metabolites.[103] *H pylori* is the most important microbial risk factor that has been recognized by the International Agency for Research on Cancer as a class I carcinogen due its role in development of gastric cancer.[104] However, recent evidence shows that other gastric microbiota may also be involved in gastric carcinogenesis. 16S rRNA gene sequencing analysis of the gastric mucosa of patients with gastric cancer showed a higher prevalence of *Lactobacillus, Streptococcus mitis, Streptococcus parasanguinis, Prevotella*, and *Veillonella*.[44]

Patients with nonatrophic gastritis, intestinal metaplasia, and gastric cancer were studied using a microarray G3 PhyloChip. A lower diversity and a greater abundance of *Pseudomonas* were found in patients with gastric cancer compared with patients with nonatrophic gastritis.[105] Interestingly, this study also found a gradual decrease in 2 *Porphyromonas* species from the TM7 phylum, *Neisseria* spp and *Streptococcus* spp, while showing a gradual increase in *Lactobacillus coleohominis* and Lachnospiraceae from gastritis to gastric metaplasia and cancer. Another study using a high-throughput sequencing platform (454 GS FLX Titanium) showed a greater bacterial diversity, a relative increase of Bacilli and the *Streptoccocci spp*, and a relative reduction of Helicobacteraceae in the cancer group compared with other groups.[43]

Although these results are apparently different, this might indicate a change in gastric microbiota with the stepwise progression to gastric cancer from gastritis. In a recent study in 315 patients, including 212 with chronic gastritis and 103 with gastric cancer, the amount of bacteria per gram of gastric mucosa was determined using quantitative PCR.[106] The bacterial load in the gastric mucosa was higher in *H pylori*–infected patients ($7.80 \pm 0.71 \times 10^8$ per gram) as compared with those who were uninfected ($7.59 \pm 0.57 \times 10^8$ per gram) ($P = .005$). An increased bacterial load was also detected in gastric cancer ($7.85 \pm 0.70 \times 10^8$ per gram) as compared with those in patients with chronic gastritis ($P = .001$). The presence of *H pylori* markedly altered the structure of microbial communities, but the relative proportions of the other members in the microbiota were not markedly changed. Patients with gastric cancer were found to have an enriched population of 5 genera of bacteria. These bacteria are all known to have the potential for cancer promotion and included *Lactobacillus, Escherichia, Shigella, Nitrospirae, Burkholderia fungorum*, and Lachnospiraceae, which were not cultured. *Nitrospirae* in particular was present in all patients with gastric cancer, but not found in patients with chronic gastritis.[106]

Bacterial diversity decreases with the transition from nonatrophic gastritis to intestinal metaplasia and then to gastric cancer, with a decrease in the number of *Porphyromonas, Neisseria, TM7* group, and *Streptococcus sinensis* but with a relative increase in *L coleohominis* and Lachnospiraceae.[105] *Pseudomonas* was significantly more prevalent in gastric cancer than in nonatrophic gastritis.[105] The presence of *H pylori* had little influence on the relative proportions of other members in the microbiota.[106] In *H pylori* carriers, normal gastric mucosa had larger populations of *Propionibacterium* spp, *Staphylococcus* spp, and *Corynebacterium* spp with smaller populations of *Clostridium* and *Prevotella*.[57]

Non–*H pylori* microbiota may also play a role in the development of gastric cancer. Studies showed that in male mice with intestinal microbiota in their gastric samples, gastric pathology developed chronic gastritis extending to atrophy and dysplasia, independent of *H pylori* infection. The presence of commensal microbiota accelerated the progression to gastric intraepithelial neoplasia in *H pylori*–infected mice,[107,108] although antibiotic therapy significantly delayed the onset of gastric neoplasia in *H pylori*–negative mice.[109] Another study compared the human gastric microbiota in gastric cancer with controls by analyzing 63 antral mucosal and 18 corpus mucosal specimens by rRNA gene sequencing. Nitrosating or nitrate-reducing bacteria were found to be 2 times higher in the cancer groups than in the control groups, but this was not statistically significant, and the investigators concluded no significant difference of microbial composition between cancer and control groups.[110]

Some studies have shown that the microbiota in gastric cancer have increased bacterial diversity, but bacterial overgrowth in the stomach has been reported in various precancerous conditions,[32,111] including hypochlorhydria and gastric mucosal atrophy. Some investigators have suggested that the gastric microbiota is involved in the production of carcinogens through the promotion of inflammation.[112,113] However, it is not clear if bacterial overgrowth is a consequence of the carcinogenic process by generating an environment that favors bacterial proliferation. Further research is required to clarify the mechanisms by which these changes occur, and the possible relationship to cause or effect.

Other data suggest that differences in the gastric microbiota might be responsible for a higher prevalence of gastric cancer in some regions. One case-control study in Colombia used deep sequencing of amplified 16S rDNA, in 2 age- and gender-matched populations, to compare the composition of the gastric microbiota in a high gastric cancer risk area in the Andes, which has a 25-fold greater risk than the comparator coastal low-risk area.[114] The composition of the microbiota was highly variable between individuals, but showed a significant correlation with their area of origin. Multiple operational taxonomic units (OTUs) were detected exclusively in both areas. Two OTUs, *Leptotrichia wadei* and a *Veillonella* sp, were significantly more abundant in the high-risk Andes mountain area, and 16 OTUs, including a *Staphylococcus* sp, were significantly more frequent in the low-risk coastal area. There was no significant correlation with the *H pylori* population or carriage of the cagPAI pathogenicity island with the composition of the microbiota.

Atrophic Gastritis

Gastric acidity is a barrier to microbes in saliva and ingested food, mainly due to the acidity and digestive activity of gastric juice.[115,116] The reduction of gastric acid secretion in patients with atrophic gastritis allows colonization of the stomach by more microbes. Although a reduction in acidity is not universal with old age, in one study 80% of healthy individuals were reported to have hypochlorhydria[117] with 105 to 108 CFU/mL bacteria in a fasting gastric aspirate. Data on gastric microbiota composition in patients with atrophic gastritis are limited. In one study, microbial quantity was positively correlated with serum pepsinogen I/pepsinogen II ratio in Asian patients.[22] In another study, *Streptococcus* species were replaced by *Prevotella* species in patients with atrophic gastritis.[75] Current evidence is too limited to comment on the overall change in gastric microbiota in atrophic gastritis, and further studies are needed to evaluate this question.

Postinfectious Dyspepsia

Acute gastrointestinal infection can lead to persistent low-grade mucosal inflammation, followed by the onset of postinfectious irritable bowel syndrome.[118–122] Several organisms are known to be responsible, including *Campylobacter*, *Salmonella*, *E coli*, and *Shigella*. Functional dyspepsia (FD) may also follow an infection that is currently recognized as postinfectious FD (PIFD).[123,124] One study reported that 17% of patients with FD had experienced an episode of acute gastroenteritis, whereas the onset of PIFD was not correlated with *H pylori* infection.[125] A prospective observational study found the incidence of FD significantly higher in patients 1 year after acute *Salmonella* gastroenteritis (13.4%) compared with controls (2%).[126] A meta-analysis found the mean prevalence of FD following acute gastroenteritis was 9.55% in the adult population and the OR for PIFD was 2.54 (95% confidence interval: 1.76–0.65).[127] The pathogenesis of PIFD is not clearly understood but might be explained by the altered immune response to dysbiosis in the upper gastrointestinal tract. However, it is not yet clear if acute gastroenteritis directly induces change in the gastric microbiota or only influences the development of postinfectious dyspepsia. Further studies in FD are underway and awaited with interest.

EFFECT OF ACID SUPPRESSION ON THE GASTRIC MICROBIOME
Effect on the Gastric Microbiota

There is a logarithmic relationship between intragastric pH and the median bacterial counts in gastric juice, with rising pH increasing the risks for enteric infections and bacterial-induced diarrhea.[50,128] Previously held concerns over the effects of therapeutic acid suppression, with histamine-2 receptor antagonists (H_2RA) and the proton pump inhibitors (PPI), has centered on the potential for proliferation of nitrate-reducing bacteria in the stomach. Increased nitrite concentrations result in faster nitrosation of dietary amines and consequently higher concentrations of N-nitroso compounds, some of which have potential for mutagenicity and carcinogenicity.[129–131]

In a 2-week study with the H_2RA, cimetidine, intragastric acidity, intragastric bacteria, nitrite, and N-nitroso compounds were evaluated before, during, and after treatment.[34] Bacteria were isolated by anaerobic culture and included *Neisseria*, *Corynebacterium*, *Streptococcus*, *Staphylococcus*, *Acetinobacter*, *Lactobacillus*, *Fusobacterium*, *Bacteroides*, *Veilonella*, and *Bifidobacterium*, and *Candida* spp were also isolated. No significant differences were found in bacterial counts or bacterial species between the 3 time periods. Bacterial counts and nitrite concentrations tended to increase with pH, but N-nitroso compounds did not. As pH became more acidic, bacterial counts decreased. PPIs elevate intragastric pH levels to a greater degree than H_2RA,[132] and intragastric bacterial activity and nitrosation were studied before, during, and after omeprazole treatment.[113] A short-lived increase in the bacterial flora with a profile similar to that reported by Milton-Thompson and colleagues[34] was found with a similar effect on endogenous N-nitroso compounds.[113] In a recent study,[133] 45 subjects, including 18 patients taking PPI, were evaluated using bacterial 16S rRNA gene profiling by pyrosequencing. Stimulated saliva, gastric fluid, and feces were examined. Salivary and gastric fluid microbiota were similar but both were markedly different from the fecal microbiota. In PPI users compared with PPI nonusers, bacterial cell numbers increased ~1000 fold in the gastric fluid of PPI users as measured by culture methods. However, between the PPI users and nonusers, bacterial numbers and composition were almost identical when measured by quantitative PCR and a similarity search using 16S profiling. The investigators concluded that the microbiota in gastric fluid had recently migrated from saliva and that bacterial overgrowth might be a consequence of acid suppression leading to a lack of bacterial killing rather than bacterial proliferation.[133]

The conclusion of several reviews addressing the adverse effects of acid suppression[132,134,135] is the modest increase in risk of enteric infection with a trend to *Salmonella*, *Campylobacter*, and *Shigella* being associated with a greater risk. *C difficile* is also a significant risk as shown in a meta-analysis of 39 studies.[136]

Nevertheless, it has long been considered that after long-term antisecretory treatment or particularly in the presence of atrophic gastritis, there is an increase in nitrosating bacteria that can convert, depending on the pH, nitrite, and other nitrogen compounds in gastric juice to potentially carcinogenic N-nitroso compounds.[41]

An important recent review of the role of ingested nitrite and nitrate and the risk of gastric cancer has concluded that research over the past 15 to 20 years has led to a paradigm change in the view of the role and risks of both nitrite and nitrate.[134] These food compounds, long considered harmful, are no longer looked on with such concern but are now thought to be indispensable for cardiovascular health. The investigators reviewed the animal toxicology of nitrite and concluded that, in the absence of a coadministered carcinogenic nitrosamine precursor, there is no evidence to support carcinogenesis. Moreover, prospective epidemiology cohort studies show no association between the estimated dietary nitrate or nitrite intake and gastric cancer.[137]

Epidemic or Spontaneous Hypochlorhydria

The spontaneous appearance of hypochlorhydria or on occasion complete achlorhydria is well documented in both individual case reports and subjects undergoing sequential gastric secretory studies, usually when participating in research protocols.[138–141]

These studies and accompanying reviews of the literature suggest that most of these cases were associated with *H pylori* infection for which the 2 group studies[138,139] and the report by Graham[140] provide some supportive evidence. The mechanisms involved, however, remain unclear, although studies on isolated parietal cells demonstrated inhibition of acid secretion by the *Campyobacter pylori* (as it was then known)[142] and by a protein obtained from *C pylori*.[143]

Bacterial infections that cause a fever are known to be associated with a reduction of acid secretion, including typhoid and paratyphoid, pulmonary TB, lung abscess, and bronchopneumonia.[28,35,144,145] It seems probable that fever rather than the infection is the cause when fever is present, but in some other instances, the organism or an expressed product may be involved.[35] The fish tapeworm *Diphyllobothrium latum* might be one example,[146] or in Chagas disease, due to *Trypanosoma cruzei*, other factors such as parasympathetic denervation may be involved.[147] Reduced acid secretion has also been observed in patients with *Ankylostoma duodenale*, but the mechanism is not known.[148]

Summary

Evolving technologies and new concepts are improving the ability to understand the complex systems that make up the gastrointestinal microbiome of the esophagus and stomach. Studies have increased the knowledge and understanding in recent years, although many studies are small and, as mentioned as a caveat in the introduction, to date have presented phenomenological observations and clinical associations rather than studies of immune, physiologic, or pathologic mechanisms, which are still in their infancy. There is also confusion between the interpretation of animal and human studies. Moreover, reports relating to changes in the gastrointestinal microbiota often focus on changes in the fecal microbiota rather than the esophageal or gastric mucosa, even when PPIs are studied. Thus, reports raise more questions than answers, and one should be particularly cautious about drawing conclusions regarding cause and effect. This argues for further studies into the microbiota of the stomach and esophagus, where exploration of host immunity and dysbiosis of the microbiota are likely to be especially fruitful.

Finally, it is probably naive to imagine that other individual bacteria with selective pathogenicity will be found, such as discovered with *H pylori* infection, where research has revealed just how complex this bacterium is and the host response to it. Indeed, a recent review comments that to date no evidence for adherence or cellular invasion has been reported for other bacteria in the stomach.[149] However, disease may result from dysbiosis not requiring adherence or invasion as a prerequisite for pathogenesis.

H.pylori research has undoubtedly become a gold standard for future research into microbes in the gastrointestinal tract and has changed the understanding and concepts of the microbiome throughout the gut. Study of how gastric acidity influences and is influenced by the microbiota is an important new direction for the whole gastrointestinal microbiome and the long-held concept that gastric acidity acts to "sterilize" the stomach is increasingly questioned. One thoughtful paper reports a systematic review of gastric acidity across 68 species, including 25 birds and 43 mammals. Scavengers and carnivores were found to have significantly greater intragastric acidity when compared with herbivores or carnivores ingesting phylogenetically distant prey.[150] Humans appear, among the primates evaluated, to have a gastric juice pH closer to carrion feeders than most carnivores and omnivores. The authors found that a general linear model, which was based on diet, explained much of the variation in pH and concluded that gastric acidity has a role in filtering novel microbial taxa before entering the intestines. They suggest humans with a low ambient pH can be protected from pathogen exposure but argue that this reduces the probability of recolonization of the gut by beneficial microbes, and they advocate measuring intragastric pH when studying gastrointestinal microbial dynamics.[150] Human gastric secretion has increased in several populations over recent decades[151–154] which may, in part, be due to the decline of H pylori infection in the population, but other factors are involved, including body weight. There is a global obesity crisis and the causes are not yet known.[155] The possible gastric mechanisms involved in the shifting diversity of the gastrointestinal microbiota should be considered in future research. They may be important if, as has been suggested, the low pH of the human stomach is contributing to a reduction in microbial diversity and a reduced probability of recolonizing with beneficial microbes.[150] These observations may be particularly relevant in an era of antibiotic and PPI overuse.

REFERENCES

1. Marshall BJ, Warren JR. Unidentified curved bacilli on gastric epithelium in active chronic gastritis. Lancet 1983;321:1273–5.
2. Warren JR, Marshall BJ. Unidentified curved bacilli on gastric epithelium in active chronic gastritis. Lancet 1983;1:1273–5.
3. Marshall BJ, Warren JR. Unidentified curved bacilli in the stomach of patients with gastritis and peptic ulceration. Lancet 1984;1:1311–5.
4. Modlin I, Sachs G. Acid related diseases—biology and treatment. Philadelphia: Lippincott Williams & Wilkins; 2004.
5. Hunt RH, Camilleri M, Crowe SE, et al. The stomach in health and disease. Gut 2015;64:1650–68.
6. Nardone G, Compare D. The human gastric microbiota: Is it time to rethink the pathogenesis of stomach diseases? United European Gastroenterol J 2015;3: 255–60.
7. Sheh A, Fox JG. The role of the gastrointestinal microbiome in Helicobacter pylori pathogenesis. Gut Microbes 2013;4(6):505–31.
8. Gagliardi D, Makihara S, Corsi PR, et al. Microbial flora of the normal esophagus. Dis Esophagus 1998;11:248–50.
9. Norder Grusell E, Dahlén G, Ruth M, et al. Bacterial flora of the human oral cavity, and the upper and lower esophagus. Dis Esophagus 2013;26(1):84–90.
10. Pei Z, Yang L, Peek RM Jr, et al. Bacterial biota in reflux esophagitis and Barrett's esophagus. World J Gastroenterol 2005;11:7277–83.
11. Fillon SA, Harris JK, Wagner BD, et al. Novel device to sample the esophageal microbiome–the esophageal string test. PLoS One 2012;7:e42938.
12. Yang L, Francois F, Pei Z. Molecular pathways: pathogenesis and clinical implications of microbiome alteration in esophagitis and Barrett esophagus. Clin Cancer Res 2012;18:2138–44.
13. Harris JK, Fang R, Wagner BD, et al. Esophageal microbiome in eosinophilic esophagitis. PLoS One 2015;10(5):e0128346.
14. Yang L, Lu X, Nossa CW, et al. Inflammation and intestinal metaplasia of the distal esophagus are associated with alterations in the microbiome. Gastroenterology 2009;137:588–97.
15. Benitez AJ, Hoffman C, Muir AB, et al. Inflammation associated microbiota in pediatric eosinophilic esophagitis. Microbiome 2015;3:23.
16. Dunbar KB, Agoston AT, Odze RD, et al. Association of acute gastroesophageal reflux disease with esophageal histologic changes. JAMA 2016;315(19): 2104–12.

17. Gall A, Fero J, McCoy C, et al. Bacterial composition of the human upper gastro-intestinal tract microbiome is dynamic and associated with genomic instability in a Barrett's esophagus cohort. PLoS One 2015;10(6):e0129055.

18. MacFarlane S, Furrie E, MacFarlane GT, et al. Microbial colonization of the upper gastrointestinal tract in patients with Barrett's esophagus. Clin Infect Dis 2007; 45:29–38.

19. Blackett KL, Siddhi SS, Cleary S, et al. Oesophageal bacterial biofilm changes in gastro-oesophageal reflux disease, Barrett's and oesophageal carcinoma: association or causality? Aliment Pharmacol Ther 2013;37:1084–92.

20. Rustgi AG, El-Serag HB. Esophageal carcinoma. N Engl J Med 2014;371: 2499–509.

21. Wang C, Yuan Y, Hunt RH. Helicobacter pylori infection and Barrett's esophagus: a systematic review and meta-analysis. Am J Gastroenterol 2009; 104(2):492–500 [quiz: 491, 501].

22. Yu G, Gail MH, Shi J, et al. Association between upper digestive tract microbiota and cancer-predisposing states in the esophagus and stomach. Cancer Epidemiol Biomarkers Prev 2014;23:735–41.

23. Nasrollahzadeh D, Malekzadeh R, Ploner A, et al. Variations of gastric corpus microbiota are associated with early esophageal squamous cell carcinoma and squamous dysplasia. Sci Rep 2015;5:8820.

24. Lozupone CA, Stombaugh JI, Gordon JI, et al. Diversity, stability and resilience of the human gut microbiota. Nature 2012;489:220–30.

25. Jaworski W. Podrêcznik chorób ¿o³dka (Handbook of gastric diseases). Wydawnictwa Dzie³ Lekarskich Polskich; 1899. p. 30–47.

26. Theisen J, Nehra D, Citron D, et al. Suppression of gastric acid secretion in patients with gastroesophageal reflux disease results in gastric bacterial overgrowth and deconjugation of bile acids. J Gastrointest Surg 2000;4:50–4.

27. Carr FJ, Chill D, Maida N. The lactic acid bacteria: a literature survey [Review] [296 refs]. Crit Rev Microbiol 2002;28(4):281–370.

28. Cotter PD, Hill C. Surviving the acid test: responses of gram-positive bacteria to low pH [Review] [263 refs]. Microbiol Mol Biol Rev 2003;67(3):429–53.

29. Azcarate-Peril MA, Altermann E, Hoover-Fitzula RL, et al. Identification and inactivation of genetic loci involved with Lactobacillus acidophilus acid tolerance. Appl Environ Microbiol 2004;70(9):5315–22.

30. Fujimura S, Kato S, Oda M, et al. Detection of Lactobacillus gasseri OLL2716 strain administered with yogurt drink in gastric mucus layer in humans. Lett Appl Microbiol 2006;43(5):578–81.

31. Sachs G, Weeks DL, Wen Y, et al. Acid acclimation by Helicobacter pylori [Review] [63 refs]. Physiology (Bethesda) 2005;20:429–38.

32. Delgado S, Cabrera-Rubio R, Mira A, et al. Microbiological survey of the human gastric ecosystem using culturing and pyrosequencing methods. Microb Ecol 2013;65:763–72.

33. Draser BS, Shiner M, McLeod GM. Studies of the intestinal flora 1. The bacterial flora of the gastrointestinal tract in healthy and achlorhydric patients. Gastroenterology 1969;56:71–9.

34. Milton-Thompson GJ, Lightfoot NF, Ahmet Z, et al. Intragastric acidity, bacteria, nitrite, and N-nitroso compounds before, during, and after cimetidine treatment. Lancet 1982;1(8281):1091–5.

35. Howden CW, Hunt RH. Progress report: relationship between gastric secretion and infection. Gut 1987;28:96–107.

36. Martinsen TC, Bergh K, Waldum HL. Gastric juice: a barrier against infectious diseases. Basic Clin Pharmacol Toxico 2005;96:94–102.

37. Corfield AP, Carroll D, Myerscough N, et al. Mucins in the gastrointestinal tract in health and disease. Front Biosci 2001;6:D1321–57.

38. Atuma C, Strugala V, Allen A, et al. The adherent gastrointestinal mucus gel layer: thickness and physical state in vivo. Am J Physiol Gastrointest Liver Physiol 2001;280:G922–9.

39. Manson JM, Rauch M, Gilmore MS. The commensal microbiology of the gastrointestinal tract. Adv Exp Med Biol 2008;635:15–28.

40. Bhaskar KR, Garik P, Turner BS, et al. Viscous fingering of HCl through gastric mucin. Nature 1992;360:458–61.

41. Correa P. Human gastric carcinogenesis: a multistep and multifactorial process—First American Cancer Society Award Lecture on Cancer Epidemiology and Prevention. Cancer Res 1992;52:6735–40.

42. Bik EM, Eckburg PB, Gill SR, et al. Molecular analysis of the bacterial microbiota in the human stomach. Proc Natl Acad Sci U S A 2006;103:732–7.

43. Eun CS, Kim BK, Han DS, et al. Differences in gastric mucosal microbiota profiling in patients with chronic gastritis, intestinal metaplasia, and gastric cancer using pyrosequencing methods. Helicobacter 2014;19:407–16.

44. Dicksved J, Lindberg M, Rosenquist M, et al. Molecular characterization of the stomach microbiota in patients with gastric cancer and in controls. J Med Microbiol 2009;58(Pt 4):509–16.

45. Bauerfeind P, Garner R, Dunn BE, et al. Synthesis and activity of Helicobacter pylori urease and catalase at low pH. Gut 1997;40:25–30.

46. Wen Y, Feng J, Scott DR, et al. The HP0165-HP0166 two-component system (ArsRS) regulates acid-induced expression of HP1186 alpha-carbonic anhydrase in Helicobacter pylori by activating the pH-dependent promoter. J Bacteriol 2007;189:2426–34.

47. Crowe SE, Alvarez L, Dytoc M, et al. Expression of interleukin 8 and CD54 by human gastric epithelium after Helicobacter pylori infection in vitro. Gastroenterology 1995;108(1):65–74.

48. Kusters JG, van Vliet AH, Kuipers EJ. Pathogenesis of Helicobacter pylori infection. Clin Microbiol Rev 2006;19:449–90.

49. Zilberstein B, Quintanilha AG, Santos MA, et al. Digestive tract microbiota in healthy volunteers. Clinics (Sao Paulo) 2007;62:47–54.

50. Sanduleanu S, Jonkers D, De Bruine A, et al. Non-Helicobacter pylori bacterial flora during acid-suppressive therapy: differential findings in gastric juice and gastric mucosa. Aliment Pharmacol Ther 2001;15:379–88.

51. Delgado S, Suarez A, Mayo B. Identification, typing and characterization of Propionibacterium strains from healthy mucosa of the human stomach. Int J Food Microbiol 2011;149:65–72.

52. Ryan KA, Jayaraman T, Daly P, et al. Isolation of lactobacilli with probiotic properties from the human stomach. Lett Appl Microbiol 2008;47:269–74.

53. Roos S, Engstrand L, Jonsson H. Lactobacillus gastricus sp. nov., Lactobacillus antri sp. nov., Lactobacillus kalixensis sp. nov. and Lactobacillus ultunensis sp. nov., isolated from human stomach mucosa. Int J Syst Evol Microbiol 2005;55:77–82.

54. Vartoukian SR, Palmer RM, Wade WG. Strategies for culture of "unculturable" bacteria. FEMS Microbiol Lett 2010;309:1–7.

55. Fraher MH, O'Toole PW, Quigley EM. Techniques used to characterize the gut microbiota: a guide for the clinician. Nat Rev Gastroenterol Hepatol 2012;9: 312–22.

56. Li XX, Wong GL, To KF, et al. Bacterial microbiota profiling in gastritis without Helicobacter pylori infection or non-steroidal anti-inflammatory drug use. PLoS One 2009;4:e7985.

57. Seo I, Jha BK, Suh SI, et al. Microbial profile of the stomach: comparison between normal mucosa and cancer tissue in the same patient. J Bacteriol Virol 2014;44:162–9.

58. Andersson AF, Lindberg M, Jakobsson H, et al. Comparative analysis of human gut microbiota by barcoded pyrosequencing. PLoS One 2008;3:e2836.

59. Khosravi Y, Dieye Y, Poh BH, et al. Culturable bacterial microbiota of the stomach of Helicobacter pylori positive and negative gastric disease patients. ScientificWorldJournal 2014;2014:610421.

60. Maldonado-Contreras A, Goldfarb KC, Godoy-Vitorino F, et al. Structure of the human gastric bacterial community in relation to Helicobacter pylori status. ISME J 2011;5:574–9.

61. Stearns JC, Lynch MD, Senadheera DB, et al. Bacterial biogeography of the human digestive tract. Scientific Rep 2011;1:170.

62. Persson C, Canedo P, Machado JC, et al. Polymorphisms in inflammatory response genes and their association with gastric cancer: a HuGE systematic review and meta-analyses. Am J Epidemiol 2011;173:259–70.

63. Ericksen RE, Rose S, Westphalen CB, et al. Obesity accelerates Helicobacter felis-induced gastric carcinogenesis by enhancing immature myeloid cell trafficking and TH17 response. Gut 2014;63:385–94.

64. Monstein HJ, Tiveljung A, Kraft CH, et al. Profiling of bacterial flora in gastric biopsies from patients with Helicobacter pylori-associated gastritis and histologically normal control individuals by temperature gradient gel electrophoresis and 16S rDNA sequence analysis. J Med Microbiol 2000;49:817–22.

65. Osaki T, Matsuki T, Asahara T, et al. Comparative analysis of gastric bacterial microbiota in Mongolian gerbils after long-term infection with Helicobacter pylori. Microb Pathog 2012;53:12–8.

66. Zaman C, Osaki T, Hanawa T, et al. Analysis of the microbial ecology between Helicobacter pylori and the gastric microbiota of Mongolian gerbils. J Med Microbiol 2014;63:129–37.

67. Khosravi Y, Dieye Y, Loke MF, et al. Streptococcus mitis induces conversion of Helicobacter pylori to coccoid cells during co-culture in vitro. PLoS One 2014;9: e112214.

68. Delgado S, Leite AM, Ruas-Madiedo P, et al. Probiotic and technological properties of Lactobacillus spp. strains from the human stomach in the search for potential candidates against gastric microbial dysbiosis. Front Microbiol 2015;5: 766.

69. Hornsby MJ, Huff JL, Kays RJ, et al. Helicobacter pylori induces an antimicrobial response in rhesus macaques in a cag pathogenicity island-dependent manner. Gastroenterology 2008;134:1049–57.

70. Pütsep K, Normark S, Boman HG. The origin of cecropins; implications from synthetic peptides derived from ribosomal protein L1. FEBS Lett 1999;451: 249–52.

71. Blaser MJ, Atherton JC. Helicobacter pylori persistence: biology and disease. J Clin Invest 2004;113:321–33.

72. Müller A, Solnick JV. Inflammation, immunity, and vaccine development for Helicobacter pylori. Helicobacter 2011;16(Suppl 1):26–32.

73. Oh JD, Kling-Bäckhed H, Giannakis M, et al. Interactions between gastric epithelial stem cells and Helicobacter pylori in the setting of chronic atrophic gastritis. Curr Opin Microbiol 2006;9:21–7.

74. Wroblewski LE, Peek RM. Targeted disruption of the epithelial barrier by Helicobacter pylori. Cell Commun Signal 2011;9:29.

75. Engstrand L, Lindberg M. Helicobacter pylori and the gastric microbiota. Best Pract Res Clin Gastroenterol 2013;27:39–45.

76. Pizzi M, Saraggi D, Fassan M, et al. Secondary prevention of epidemic gastric cancer in the model of Helicobacter pylori-associated gastritis. Dig Dis 2014;32:265–74.

77. Bernhardt H. Zentralblatt fur Bakteriologie, Parasitenkunde, Infektionskrankheiten und Hygiene—Erste Abteilung Originale—Reihe A: Medizinische Mikrobiologie und Parasitologie. [Presence of the genus Lactobacillus (Beijerinck) in the human stomach (author's transl)]. Zentralbl Bakteriol Orig A 1974;226(4):479–90 [in German].

78. Valeur N, Engel P, Carbajal N, et al. Colonization and immunomodulation by Lactobacillus reuteri ATCC 55730 in the human gastrointestinal tract. Appl Environ Microbiol 2004;70(2):1176–81.

79. Saeed A, Heczko PB. Surface properties of Lactobacilli isolated from healthy subject. Folia Med Cracov 2007;48(1–4):99–111.

80. Hakalehto E, Vilpponen-Salmela T, Kinnunen K, et al. Lactic acid bacteria enriched from human gastric biopsies. ISRN Gastroenterol 2011;2011:109183.

81. Moreau MC, Ducluzeau R, Raibaud P. Hydrolysis of urea in the gastrointestinal tract of "monoxenic" rats: effect of immunization with strains of ureolytic bacteria. Infect Immun 1976;13(1):9–15.

82. Suzuki K, Benno Y, Mitsuoka T, et al. Urease-producing species of intestinal anaerobes and their activities. Appl Environ Microbiol 1979;37(3):379–82.

83. Fordtran JS, Walsh JH. Gastric acid secretion rate and buffer content of the stomach after eating. Results in normal subjects and in patients with duodenal ulcer. J Clin Invest 1973;52(3):645–57.

84. Walsh JH, Richardson CT, Fordtran JS. pH dependence of acid secretion and gastrin release in normal and ulcer subjects. J Clin Invest 1975;55(3):462–8.

85. Feldman M, Walsh JH. Acid inhibition of sham feeding-stimulated gastrin release and gastric acid secretion: effect of atropine. Gastroenterology 1980;78(4):772–6.

86. Peterson WL, Barnett C, Walsh JH. Effect of intragastric infusions of ethanol and wine on serum gastrin concentration and gastric acid secretion. Gastroenterology 1986;91(6):1390–5.

87. Mogard MH, Maxwell V, Reedy TJ, et al. Gastric acidification inhibits meal-stimulated gastric acid secretion after prostaglandin synthesis inhibition by indomethacin in humans. Gastroenterology 1987;93(1):63–8.

88. Padol IT, Hunt RH. The evolutionary impact of Lactobacilli on H. pylori and gastric acid secretion: did a century of dietary change alter the gastric microbiota? Helicobacter 2011;16(Suppl 1, P11.12):141.

89. Myllyluoma E, Kajander K, Mikkola H, et al. Probiotic intervention decreases serum gastrin-17 in Helicobacter pylori infection. Dig Liver Dis 2007;39(6):516–23.

90. Wang KY, Li SN, Liu CS, et al. Effects of ingesting Lactobacillus- and Bifidobacterium-containing yogurt in subjects with colonized Helicobacter pylori. Am J Clin Nutr 2004;80:737–41.

91. Heczko PB, Strus M, Kochan P. Critical evaluation of probiotic activity of lactic acid bacteria and their effects. J Physiol Pharmacol 2006;57(Suppl 9):5–12.

92. Uchida M, Kurakazu K. Yogurt containing Lactobacillus gasseri OLL2716 exerts gastroprotective action against [correction of agaisnt] acute gastric lesion and antral ulcer in rats. J Pharmacol Sci 2004;96:84–90.

93. Cui Y, Wang CL, Liu XW, et al. Two stomach-originated Lactobacillus strains improve Helicobacter pylori infected murine gastritis. World J Gastroenterol 2010;16(4):445–52.

94. Kim MN, Kim N, Lee SH, et al. The effects of probiotics on PPI-triple therapy for Helicobacter pylori eradication. Helicobacter 2008;13:261–8.

95. Canducci F, Cremonini F, Armuzzi A, et al. Probiotics and Helicobacter pylori eradication. Dig Liver Dis 2002;34(Suppl 2):S81–3.

96. Imase K, Tanaka A, Tokunaga K, et al. Lactobacillus reuteri tablets suppress Helicobacter pylori infection–a double-blind randomised placebo-controlled cross-over clinical study. Kansenshogaku Zasshi 2007;81(4):387–93.

97. Zou J, Dong J, Yu X. Meta-analysis: lactobacillus containing quadruple therapy versus standard triple first-line therapy for Helicobacter pylori eradication. Helicobacter 2009;14(5):97–107.

98. Bhatia SJ, Kochar N, Abraham P, et al. Lactobacillus acidophilus inhibits growth of Campylobacter pylori in vitro. J Clin Microbiol 1989;27(10):2328–30.

99. Midolo PD, Lambert JR, Hull R, et al. In vitro inhibition of Helicobacter pylori NCTC 11637 by organic acids and lactic acid bacteria. J Appl Bacteriol 1995;79(4):475–9.

100. Holz C, Busjahn A, Mehling H, et al. Significant reduction in Helicobacter pylori load in humans with non-viable lactobacillus reuteri DSM17648: a pilot study. Probiotics Antimicrob Proteins 2015;7(2):91–100.

101. Wu TS, Hu HM, Kuo FC, et al. Eradication of Helicobacter pylori infection. Kaohsiung J Med Sci 2014;30:167–72.

102. Aiba Y, Nakano Y, Koga Y, et al. A highly acid-resistant novel strain of Lactobacillus johnsonii No. 1088 has antibacterial activity, including that against Helicobacter pylori, and inhibits gastrin-mediated acid production in mice. Microbiologyopen 2015;4(3):465–74.

103. Abreu MT, Peek RM Jr. Gastrointestinal malignancy and the microbiome. Gastroenterology 2014;146:1534–46.e3.

104. Schistosomes, liver flukes and Helicobacter pylori. IARC Working Group on the Evaluation of Carcinogenic Risks to Humans. Schistosomes, liver flukes and Helicobacter pylori. Lyon, 7-14 June 1994. IARC Monogr Eval Carcinog Risks Hum 1994;61:1–241.

105. Aviles-Jimenez F, Vazquez-Jimenez F, Medrano-Guzman R, et al. Stomach microbiota composition varies between patients with non-atrophic gastritis and patients with intestinal type of gastric cancer. Sci Rep 2014;4:4202.

106. Wang L, Zhou J, Xin Y, et al. Bacterial overgrowth and diversification of microbiota in gastric cancer. Eur J Gastroenterol Hepatol 2016;28(3):261–6.

107. Lofgren JL, Whary MT, Ge Z, et al. Lack of commensal flora in Helicobacter pylori-infected INS-GAS mice reduces gastritis and delays intraepithelial neoplasia. Gastroenterology 2011;140:210–20.

108. Lertpiriyapong K, Whary MT, Muthupalani S, et al. Gastric colonisation with a restricted commensal microbiota replicates the promotion of neoplastic lesions

by diverse intestinal microbiota in the Helicobacter pylori INS-GAS mouse model of gastric carcinogenesis. Gut 2014;63:54–63.

109. Lee CW, Rickman B, Rogers AB, et al. Combination of sulindac and antimicrobial eradication of Helicobacter pylori prevents progression of gastric cancer in hypergastrinemic INS-GAS mice. Cancer Res 2009;69:8166–74.

110. Jo HJ, Kim J, Kim N, et al. Analysis of gastric microbiota by pyrosequencing: minor role of bacteria other than Helicobacter pylori in the gastric carcinogenesis. Helicobacter 2016;21(5):364–74.

111. Forsythe SJ, Dolby JM, Webster AD, et al. Nitrate- and nitrite-reducing bacteria in the achlorhydric stomach. J Med Microbiol 1988;25:253–9.

112. Forsythe SJ, Cole JA. Nitrite accumulation during anaerobic nitrate reduction by binary suspensions of bacteria isolated from the achlorhydric stomach. J Gen Microbiol 1987;133:1845–9.

113. Sharma BK, Santana IA, Wood EC, et al. Intragastric bacterial activity and nitrosation before, during, and after treatment with omeprazole. Br Med J 1984;289:717–9.

114. Yang I, Woltemate S, Piazuelo MB, et al. Different gastric microbiota compositions in two human populations with high and low gastric cancer risk in Colombia. Sci Rep 2016;6:18594.

115. Hunt RH. The protective role of gastric acid. Scand J Gastroenterol 1988;23(Suppl 146):34–9.

116. Yoshiyama H, Nakazawa T. Unique mechanism of Helicobacter pylori for colonizing the gastric mucus. Microbes Infect 2000;2:55–60.

117. Husebye E, Skar V, Høverstad T, et al. Fasting hypochlorhydria with gram positive gastric flora is highly prevalent in healthy old people. Gut 1992;33:1331–7.

118. Ishihara S, Tada Y, Fukuba N, et al. Pathogenesis of irritable bowel syndrome-review regarding associated infection and immune activation. Digestion 2013;87:204–11.

119. Ishihara S, Aziz M, Oshima N, et al. Irritable bowel syndrome and inflammatory bowel disease: infectious gastroenteritis-related disorders? Clin J Gastroenterol 2009;2:9–16.

120. Spiller R, Aziz Q, Creed F, et al. Guidelines on the irritable bowel syndrome: mechanisms and practical management. Gut 2007;56:1770–98.

121. Ohman L, Simrén M. Pathogenesis of IBS: role of inflammation, immunity and neuroimmune interactions. Nat Rev Gastroenterol Hepatol 2010;7:163–73.

122. El-Salhy M. Irritable bowel syndrome: diagnosis and pathogenesis. World J Gastroenterol 2012;18:5151–63.

123. Miwa H, Watari J, Fukui H, et al. Current understanding of pathogenesis of functional dyspepsia. J Gastroenterol Hepatol 2011;26(Suppl 3):53–60.

124. Lee KJ, Tack J. Duodenal implications in the pathophysiology of functional dyspepsia. J Neurogastroenterol Motil 2010;16:251–7.

125. Tack J, Demedts I, Dehondt G, et al. Clinical and pathophysiological characteristics of acute-onset functional dyspepsia. Gastroenterology 2002;122:1738–47.

126. Mearin F, Pérez-Oliveras M, Perelló A, et al. Dyspepsia and irritable bowel syndrome after a Salmonella gastroenteritis outbreak: one-year follow-up cohort study. Gastroenterology 2005;129:98–104.

127. Futagami S, Itoh T, Sakamoto C. Systematic review with metaanalysis: postinfectious functional dyspepsia. Aliment Pharmacol Ther 2015;41:177–88.

128. Yeomans ND, Brimblecombe RW, Elder J, et al. Effects of acid suppression on microbial flora of upper gut. Dig Dis Sci 1995;40(2 Suppl):81S–95S.

129. Stockbrugger RW. Bacterial overgrowth as a consequence of reduced gastric acidity. Scand J Gastroenterol Suppl 1985;111:7–16.
130. Svendsen JH, Dahl C, Svendsen LB, et al. Gastric cancer risk in achlorhydric patients. A long-term follow-up study. Scand J Gastroenterol 1986;21:16–20.
131. Ahn JS, Eom CS, Jeon CY, et al. Acid suppressive drugs and gastric cancer: a meta-analysis of observational studies. World J Gastroenterol 2013;19:2560–8.
132. Williams C, McColl KE. Review article: proton pump inhibitors and bacterial overgrowth. Aliment Pharmacol Ther 2006;23:3–10.
133. Tsuda A, Suda W, Morita H, et al. Influence of proton-pump inhibitors on the luminal microbiota in the gastrointestinal tract. Clin Transl Gastroenterol 2015; 6:e89.
134. Laine L, Ahnen D, McClain C, et al. Review article: potential gastrointestinal effects of long-term acid suppression with proton pump inhibitors. Aliment Pharmacol Ther 2000;14(6):651–68.
135. Walker MM, Talley NJ. Review article: bacteria and pathogenesis of disease in the upper gastrointestinal tract–beyond the era of Helicobacter pylori. Aliment Pharmacol Ther 2014;39(8):767–79.
136. Kwok CS, Arthur AK, Anibueze CI, et al. Risk of Clostridium difficile infection with acid suppressing drugs and antibiotics: meta-analysis. Am J Gastroenterol 2012;107:1011–9.
137. Bryan NS, Alexander DD, Coughlin JR, et al. Ingested nitrate and nitrite and stomach cancer risk: an updated review. Food Chem Toxicol 2012;50:3646–65.
138. Ramsey EJ, Carey KV, Peterson WL, et al. Epidemic gastritis with hypochlorhydria. Gastroenterology 1979;76:1449–57.
139. Gledhill T, Leicester RJ, Addis B, et al. Epidemic hypochlorhydria. Br Med J 1985;289:1383–6.
140. Graham DY, Alpert LC, Smith JL, et al. Iatrogenic Campylobacter pylori infection is a cause of epidemic achlorhydria. Am J Gastroenterol 1988;83(9):974–80.
141. Hunt RH. Helicobacter pylori and spontaneous hypochlohydria. In: Rathbone BJ, Heatley RV, editors. Helicobacter pylori and gastroduodenal disease. 2nd edition. London: Blackwell Scientific Publications; 1992. p. 187–97.
142. Defize J, Goldie J, Hunt RH. Effect of Campylobacter pylori on, and production by, isolated guinea pig parietal cells. Gut 1988;29:A1435.
143. Cave DR, Vargas M. Effect of Campylobacter pylori on acid production by parietal cells. Lancet 1989;i:187–9.
144. Beaumont W. Experiments and observations on the gastric juice and the physiology of digestion. 1833. Boston: Harvard University Press; 1929. p. 107.
145. Berglund H, Chang HC. Transitory character of the achlorhydria during fever demonstrated by the histamine test. Proc R Soc Exp Biol Med 1929;26:422–3.
146. Salokannel J. Intrinsic factor in tapeworm anaemia. Acta Med Scand 1970; 188(Suppl 517):1–51.
147. Padovan W, Godoy RA, Meneghelli UG, et al. Acid and pepsin secretion in chronic Chagas' disease patients in response to graded doses of pentagastrin and bethanochol. Digestion 1982;23:48–56.
148. Pimparkar BD, Sharma P, Satoskar RS, et al. Anaemia and gastrointestinal function in ancylostomiasis. Postgrad J Med 1982;28:51–63.
149. Schulz C, Schütte K, Malfertheiner P. Helicobacter pylori and other gastric microbiota in gastroduodenal pathologies. Dig Dis 2016;34(3):210–6.
150. Beasley DE, Koltz AM, Lambert JE, et al. The evolution of stomach acidity and its relevance to the human microbiome. PLoS One 2015;10(7):e0134116.

151. Kinoshita Y, Kawanami C, Kishi K, et al. Helicobacter pylori independent chronological change in gastric acid secretion in the Japanese. Gut 1997;41:452–8.
152. Kekki M, Sipponen P, Siurala M. Age behaviour of gastric acid secretion in males and females with a normal antral and body mucosa. Scand J Gastroenterol 1983;18(8):1009–16.
153. Iijima K, Koike T, Abe Y, et al. Time series analysis of gastric acid secretion over a 20-year period in normal Japanese men. J Gastroenterol 2015;50(8):853–61.
154. Di Mario F, Goni E. Gastric acid secretion: changes during a century. Best Pract Res Clin Gastroenterol 2014;28(6):953–65.
155. Gortmaker SL, Swinburn B, Levy D, et al. Changing the future of obesity: science, policy and action. Lancet 2011;378(9793):838–47.

The Gut Microbiota in Inflammatory Bowel Disease

Donal Sheehan, MB, Fergus Shanahan, MD, DSc*

KEYWORDS

- Ulcerative colitis • Crohn's disease • Microbiota • Fecal microbial transplantation
- Inflammatory bowel disease

KEY POINTS

- Environmental factors that shape the composition and function of the microbiota are maximally active during the earliest perinatal and postnatal phase of life.
- The neonatal and infant microbiota shapes the development and maturation of the immune system.
- Most of the genetic risk factors for inflammatory bowel disease code for proteins that sense or regulate the host response to the microbiota.
- The molecular mechanisms by which genes, microbes, and the immune system interact in the pathogenesis of inflammatory bowel disease are becoming clarified.
- Strategies for manipulating the microbiota have been remarkably effective in experimental animals but attempts to translate these to the human context have been resoundingly disappointing.

INTRODUCTION

Therapeutic strategies for inflammatory bowel disease (IBD) have increased over the past decade, but considerable unmet needs remain. Increasingly, patients seek safer, long-term options and alternatives to immunomodulatory and immunosuppressive drugs. The prospect of modulating the microbiota in both Crohn's disease and ulcerative colitis is conceptually appealing and is based on sound rationale.[1–4] However,

Conflict of Interest Statement: F. Shanahan is a founder shareholder in Atlantia Food Clinical Trials and Alimentary Health Ltd. He is director of the *APC Microbiome Institute*, a research center funded in part by Science Foundation Ireland (APC/SFI/12/RC/2273) and which is/has recently been in receipt of research grants from Abvie, Alimentary Health, Cremo, Danone, Janssen, Friesland Campina, General Mills, Kerry, Mead Johnson, Nutricia, 4D pharma and Second Genome, and Sigmoid pharma.
Department of Medicine, APC Microbiome Institute, University College Cork, National University of Ireland, Ireland
* Corresponding author.
E-mail address: F.Shanahan@ucc.ie

clinicians wait expectantly for translation of advances in understanding the gut micro-biota to clinical therapeutics and some may feel blinded by a blizzard of inconclusive publications. In this overview, we try to make clinical sense of a large body of factual data, explore the clinical implications of the relationship between the microbiota and IBD and summarise the lessons learned.

BROKEN BIOME OR BROKEN HOST?

For many years, the cardinal question surrounding the pathogenesis of IBD has been: Is this an abnormal immune response to a normal microbiota or is this an appropriate response to an abnormal microbiota? It is now clear from various animal models that both situations may arise and may overlap.[5,6] Genetically determined anomalies of the innate immune system can lead to a modification of the microbiota, which becomes colitogenic upon transfer to an otherwise normal recipient. In addition, because the microbiota shapes the maturation of the immune system in early life,[7] any disruption of the microbiota such as that caused by antibiotic exposure may lead to suboptimal immunity and/or risk of IBD in later life.[5]

THE ENVIRONMENTAL INFLUENCE ON INFLAMMATORY BOWEL DISEASE

Despite much focus on genetics within the past decade, 2 lines of evidence confirm the environment as a risk factor for IBD. First, the concordance rate in genetically iden-tical twins (approximately 40%-50% for Crohn's disease and approximately 10% for ulcerative colitis) suggests a substantial environmental influence, particularly in ulcer-ative colitis. Second, the increasing frequency of both conditions has occurred over too short a period to be owing to changes in the population pool of genetic risk factors. Indeed, the known genetic risk factors are relatively common in society and, in most instances, are insufficient alone to cause disease.

Clinicians might despair at inconclusive and occasionally futile epidemiologic sur-veys chasing putative environmental risks, such as notional north/south and east/west gradients but amid this fog one can make cogent epidemiologic conclusions. First, the environmental influences on Crohn's and ulcerative colitis seem to be similar but with 2 noteworthy exceptions. Cigarette smoking has a polarizing influence on the 2 main forms of IBD, whereby smoking is both a risk and aggravating influence for Crohn's disease, whereas in ulcerative colitis, the cessation of smoking is a risk factor for relapse and active smoking has a modest beneficial influence. In addition, an episode of acute appendicitis, particularly in childhood or early adolescence, has a protective influence on the risk of developing ulcerative colitis but not Crohn's disease or celiac disease. Second, like many immunoallergic disorders, both forms of IBD may be considered as diseases of a modern lifestyle. As countries undergo socioeconomic development, the incidence and prevalence of ulcerative colitis increases first and then is followed by similar trends in Crohn's disease. Thus, many of the epidemiologic observations of the past actually represent the variable influence of socioeconomic development.[5,8]

MICROBIOTA AS A PROXY MARKER OF ENVIRONMENTAL INFLUENCE IN INFLAMMATORY BOWEL DISEASE

Although some environmental and lifestyle factors such as stress, drug therapy, pollu-tion and radiation might have independent influences on disease activity, most, if not all, of the elements of a modern lifestyle in socioeconomically developed countries shape the composition and functional activity of the gut microbiota. Because the microbiota is critical for maturation of the host immune–inflammatory response, it is plausible that the microbiota is the predominant and proximate environmental influence on the risk of developing chronic inflammatory disorders in later life such as IBD (**Fig. 1**). The same seems to be true of obesity and metabolic disorders.[9] In particular, there is persuasive evidence for the adverse influence of diet and antibiotics on the progressive reduction in microbial diversity and loss of certain protective microbial species ("old friends"). In contrast with the earlier hygiene hypothesis, the old friends concept proposes that the key microbial exposures in early life are not the crowd infections such as childhood viral infections, but rather ancestral microbes that were present during the hunter–gatherer phase of mankind's existence when the immune system was evolving. Such ancestral old friends include the indigenous microbiota, *Helicobacter pylori*, helminths, and hepatitis A virus.[10]

THE EARLY LIFE WINDOW OF INFLUENCE

Environmental or lifestyle risk factors for developing IBD exert their influence early in life. This has been well-demonstrated by studies of human migrants from low-incidence developing countries to high-incidence developed countries. The earlier one migrates from a low-risk, developing country to a modern society with a high incidence of IBD, the greater the risk of acquiring the risk of the new country.[5] This window of time in early perinatal and postnatal life is when the microbiota is developing and becoming stabilized. It is also a critical period of maturation of the immune system, inflammatory response, mucosal barrier and several extraintestinal systems including the brain–gut axis, stress responses, and adipogenesis.[9] The central role of the microbiota in promoting optimal maturation of the host immune and

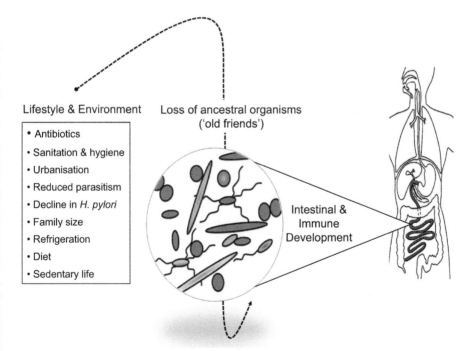

Fig. 1. Linking modern lifestyle and environment with chronic inflammatory disease with the microbiota serving as the proximate environmental risk factor.

metabolic function has been in evidence since the first comparative studies of germ-free and conventionally raised animals. One implication of this early window of influence is that preventive strategies for IBD based on microbial manipulation should focused on early life, perhaps even prenatally at the level of the maternal microbiome. In addition, microbial manipulation after the onset of the disease may be futile, too late.

A NEXUS OF GENES, IMMUNITY, AND MICROBES

The 3 main contributors to the pathogenesis of IBD are genes (which provide predisposition), immunity (mechanism of tissue injury) and, microbes (environmental stimuli; **Fig. 2**). The molecular mechanisms by which they interact are beginning to emerge.[1–4] Most of the risk genes for IBD code for intracellular sensors of the microbiota (eg, NOD2) or code for regulators of the host response to the microbiota (eg, interleukin [IL]-12/IL23R pathway), including barrier function and autophagy. Thus, susceptibility might arise when mutant genes lead to inappropriate or inadequate clearance of bacteria from the mucosa. Alternatively, there may be a loss of protective organisms and their antiinflammatory metabolites or defective sensing of protective signals. In some individuals, there seems to be loss of *Faecalobacter prausnitzii*, which produces an antiinflammatory protein that inhibits the nuclear factor-κB pathway in the intestinal epithelium.[11] Furthermore, the commensal bacterium *Bacteroides fragilis* has immunoregulatory properties by which its capsular polysaccharide A is presented to the host immune system packaged within outer membrane vesicles and leads to the generation of regulatory T cells. In susceptible humans with the genetic risk variant in ATG16L1, there is defective sensing and failure of the protective T regulatory response to the outer membrane vesicles.[12]

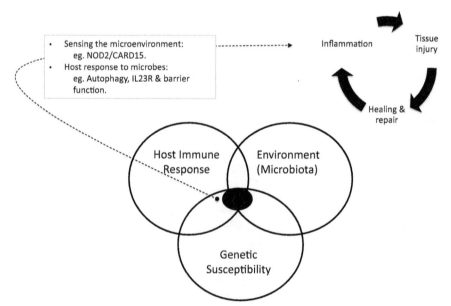

Fig. 2. A cycle of inflammation, injury, and repair is initiated and driven by abnormal interactions among genetic risk factors, environmental triggers and modifiers and the host immune system. IL, interleukin.

WHO GETS SICK?

Because the genetic and environmental/microbial risk factors for IBD are both common in socioeconomically developed societies, it is puzzling as to why these conditions are not more common and what determines who manifests clinical disease. In a highly insightful animal model, it was shown that both genetic susceptibility and the indigenous microbiota were required for pathogenesis of IBD but a combination of environmental triggers, such as chemicals and viruses determined the timing of onset of disease.[13] The human analogy of this might be coincidental smoking and intestinal viral infection in a predisposed person. Insight into the role of infections has also been gained from animal models. Thus, when infectious or other environmental agents create a temporary break in the mucosal barrier, they expose the host immune system to the indigenous microbiota and lead to proliferation of long-lived commensal-specific effector T cells in addition to pathogen-specific T cells. Accumulation of the former may eventually tip the balance from physiologic to pathologic inflammation and the onset of IBD.[14,15]

THE MICROBIOTA AT DIFFERENT PHASES OF DISEASE

In addition to the conditioning influence of the microbiota on the developing immune and inflammatory response, the microbiota also influences the clinical course of IBD at various phases of the disease.[16] Bacteria and their metabolites have been shown to contribute to the development of adhesions and cicatrization, translocation and abscess formation, extraintestinal associations including liver disease, and colitis-associated cancer.[17–21] In addition, the microbiota is implicated in obesity-related and other metabolic disorders increasingly linked with IBD.[9]

THE MICROBIOTA IN INFLAMMATORY BOWEL DISEASE

Although many investigators have reported changes in the microbiota of patients with both ulcerative colitis and Crohn's disease, a specific microbial signature or consistent pattern of change has not been identified and certainly nothing that is of diagnostic precision. Changes in total bacterial numbers within the mucosa and reduced bacterial diversity have been reported consistently along with changes in composition.[1] Many studies have been confounded by differences in disease duration, phase of disease, previous treatment, and variations in analysis. However, a particularly informative study of pediatric patients with Crohn's disease is the largest to date and confirms the association between the disease state, alterations to bacterial taxa and reduction in species diversity in treatment-naïve cohort with new onset disease.[22] Luminal and mucosal microbial analysis was performed. The most significant changes were seen in mucosal samples and included increased abundance of *Enterobacteriaecae, Fusobacteriaece, Pasteurelleceae,* and *Bifidobacteriaeae.* Of potential clinical relevance was the finding that microbiota profiles at diagnosis were predictive of subsequent clinical outcomes based on the Pediatric Crohn's Disease Activity Index. Specifically, *Enterobacteriaeceae* correlated negatively with future Pediatric Crohn's Disease Activity Index and *Fusobacterium* and *Haemophilus* positively. Interestingly, the possible use of rectal biopsies as a marker of the overall microbiota profile was suggested by the finding that disease location—colonic, ileocolonic, or ileal—did not offset the similarity between rectal and ileal biopsy-associated microbiota profiles. Thus, the more readily accessible rectal biopsies may be of use to characterize the microbiota profile regardless of disease phenotype.[22]

The more consistent shifts in bacterial species reported in Crohn's disease and colitis are summarized in **Table 1**. Research strategies are moving away from correlative

Table 1
Representative examples of the more consistent disturbances of microbiota reported in patients with Crohn's disease and ulcerative colitis

Increased in IBD	Decreased in IBD
• Mucosal bacterial numbers	• Diversity
• Adherent–invasive *Escherichia coli*	• Bacteriodes
• *Enterobacteriaceae*	• Clostridia
• *Fusobacteriaceae*	• *Bifidobacteriaceae*
• *Mycobacterium avium paratuberculosis*	• *Faecalibacterum prausnitizi*
• *Clostridium difficile*	

Abbreviation: IBD, inflammatory bowel disease.

studies to those aiming to provide mechanistic insights. For example, pathogenic strains of adherent invasive *Escherichia coli* have been the focus of particular attention with consistent findings of increased mucosal levels in ileal Crohn's disease.[23–25] An inflamed ileum provides a niche environment for these pathabionts to propagate.[26] They may trigger or promote further inflammation via lipopolysaccharide-mediated activation of the inflammatory cascade or through their effect on autophagy. Autophagy genes have been shown to play a key role in human intestinal Paneth cell function[13] and mutations in autophagy genes are linked with Crohn's disease. Individuals with genetic risk that impairs autophagy function may be particularly susceptible to the replication of adherent invasive *Escherichia coli* within the ileal mucosa[27] and lack the ability to clear them effectively.[28]

The protective effect of some bacteria is owing to their ability to use dietary fiber to produce short chain fatty acids (SCFA) that serve as an energy source for colonic epithelium. *Faecalibacterium prausnitizi*, discussed for its capacity to produce an anti-inflammatory protein, is also a producer of the SCFA butyrate is reduced in ileal CD[24] and depletion of *F prousnitzii* is associated with an increased risk of postoperative recurrence of ileal Crohn's disease.[29] *Roseburia*, a clade IV *Clostridia*, is associated with antiinflammatory T-cell production and butyrate is reduced in IBD subgroups.[24] Another SCFA producer, *Oridobacter*, of the Bacteriodes phylum, has been reported to be reduced in both pancolitis and ileal Crohn's disease.[24]

It is noteworthy that the functional capacity is probably more variable and less stable than the composition of the microbiota and is particularly shaped by dietary factors such as dietary fiber. Low-fiber diets, often recommended for patients with cicatrizing Crohn's disease, may have a secondary impact on the microbiota of these patients. Reduced dietary fiber, already a feature of modern diets, has been linked with a progressive loss of diversity, which may not be recoverable after the restoration of dietary fiber.[30]

THE GUT VIROME AND INFLAMMATORY BOWEL DISEASE

Most studies have focused exclusively on the bacterial component of the gut microbiota with little attention to the gut virome in IBD. Viruses are actually the most abundant biological entities within the gut, greatly outnumbering bacteria.[31] The biological function of viruses within the gut is unclear but, like bacteria, they have the capacity to shape mucosal immunity and support intestinal homeostasis. The common enteric RNA virus, murine norovirus has been shown to replace the beneficial function of commensal bacteria in the gut.[32] Infection of germ-free or antibiotic-treated mice with murine norovirus restored lymphocyte function and intestinal morphology without inducing inflammation. Of particular relevance to patients with IBD is that the presence of environmental murine norovirus is necessary for the Crohn's disease susceptibility gene *ATG16L1* to disrupt Paneth cell function.[13] This suggests that virus–gene interactions could be as important as bacteria–host gene interactions in determining risk of IBD development.

Bacteriophages are a subset of viruses which may have potential for exploitation for disease monitoring and as therapeutic agents in IBD.[33] Phage can bind to and kill a narrow range of bacteria with exquisite specificity and may play a key role in shaping microbial population structure, maintaining microbial diversity within the gut ecosystem.[34] Whether this can be deployed therapeutically in IBD is intriguing but uncertain.

In mucosal biopsies from patients with Crohn's disease, phage numbers were significantly higher than controls.[35] Increased diversity and richness of phage have been found in patients with IBD.[36,37] This increased diversity was in contrast to the reduced diversity of bacteria seen in the same patients. Phage populations have also been shown to be susceptible to environmental influences including diet[38] and antibiotics,[39] both of which are modifiers of disease risk for IBD.

THE MYCOBIOME AND INFLAMMATORY BOWEL DISEASE

The fungal components (mycobiome) of the gut, has largely been neglected,[40] although *Aspergillus, Cryptococcus, Penicillium, Pneumocystis,* and *Saccharomycetaceae* yeasts (*Candida* and *Saccharomyces*) have been found in health individuals.[41] A diet rich in carbohydrates has been linked to fungal abundance.[42] *Candida* was positively correlated with carbohydrate consumption and negatively correlated with total saturated fatty acids. *Aspergillus* was negatively correlated with SCFA levels in people on a carbohydrate-rich diet. A study of patients with IBD did not show disease-specific fungal species in the Crohn's disease or colitis, but revealed greater fungal diversity in patients with Crohn's disease in comparison with controls.[43]

IS THE MICROBIOTA A PLAUSIBLE TARGET FOR THERAPY OR PROPHYLAXIS?

From first principles, it seems that the rationale for modifying the microbiota as one of the main contributors to the pathogenesis of IBD is sound in both Crohn's disease and ulcerative colitis. However, there are significant caveats that temper enthusiasm. First, there is the high degree of heterogeneity of both Crohn's disease and ulcerative colitis. Genetic heterogeneity may translate to therapeutic heterogeneity if different genetic risk factors are linked with different microbiota signatures. Second, the topographic distribution of disease may influence responsiveness to microbial manipulation; it has been known since the earliest trials with antibiotics such as metronidazole in Crohn's disease, that colonic but not small bowel disease is responsive. Third, the therapeutic window of time for microbiota manipulation may be in the earliest phase of life when the microbiota is becoming established and exerting its influence on the maturing immune system. Attempts to influence host–microbe interactions in later life may be too late. Fourth, there is a remarkable discordance between the encouraging results for all forms of microbial manipulation in animal models and the disappointing results in humans, to date. Results with probiotics and prebiotics have been reviewed extensively by us elsewhere,[16] with broad conclusions presented in **Box 1**. Of course, the ultimate host–microbe experiment is microbial transplantation, which is addressed elsewhere in this issue and summarized below in relation to IBD.

FECAL MICROBIOTA TRANSPLANTATION

The efficacy of fecal microbiota transplantation (FMT) in patients with recurrent *Clostridium difficile* has engendered optimism for its use in IBD and other conditions.

Box 1
What clinicians should know about probiotics in IBD

Probiotics and prebiotics, which have been consistently effective in experimental animal models of IBD, have seldom been translated with equivalent success to humans.

None of the present generation of probiotic has been beneficial in Crohn's disease; results have been more encouraging in ulcerative colitis, particularly patients with pouchitis.

Probiotics are not created equally; they should be considered on a strain-by-strain basis and interstrain extrapolations are not valid. Bifidobacteria tend to be more effective than lactobacilli in ulcerative colitis.

In the absence of compelling evidence, consumers should select a reputable supplier to offset concerns surrounding variability in quality control of probiotic products.

Probiotics are supplements, not substitutes or alternatives for conventional therapy. Their effects should be anticipated to be modest. Major physiologic changes are neither expected nor desirable.

In adulthood, probiotics usually do not colonize the host and, therefore, must be taken indefinitely to achieve the desired effect.

Combinations of probiotics are not necessarily additive or synergistic, they may be competitive.

There is a long safety record with probiotics and prebiotics but there is no such thing as zero risk.

Studies of next generation (non–lactic acid bacteria) probiotics or beneficial microbes are awaited.

Abbreviation: IBD, inflammatory bowel disease.

Curiously, FMT and other strategies that aim to restore a healthy gut ecosystem is acceptable and conceptually appealing to many patients. Gastroenterologists will be familiar with requests for FMT from patients who desire a treatment that they view as a more natural approach than long-term immunosuppression therapy. There is, however, a need to manage expectations, and convincing evidence in support of FMT in IBD is lacking. FMT at present is an experimental treatment. Two randomized control trials of FMT in patients with ulcerative colitis have been published. In the first,[24] 70 patients with active colitis were randomly assigned to receive FMT by enema once weekly for 6 weeks or placebo consisting of a water enema.[44] The primary endpoint was remission at 7 weeks. Nine patients (24%) who underwent FMT and 2 (5%) who received placebo were in remission at 7 weeks. This result was statistically significant; however, the plan to rerandomize responders to open-label placebo or weekly FMT for 12 months was abandoned owing to the small number of responders. Importantly, no significant difference in adverse events in FMT or placebo groups was seen. It may be noteworthy for future FMT studies that 7 of the 9 patients in remission after FMT used a single donor and that 3 of 4 patients with UC for less than 1 year compared with 6 of 34 with UC greater than 1 year entered remission. The second randomized control trial administered the FMT by nasodoudenal tube at the start of the study and 3 weeks later, the placebo group received autologous FMT.[45] Seven of 23 patients who received healthy donor stool compared with 5 of 25 placebo patients achieved the primary outcome of clinical remission at 12 weeks, a nonsignificant difference. Analysis showed that the fecal microbial composition of responders in the treatment group initially overlapped with that of nonresponders at baseline and then altered toward that of healthy donors at week 12; this was attributed primarily to restoration of *Clostridium* clusters IV, XIVa and XVIII and reduced bacteriodes. This finding is important, because it suggests that FMT responders achieve restoration of their microbiota and raises questions regarding donor selection as well as optimizing patient selection based on baseline microbiota composition.

Studies of FMT in Crohn's disease are more limited. A small study of 9 pediatric patients age 12 to 19 years[46] with mild to moderate symptoms found 7 of 9 patients at 2 weeks and 5 of 9 at 12 weeks were in clinical remission based on Pediatric Crohn's Disease Activity Index scores. Donors in this study were parents of the patients and FMT was administered by via nasogastric tube. It seemed that the responders tended to achieve engraftment whereas the nonresponders did not.

Host–microbe interactions in IBD are much more complex than the "1 microbe–1 disease" model that applies to *C difficile* and *Helicobacter*-related peptic ulcer disease. Thus, there is no single target for FMT in IBD; rather, the objective is to restore microbiological diversity and community structures. Clinical efficacy with FMT in IBD may depend on underlying host susceptible, including genetic risk. Significant uncertainties also remain in terms of timing, frequency, and route of administration of FMT. The optimum time for manipulation of microbial composition maybe in early life when gut colonization is occurring in concert with immune development. Thus, those with established IBD may have long missed their window of opportunity. This window of opportunity may also lie within the early stages or first year of IBD development. The role of FMT may not be to replace current treatments for induction of remission, but as an adjunct to restore gut microbial diversity and improve long-term outcomes in those who have achieved control of disease by conventional means.

Although FMT to date is considered safe[47] and transmission of known infectious agents should be preventable with appropriate screening, there remains the possibility of a pathogen in IBD that is waiting to be discovered. In addition, the transfer of undesirable immunologic, physiologic, or metabolic phenotypes has been demonstrated in animals and seems likely in humans.[16,48] This implies that donor selection a key safety priority with focus not just on the exclusion of infectious risk, but also on the donor phenotype and the composition and diversity of the donor microbiota. It seems likely that donor microbiota may have to be matched to the recipient's microbial composition and possibly selected specifically for the recipient's genotype and disease subset.[49] The future promises the deployment of more sophisticated and designer approaches, with specific microbial mixtures being deployed.[50]

SUMMARY

Disturbances of host–microbe interactions in genetically susceptible individuals are fundamental to the pathogenesis of IBD. However, despite remarkable advances in understanding the microbiota, translation to new treatments for patients with either Crohn's disease or ulcerative colitis has proved to be more complex than previously considered. Clarification of the molecular mechanisms by which genes, microbes, and the immune system interact promises to yield new therapeutic targets and perhaps the prospect of truly personalized medicine in which the host genome is reconciled with the appropriate manipulation of the host microbiome.

REFERENCES

1. Kostic AD, Xavier RJ, Gevers D. The microbiome in inflammatory bowel disease: current status and the future ahead. Gastroenterology 2014;146:1489–99.
2. Huttenhower C, Kostic AD, Xavier RJ. Inflammatory bowel disease as a model for translating the microbiome. Immunity 2014;40:843–54.

3. Dalal SR, Chang EB. The microbial basis of inflammatory bowel diseases. J Clin Invest 2014;124:4190–6.
4. de Souza HS, Fiocchi C. Immunopathogenesis of IBD: current state of the art. Nat Rev Gastroenterol Hepatol 2016;13:13–27.
5. Shanahan F. The gut microbiota-a clinical perspective on lessons learned. Nat Rev Gastroenterol Hepatol 2012;9:609–14.
6. Buttó LF, Haller D. Dysbiosis in intestinal inflammation: cause or consequence. Int J Med Microbiol 2016;306(5):302–9.
7. Gensollen T, Iyer SS, Kasper DL, et al. How colonization by microbiota in early life shapes the immune system. Science 2016;352(6285):539–44.
8. Bernstein CN, Shanahan F. Disorders of a modern lifestyle: reconciling the epidemiology of inflammatory bowel diseases. Gut 2008;57(9):1185–91.
9. Shanahan F, Sheehan D. Microbial contributions to chronic inflammation and metabolic disease. Curr Opin Clin Nutr Metab Care 2016;19:257–62.
10. Bloomfield SF, Rook GA, Scott EA, et al. Time to abandon the hygiene hypothesis: new perspectives on allergic disease, the human microbiome, infectious disease prevention and the role of targeted hygiene. Perspect Public Health 2016;136: 213–24.
11. Quévrain E, Maubert MA, Michon C, et al. Identification of an anti-inflammatory protein from Faecalibacterium prausnitzii, a commensal bacterium deficient in Crohn's disease. Gut 2016;65:415–25.
12. Chu H, Khosravi A, Kusumawardhani IP, et al. Gene-microbiota interactions contribute to the pathogenesis of inflammatory bowel disease. Science 2016; 352:1116–20.
13. Cadwell K, Liu JY, Brown SL, et al. A key role for autophagy and the autophagy gene Atg16l1 in mouse and human intestinal Paneth cells. Nature 2008;456: 259–63.
14. Hand TW, Dos Santos LM, Bouladoux N, et al. Acute gastrointestinal infection induces long-lived microbiota-specific T cell responses. Science 2012;337(6101): 1553–6.
15. Fonseca DM, Hand TW, Han SJ, et al. Microbiota-dependent sequelae of acute infection compromise tissue-specific immunity. Cell 2015;163(2):354–66.
16. Shanahan F, Quigley EM. Manipulation of the microbiota for treatment of IBS and IBD-challenges and controversies. Gastroenterology 2014;146:1554–63.
17. Bothin C, Midtvedt T. The role of gastrointestinal microflora in postsurgical adhesion formation–a study in germfree rats. Eur Surg Res 1992;24:309–12.
18. Mourelle M, Salas A, Guarner F, et al. Stimulation of transforming growth factor beta1 by enteric bacteria in the pathogenesis of rat intestinal fibrosis. Gastroenterology 1998;114:519–26.
19. Van Tol EAF, Holt L, Ling Li F, et al. Bacterial cell wall polymers promote intestinal fibrosis by direct stimulation of myofibroblasts. Am J Physiol 1999;277:G245–55.
20. Rigby RJ, Hunt MR, Scull BP, et al. A new animal model of postsurgical bowel inflammation and fibrosis: the effect of commensal microflora. Gut 2009;58: 1104–12.
21. Shanahan F. The colonic microbiota in health and disease. Curr Opin Gastroenterol 2013;29:49–54.
22. Gevers D, Kugathasan S, Denson LA, et al. The treatment-naive microbiome in new-onset Crohn's disease. Cell Host Microbe 2014;15:382–92.
23. Darfeuille-Michaud A, Boudeau J, Bulois P, et al. High prevalence of adherent-invasive Escherichia coli associated with ileal mucosa in Crohn's disease. Gastroenterology 2004;127:412–21.

24. Morgan XC, Tickle TL, Sokol H, et al. Dysfunction of the intestinal microbiome in inflammatory bowel disease and treatment. Genome Biol 2012;13:R79.
25. Martinez-Medina M, Aldeguer X, Lopez-Siles M, et al. Molecular diversity of Escherichia coli in the human gut: new ecological evidence supporting the role of adherent-invasive E. coli (AIEC) in Crohn's disease. Inflamm Bowel Dis 2009; 15:872–82.
26. Chassaing B, Rolhion N, de Vallee A, et al. Crohn disease–associated adherent-invasive E. coli bacteria target mouse and human Peyer's patches via long polar fimbriae. J Clin Invest 2011;121:966–75.
27. Lapaquette P, Glasser AL, Huett A, et al. Crohn's disease-associated adherent-invasive E. coli are selectively favoured by impaired autophagy to replicate intracellularly. Cell Microbiol 2010;12:99–113.
28. Sadaghian Sadabad M, Regeling A, de Goffau MC, et al. The ATG16L1-T300A allele impairs clearance of pathosymbionts in the inflamed ileal mucosa of Crohn's disease patients. Gut 2015;64:1546–52.
29. Sokol H, Pigneur B, Watterlot L, et al. Faecalibacterium prausnitzii is an anti-inflammatory commensal bacterium identified by gut microbiota analysis of Crohn disease patients. Proc Natl Acad Sci U S A 2008;105:16731–6.
30. Sonnenburg ED, Smits SA, Tikhonov M, et al. Diet-induced extinctions in the gut microbiota compound over generations. Nature 2016;529:212–5.
31. Dalmasso M, Hill C, Ross RP. Exploiting gut bacteriophages for human health. Trends Microbiol 2014;22:399–405.
32. Kernbauer E, Ding Y, Cadwell K. An enteric virus can replace the beneficial function of commensal bacteria. Nature 2014;516:94–8.
33. Weinbauer MG. Ecology of prokaryotic viruses. FEMS Microbiol Rev 2004;28: 127–81.
34. Rodriguez-Valera F, Martin-Cuadrado AB, Rodriguez-Brito B, et al. Explaining microbial population genomics through phage predation. Nat Rev Microbiol 2009;7: 828–36.
35. Lepage P, Colombet J, Marteau P, et al. Dysbiosis in inflammatory bowel disease: a role for bacteriophages? Gut 2008;57:424–5.
36. Wagner J, Maksimovic J, Farries G, et al. Bacteriophages in gut samples from pediatric Crohn's disease patients: metagenomic analysis using 454 pyrosequencing. Inflamm Bowel Dis 2013;19:1598–608.
37. Norman JM, Handley SA, Baldridge MT, et al. Disease-specific alterations in the enteric virome in inflammatory bowel disease. Cell 2015;160:447–60.
38. Minot S, Sinha R, Chen J, et al. The human gut virome: inter-individual variation and dynamic response to diet. Genome Res 2011;21:1616–25.
39. Modi SR, Lee HH, Spina CS, et al. Antibiotic treatment expands the resistance reservoir and ecological network of the phage metagenome. Nature 2013;499: 219–22.
40. Mukherjee PK, Sendid B, Hoarau G, et al. Mycobiota in gastrointestinal diseases. Nat Rev Gastroenterol Hepatol 2015;12:77–87.
41. Dollive S, Peterfreund GL, Sherrill-Mix S, et al. A tool kit for quantifying eukaryotic rRNA gene sequences from human microbiome samples. Genome Biol 2012;13: R60.
42. Hoffmann C, Dollive S, Grunberg S, et al. Archaea and fungi of the human gut microbiome: correlations with diet and bacterial residents. PLoS One 2013;8: e66019.
43. Ott SJ, Kuhbacher T, Musfeldt M, et al. Fungi and inflammatory bowel diseases: alterations of composition and diversity. Scand J Gastroenterol 2008;43:831–41.

44. Moayyedi P, Surette MG, Kim PT, et al. Fecal microbiota transplantation induces remission in patients with active ulcerative colitis in a randomized controlled trial. Gastroenterology 2015;149:102–9.e6.

45. Rossen NG, Fuentes S, van der Spek MJ, et al. findings from a randomized controlled trial of fecal transplantation for patients with ulcerative colitis. Gastroenterology 2015;149:110–8.e4.

46. Suskind DL, Brittnacher MJ, Wahbeh G, et al. Fecal microbial transplant effect on clinical outcomes and fecal microbiome in active Crohn's disease. Inflamm Bowel Dis 2015;21:556–63.

47. Gough E, Shaikh H, Manges AR. Systematic review of intestinal microbiota transplantation (fecal bacteriotherapy) for recurrent Clostridium difficile infection. Clin Infect Dis 2011;53:994–1002.

48. Kelly CR, Kahn S, Kashyap P, et al. Update on fecal microbiota transplantation 2015: indications, methodologies, mechanisms, and outlook. Gastroenterology 2015;149:223–37.

49. Vermeire S, Joossens M, Verbeke K, et al. Donor species richness determines faecal microbiota transplantation success in inflamm bowel disease. J Crohns Colitis 2016;10:387–94.

50. Petrof EO, Gloor GB, Vanner SJ, et al. Stool substitute transplant therapy for the eradication of Clostridium difficile infection: 'RePOOPulating' the gut. Microbiome 2013;1:3.

Gut Microbiota and Complications of Liver Disease

Chathur Acharya, MBBS[a], Jasmohan S. Bajaj, MD, MS[b,*]

KEYWORDS

- Cirrhosis • Bile acids • Nonalcoholic steatohepatitis • Alcoholic liver disease
- Dysbiosis • Microbiome • Firmicutes • Bacteroidetes

KEY POINTS

- Intestinal microbial dysbiosis has a large role in the progression of liver disease toward cirrhosis via endotoxemia, intestinal barrier dysfunction, and bile acid changes.
- Decompensation of cirrhosis results in significant changes to the gut microbiome that correlates with complications.
- Dysbiosis predicts decompensation and acute chronic liver failure; hence, every attempt has to be made to modulate this dysbiosis to prevent these outcomes.
- Bile acid changes are an important tool to study microbial function, and the microbiota-modulated bile acid profile plays an important role in progression of human liver disease.

INTRODUCTION

The fundamental understanding of liver disease, especially cirrhosis and its complications, has changed dramatically over the last decade with the introduction of the culture-independent microbiome analysis. Cirrhosis is estimated to affect 0.27% of the general population.[1] Hepatitis C cirrhosis, alcoholic cirrhosis, and nonalcoholic steatohepatitis (NASH)-related cirrhosis are the most common causes, accounting for 53.5%. With the changing demography and increasing obesity, NASH-related cirrhosis is projected to be the most prevalent cause in the future.[2]

There are multiple initial insults spanning from viral hepatitides, fatty liver (alcoholic and nonalcoholic), and biliary stasis to name a few. These initial insults result in

Disclosures: None.
Grant Support: CX10076 VA Merit Review and NIDDK RO1DK089713 (J.S. Bajaj).
[a] Division of General Internal Medicine, Virginia Commonwealth University, 1200 E Broad St, Richmond, VA 23298, USA; [b] Division of Gastroenterology, Hepatology, and Nutrition, McGuire VA Medical Center, Virginia Commonwealth University, 1201 Broad Rock Boulevard, Richmond, VA 23249, USA
* Corresponding author.
E-mail address: jsbajaj@vcu.edu

Gastroenterol Clin N Am 46 (2017) 155–169
http://dx.doi.org/10.1016/j.gtc.2016.09.013
0889-8553/17/© 2016 Elsevier Inc. All rights reserved.

gastro.theclinics.com

inflammation, which is clinically detected by fatigue, malaise, and elevated liver functions. With repeated insult, the inflammation translates to fibrosis, and with continued insults, eventually cirrhosis. Clinically, the precirrhotic state is phenotypically different from the postcirrhotic state with portal hypertension being the major driver of clinical manifestations later. Cirrhosis is associated with complications of hepatic encephalopathy (HE), spontaneous bacterial peritonitis (SBP), variceal bleeding, ascites, and other manifestations of volume overload and also renal complications. However, all cirrhotics do not progress at the same pace, and decompensation is unpredictable. The rate of decompensation for alcoholic cirrhosis is estimated to vary between 4% and 25%[3,4] for NASH cirrhosis, ∼2% over 5 years despite minimal histologic progression,[5] and with hepatitis C cirrhosis, the cumulative probability for decompensation at 1 year is ∼5%.[6,7] Continuing with the initial insult definitely leads to decompensation, but studies have noted progression of disease from fibrosis to cirrhosis despite cessation of the insulting factor.[8] To understand why certain patients remain stable while others decompensate despite control of inciting insults, investigators have evaluated the gut microbiome and its associated changes in various stages and causes of liver disease to further explain this phenomenon.

The intestinal microbiome itself is a complex composition of microorganisms that is well known to be implicated in cirrhosis and its complications.[9] The metabolic neural pathway also known as the gut-liver–brain axis is a key player in cirrhosis and particularly in HE, and this pathway is strongly regulated by the gut microbiome. Dysbiosis, or an unfavorable change in the composition of the microbiome with a reduction in autochthonous (Firmicutes) bacteria and growth of other taxa (Bacteroidetes, Actinobacteria), is well known to occur in advanced liver disease[10] and other intestinal abnormality.[11,12] Dysbiosis is thought to be central to the proposed pathophysiology of the microbiota and gastrointestinal abnormality for liver disease onset, progression, and development of complication. Typically in dysbiosis there occurs a change in the balance of native Firmicutes to Bacteroidetes species with the former decreasing and the latter increasing. These native bacteria are important for the harmony of the gastrointestinal flora, and as such, for the well-being of the entire body, which is why science now considers the human microbiome as an organ in itself. The autochthonous bacteria produce short-chain fatty acids (SCFAs) that nourish the colonic mucosal cells and reduce local colonic inflammation and also antibacterial peptides and hence help maintain the intestinal barrier.[13] Hence, dysbiosis is associated with increased inflammation and endotoxemia in multiple gastrointestinal abnormality, and in particular, liver disease. The Cirrhosis Dysbiosis Ratio (CDR) is the ratio of autochthonous to nonautochthonous taxa in cirrhosis. The lower the CDR, the more the endotoxemia and more decompensated the cirrhosis.[14]

To give a brief overview of the pathophysiology, the intestine and its barrier, that is, epithelium, Peyers patches, and its lymphoid tissue, act as the first immune system to come into contact with bacteria endotoxins or lipopolysaccharides (LPS), also known as pathogen-associated molecular patterns (PAMPs), that are produced by human microbiota. Because of changes in the intestinal barrier, there is bacterial translocation (BT), which exposes the intestinal immune system to antigens. The intestinal cells have a system of receptors, namely the membranous Toll-like receptors (TLR) and intracellular nucleotide oligomerization domain– like receptors (NLR), that recognize bacterial LPS, bacterial DNA, and peptidoglycans.[15,16] Recognition of the bacterial product by its receptors leads to upregulation of inflammatory mediators like tumor necrosis factor- (TNF-α).[17] Another integral factor in this process is the portal vein that acts as the main conduit for transfer of LPS and other bacterial products from the intestines to the liver. The final step in this chain is that the metabolites interact with hepatocytes and Kupffer cells via the hepatic TLR and NLR, resulting in changes that promote a cirrhotic morphology.[18]

In this article, the authors touch upon the proposed pathophysiology of how the microbiome is associated with different liver disease stages and microbiome, focusing mainly on human studies. In **Tables 1** and **2**, the authors provide details about the main recent clinical studies that show dysbiosis in chronic liver disease (CLD). This review focuses primarily on human nonalcoholic fatty liver disease (NAFLD)/NASH-related liver disease, and alcohol-related liver disease (ALD), because these causes are the paradigms for microbiome-related endotoxemia, dysbiosis, and related changes in the liver. The onset of cirrhosis, regardless of cause, results in changes to the microbiome, which is furthered by decompensation.

Table 1
List of human studies for nonalcoholic steatohepatitis and alcohol-related liver disease

Authors and Year	Groups Compared	Sample Used for Analysis	Results
Human studies in NAFLD/NASH			
Raman et al,[19] 2013	Healthy controls vs NASH	Stool	Increased Ruminococcaceae with reduced Lactobacillae and Lachnospiraceae
Zhu et al,[48] 2013	Adolescent health control vs obese vs NASH	Stool	Increased Bacteroidaceae and *Bifidobacterium* with reduced Ruminococcaceae and Lachnospiraceae
Mousaki et al,[20] 2013	Controls vs simple steatosis vs NASH	Stool	NASH had a lower (Bacteroidetes to total bacteria counts) compared the rest and higher fecal *Clostridium coccoides*
Bajaj et al,[14] 2014	Controls vs NASH cirrhosis	Stool	Increased Porphyromonadaceae, Bacterioidaceae, and reduced Veillonellaceae
Boursier et al,[21] 2016	Non cirrhotics— NASH vs no NASH	Stool	Increased Porphyromonadaceae, Ruminococcaceae, and Enterobacteriaceae with reduced Veillonellaceae and Ruminococcaceae
Human studies in ALD			
Mutlu et al,[74] 2012	Healthy controls vs alcohol cirrhotics	Sigmoid mucosal biopsies	Increased Bacterioidaceae
Bajaj et al,[95] 2014	Controls vs alcohol cirrhotics	Stool	Increased Enterobacteriaceae and Halomonadaceae, reduced Lachnospiraceae, Ruminococcaceae, and *Clostridiales XIV*
Kakiyama et al,[76] 2014	Nonalcoholic cirrhotics vs alcoholic cirrhotics	Stool	Increased Bacterioidaceae and reduced Veillonellaceae

Table 2
List of human studies that correlated microbiome changes to hepatic encephalopathy and acute-on-chronic liver failure

Authors and Year	Groups Compared	Sample Used for Analysis	Results
Bajaj et al,[77] 2012	Controls vs HE and no HE	Stool	Increased Veillonellaceae in OHE compared with no OHE cirrhotics, Porphyromonadaceae correlated with cognition
Bajaj et al,[78] 2012	Controls vs HE and no HE	Sigmoid mucosal biopsy	Increased *Enterococcus*, *Megasphaera*, and *Burkholderia* linked to poor cognition and higher inflammation; reduced *Enterococcus*, *Megasphaera*, and *Burkholderia*. Alcaligeneceae and Porphyromonadaceae were associated with poor cognition
Zhang et al,[89] 2013	Controls vs MHE vs without MHE	Stool	*Veillonella parvula* and *S salivarius* correlated negatively with cognitive function
Bajaj et al,[14,95] 2014	Cirrhotics of all causes studied prospectively	Stool	Increased pathogenic bacteria (Porphyromonadaceae, Bacterioidaceae) with no real change in autochthonous bacteria in OHE. ACLF was associated with increased Propionibacteriaceae and Halomonadaceae but reduced Lachnospiraceae and Veillonellaceae
Chen et al,[101] 2015	Controls vs ACLF cirrhotics all causes	Stool	ACLF was associated with increased Pasteurellaceae, Streptococcaceae, and Enterococcaceae with decreased Bacterioidaceae, Lachnospiraceae, and Ruminococcaceae
Ahluwalia et al,[90] 2016	Controls vs cirrhotics all causes	Stool	HE patients had higher relative abundance of autochthonous bacteria and higher abundance of Enterococcaaceae, Staphlyococcaceae, Porphyromonadaceae, and Lactobacillaceae. The autochthonous families correlated negatively with MRI brain and positively with pathogenic bacteria

NONALCOHOLIC FATTY LIVER DISEASE

NAFLD and its more sinister evolution, NASH, is slated to be the most common cause for CLD and liver transplantation in the near future.[22] It is estimated that one-third of the general US population has a fatty liver.[23] Up to 20% to 30% of NAFLD patients progress to NASH,[24] and 30% of NASH cases progress to cirrhosis.[25] NAFLD and NASH are commonly associated with the metabolic syndrome, and as noted in previous studies, is a proinflammatory state that is associated with higher levels of serum TNF-α, interleukin-6 (IL-6), and adipokines.[26,27] The linkages of the gut microbiome and changes with the microbiome with regards to the causation in NAFLD/NASH have been studied for a while now, and the microbiome probably has a larger role in the causation than is known.

Precirrhosis Nonalcoholic Fatty Liver Disease Microbiota Changes

In order to understand why the microbiota is tied into NAFLD and NASH, one needs to first understand how obesity and the metabolic syndrome affect the human microbiome. The human microbiome has been noted to be altered in obesity, and dysbiosis has been well documented.[28,29] A study by Mouzaki and colleagues[30] looked at 50 patients (of which 22 had NASH) to understand the obesity and dysbiosis paradigm and showed an inverse relationship existed between percentage Bacteriodetes species and the presence of NASH; this confirmed a possible role of dybiosis in NAFLD. An aspect of dysbiosis in NAFLD that is often overlooked is the effect of the microbiome in extraction of energy from the gut[31] where dysbiosis results in increased production of SCFAs in the intestine with increased monosaccharides, that on transport to the liver activates the proteins that promote hepatic lipogenesis and steatosis.[32] Type 2 diabetes mellitus (DM), an integral a component of the metabolic syndrome, has no immediate effect on the microbiome per se, but dysbiosis seems to affect the development of DM.[33] However, once DM sets in, it has a role in dysbiosis and pathogenesis of cirrhosis, as mentioned in a later section.

In humans with NAFLD/NASH, higher levels of LPS in the serum[34] and increased expression of the TNF-α gene in hepatic tissues have been noted,[27] confirming the proinflammatory state associated with these abnormalities.[27] Disruption of the intestinal barrier, that is, disruption of intercellular tight junctions, has been seen in NAFLD and could directly contribute to LPS and other bacterial products reaching the liver.[35] The mechanism underlying disruption of the barrier is thought to be from local colonic inflammation; however, the evidence for this is conflicting and indirect in adult humans, as seen in a study by Pendyala and colleagues,[36] where weight loss in obese individuals resulted in reduced colonic inflammation. Other studies to study colonic inflammation via fecal calprotectin and leptin showed no difference between obese and lean adults.[37,38] Regardless of the functionality of the intestinal barriers, it has been shown that bacterial LPS are transported out of the intestine to the liver via the portal vein along with chylomicrons that are formed during consumption of high-fat diets.[39] This step is key to aid in the passage of proinflammatory bacterial products past the intestinal barrier, to the liver, where these products interact with their corresponding TLR and induce production of proinflammatory mediators like TNF-α and then subsequent procirrhotic changes.[40,41] Hence, multiple mechanisms that underlie the development of microbial dysbiosis in NAFLD are seen.

Intestinal Barrier Dysfunction and the Microbiome in Nonalcoholic Fatty Liver Disease

Another prominent factor that could promote endotoxemia in NAFLD and NASH is small intestinal bacterial overgrowth (SIBO). For unclear reasons, the prevalence of

SIBO has been found higher in obesity and NAFLD.[42] The estimated prevalence of SIBO in NALFD ranges from 50% to 70% from various studies.[42,43] SIBO has been recognized as an independent risk factor for the severity of hepatic steatosis[35,42] because of its role in the dysfunction of the intestinal barrier. SIBO in general results in a quantitative change in the microbiome that is associated with dysbiosis, which leads to increased intestinal permeability and increased gut bacterial product translocation, essential in the transition pathway from NAFLD to NASH to cirrhosis.[44] Intestinal microbiota, apart from providing bacterial byproducts, increasing intestinal barrier permeability, also suppress small intestinal secretion of fasting-induced adipocyte factor, which results in increased triglyceride deposition in the hepatocytes.[45] Studies that have looked at the microbiome change in NAFLD have not exactly been able to classify if the changes are SIBO related, and as such, there are no microbiome studies that document the exact changes in NAFLD/NASH from SIBO.

Role of Microbiota and Their Products as a "Second Hit" for Nonalcoholic Steatohepatitis Development

The human microbiome has a strong role in progression of NAFLD to NASH. The 2-hit hypothesis proposed by Day and James[46] puts hepatic steatosis as the first hit. Multiple second hits are possible with this model. Prior papers have studied blood-ethanol concentrations in pediatric NASH subjects and obese non-NASH subjects and noted elevated levels in the former.[47,48] They deduced that the production of endogenous alcohol by *Escherichia coli* in the intestinal microbiome played a role in NASH development. Another study of 15 adult female patients placed on regulated choline content diets noted that liver fat was inversely proportional to choline deficiency in the diets.[49] Crespo and colleagues[50] studied 52 adult obese patients and looked at the relationship between TNF-α p55 and p75 (TNF-α receptors) and noted overexpression of TNF-α mRNA in NASH patients with increased overexpression with increased severity of NASH. Last, TLR-mediated signaling in Kupffer cells[51] is another proposed second hit. Whatever the second hit, given all the evidence, microbiome has an important role in NAFLD from the precirrhotic to the cirrhotic stages.

Another important mode of evaluating bacterial products is the bile acid (BA) profile. BAs are thought to regulate the microbiome by a potential detergent effect on the cell walls of the intestinal microbacteria[52] and also by interacting with the Farnesoid X receptor (FXR) in the liver, which not only induces excretion of BAs from the liver but also induces antimicrobial peptides production.[53,54]

The conjugated forms of primary acids BAs (cholic acid [CA] and chenodeoxycholic acid) have been found to be higher in the serum of NAFLD patients,[55] and similarly, the conjugated form of primary and secondary BAs (lithocolic and deoxycholic acid) were noted to be 2.4 times higher in patients with NASH compared with controls.[56] Lake and colleagues[57] studied the composition of BAs in the human livers of NAFLD patients and interestingly found a reduced level of CA and glycodeoxycholic acid and an increase in taurocholic acid and taurodeoxycholic acid. A recent study looking at the fecal composition of NAFLD and NASH adults confirmed a higher fecal BA level with a predominance of primary BAs in the stool of NASH patients (NASH > NAFLD), further clarifying the mechanism by which BAs regulate dysbiosis.[58] To further assess the interplay, Neuschwander-Tetri and colleagues[59] in a multicenter randomized trial studied the effect of obeticholic acid (BA derivative that activates FXR) in NASH patients and noted improvement in the histologic features of NASH based on the NAFLD activity score on liver biopsies.

ALCOHOLIC-RELATED LIVER DISEASE

ALD spans the spectrum of CLD from steatosis, steatohepatitis, liver fibrosis, and eventually cirrhosis, to more acute manifestations like acute alcoholic hepatitis. Along with NAFLD, it is one of the leading causes of CLD.[60] However, only about 10% of chronic alcoholics end up with CLD[61] and only 15% of chronic alcoholics end up developing cirrhosis. Hence, other factors, such as host factors, immunity, and the human microbiome, could contribute to the disease progression.

Precirrhosis Changes to the Microbiome in Alcohol-Related Liver Disease

As with NAFLD/NASH, the microbiome contributes to ALD via intestinal dysbiosis and increased BT. Bode and colleagues[62] first showed a significantly higher number of aerobic and anaerobic bacteria on jejunal aspirates of chronic alcoholics; this held true for alcoholic cirrhotics in a subsequent study.[63] In ALD, endotoxemia has also been noted well before the onset of cirrhosis, supporting the theory of BT.[64,65] The translocation of PAMPs out of the intestine in ALD would need a faulty intestinal barrier, and Bjarnason and colleagues[66] showed that with chronic alcohol intake there was increased intestinal permeability that persisted up to 2 weeks after cessation of consumption. Studies have shown that even acute alcohol intake (single dose) can lead to increased gastrointestinal permeability.[67] This intestinal permeability has been explained by small bowel injury (duodenal and jejunal), which was noted to occur with ethanol intake,[68] and further studies have shown enlarged intercellular spaces below the tight junctions of the distal duodenal mucosa.[69] In vitro studies have shown that acetaldehyde, a metabolite of ethanol, is responsible for the tight junction disruptions.[70,71] Acetaldehyde dehydrogenase, which metabolizes acetaldehyde, has a low activity in the colonic mucosa,[72] and theoretically acetaldehyde could persist in the colon and cause local damage. No human or animal studies have been done to this effect yet.

Intestinal Barrier Dysfunction and the Microbiome in Alcohol-Related Liver Disease

As mentioned in the above NALFD section, SIBO is associated with dysbiosis and increased BT, dysmotility, and eventual endotoxemia and is widely prevalent in ALD.[68] Most of the evidence for SIBO changes to the microbiome in ALD is actually from animal model studies.[73] Mutlu and colleagues[74] studied chronic alcoholics with no cirrhosis and in colonic microbiome analysis found dysbiosis with a relative lower median abundance of Bacteroidetes and higher abundance of Proteobacteria. Human studies by Leclercq and colleagues[75] showed that there is increased intestinal permeability in alcoholics, and this was associated with increased abundance of Ruminococcaceae family as well as some bacteria from the Lachnospiraceae family. Interestingly, they also noted that increased intestinal permeability correlated negatively with total number of gut bacteria, but the increased permeability was associated with dysbiosis. As with NAFLD/NASH, with chronic alcoholism, there is a change in the intestinal and serum BA concentration. Kakiyama and colleagues[76] showed that chronic alcoholics had a higher concentration of intestinal secondary BAs and also primary BAs with a higher secondary to primary BA ratio. The same study noted that there was an increase in bacteria from Firmicutes and a reduction in phyla Bacteroidetes in comparison with the non-ALD cirrhosis subjects. Further studies regarding alcoholics and BA variation with the microbiome are needed.

Postcirrhosis Microbiome Changes

Once cirrhosis has set in, the microbiome changes are often due to other mechanisms playing a larger role in promoting dysbiosis. Microbiota changes can have clinically relevant outcomes such as HE, infections such as SBP, acute-on-chronic liver failure (ACLF), and readmissions.[14,77,78] In patients with cirrhosis and SBP or HE, lower levels of Firmicutes and higher levels of Bacteroidetes correlated with higher endotoxemia and clinically a higher MELD (model for end-stage liver disease) score correlated with lower levels of autochthonous bacteria. As the liver disease progresses and decompensation ensues, the CDR ratio reduces further and dysbiosis plays a larger role.[14]

Intestinal barrier dysfunction is noted to be increased in cirrhosis and is also associated with endotoxemia similar to the precirrhotic state.[79,80] Interestingly, the level of endotoxemia was noted to be higher in alcoholic cirrhosis as compared with other causes in early studies.[81,82] The microbiome changes after cirrhosis in ALD are similar to that seen in any other cause for cirrhosis, excepting that as cirrhosis onsets the ratio of Bacteriodetes and Firmicutes changes with the former reducing. In most other causes, the opposite happens. Mutlu and colleagues[74] also showed that among the Bacteroidetes it was the *Bacteriodaceae* that were reduced in chronic alcoholics, and they had higher levels of Proteobacteria. The CDR similar to SIBO has a direct relationship with the severity of liver disease, and interestingly, alcoholic cirrhosis has been noted to have the lowest CDR.[14]

In understanding the role of BAs in cirrhosis, Kakiyama and colleagues[76] showed an increase in BAs in the serum of cirrhotics (NASH related and alcoholic), and that there was a reduced quantity of BAs entering the intestine from the liver as the severity of liver disease progressed. In another study, the same group found that the fecal levels of total BAs were higher in the stool in all alcoholic and nonalcoholic cirrhotics.[83] Last, DM, irrespective of the metabolic syndrome, has an increased prevalence in cirrhotic patients,[84] contributes to dysbiosis, and prognosticates complications in cirrhosis.[85] The presence of DM with insulin use in cirrhosis does alter the gut microbiome, causing a relative increase in Bacteroidetes and other families, but also a reduction in Firmicutes. This change is similar to what is seen in NASH cirrhosis with DM not taking insulin, but does not confer an increased risk for readmissions as seen in a prospective study.[86]

Hepatic Encephalopathy

With decompensation of cirrhosis come multiple microbiome changes. While looking at the studies, one must keep in mind that decompensated patients are generally sicker and may also be on microbiome-altering therapy (rifaximin or lactulose). With the onset of HE, there is an increased endotoxemia[14,87] and the CDR reduces, signaling microbiome changes, although in the study by Bajaj and colleagues,[88] the predominant change was increased in Bacteroidetes species with no changes in the autochthonous species. Changes to the microbiome have been noted to start with early HE or minimal HE (MHE). Salivary microbiota changes have been shown to correlate with stool microbiota changes and could be explored as a new frontier in immune profiling in cirrhosis. Stool microbiota studies in cirrhotics and MHE noted an increase in *Streptococcus salivarius* in patients with MHE and an increased blood ammonia level.[89] In another study, no difference was noted in the stool microbiome between MHE and overt HE (OHE),[78] although in a similar study by the same group, there was a significant difference in the colonic mucosal microbiome between OHE and healthy subjects with no difference in the MHE and OHE groups.[77] In more studies, Bajaj and colleagues[78] showed that certain bacterial taxa such as *Proteobacteria* correlated with endotoxemia and cognition. Ahluwalia and colleagues[90] looked at the correlation of intestinal bacteria, HE, and magnetic resonance spectroscopy (MRS) and found that pathogenic taxa (*Enterococcaaceae, Staphlyococcaceae,*

Porphyromonadaceae, and *Lactobacillaceae*) positively correlated with MRS and HE and auhochthonous taxa correlated negatively. Lactulose withdrawal in HE patients did not bring about changes to the microbiome,[91] but in another study, treatment of HE with rifaximin also induces changes to the microbiome with improved endotoxemia and cognition.[92] The changes correlated with changes in serum saturated and unsaturated fatty acids (UFA) with the UFAs increasing and possibly helping in improved brain function. The exact changes to the microbiome taxa by treatment have yet to be documented.

To alter the microbiome to prevent decompensation, prebiotics and probiotics have been studied. In healthy adults, there is no evidence of probiotics resulting in changes[93]; however, in cirrhotics, probiotics belonging to Firmicutes and Actinobacteria phyla have been studied in randomized controlled trials (RCTs) and have been proven to be beneficial. VLS#3 (mixture of multiple probiotic strains) given daily has been proven to reduce the severity of cirrhosis and reduce HE-related admissions in cirrhotics of alcoholic, NASH, and hepatitis C–related causes, although the exact microbiome changes were not noted in this study as well.[94] Lactobacillus GG (LGG) use in an RCT for cirrhotics who were diagnosed to have MHE showed those randomized to LGG reduced dysbiosis through an increased relative abundance of autochthonous taxa and a reduced relative abundance of potentially pathogenic taxa (*Enterobacteriaceae* and *Porphyromonadaceae*), along with reduction in endotoxemia.[95]

Spontaneous Bacterial Peritonitis

BT and SIBO are integral to SBP onset in cirrhosis, and hence, dysbiosis plays an important role here. A higher prevalence of gram-negative bacteria of the Enterobacteriacae family has been noted in cirrhotics with and without decompensation,[14,96] and it is bacteria from this family that are predominantly noted in SBP ascitic fluid cultures.[97] As seen earlier, with advance in liver disease, the dysbiosis typically worsens.[14] In patients with SBP or infections, the CDR ratio was noted to be lower; there was a higher degree of endotoxemia, and the CDR negatively correlated with endotoxemia. The dysbiosis, however, remained stable for cirrhotics who had not decompensated, indicating that the microbiome changes likely start after decompensation starts.

Prediction of Admissions in Cirrhosis

Bajaj and colleagues[86] studied 278 cirrhotics (all causes), looking at DM as a factor for readmission. In their prospective study with a median readmission time of 90 days, they looked at the stool and sigmoid colon microbiome and noted that cirrhotics that had a nonelective readmission had a reduction in 2 families in the Bacteroidetes phyla. Reduction of Bacteroidetes is associated with increased risk of infection,[98] and hence, on comparing this phyla between alcoholic cirrhotics and NASH cirrhotics given the relative abundance of this phyla in NASH cirrhotics, they have a lesser rate of infection compared with alcoholic cirrhotics.

Acute-on-Chronic-Liver Failure and Death

ACLF is defined as the presence of failure of 2 or more organs in cirrhotic patients. It portends a poor prognosis and has a high mortality.[99,100] Patients with ACLF have been noted to have a higher level of endotoxemia, and in a large study, patients who developed ACLF and organ failure 30 days after admission could be differentiated from those who did not based on microbiota.[14] This association between ACLF, mortality and microbiota was confirmed by Chen and colleagues,[101] who also noted that this dysbiosis is marked in ACLF and can independently predict mortality. Bajaj and colleagues also noted that there was an increase in gram-negative bacteremia on stool microbiome analysis, greater endotoxemia, and these patients had a lower CDR compared with the infected cirrhotics in their study in those who survived. These changes likely occurred well before death and decompensation and may definitively play a role in disease.

SUMMARY

To conclude, dysbiosis correlates with endotoxemia, starts early in NAFLD and ALD, and progressively worsens with increasing severity of liver disease. BAs are major proponents of dysbiosis, and alteration in BA profile could profoundly impact liver disease progression. Once cirrhosis sets in, the microbial composition and function alterations worsen and contribute to complications such as HE and ACLF, and can be a predictor of readmissions and mortality.

REFERENCES

1. Scaglione S, Kliethermes S, Cao G, et al. The epidemiology of cirrhosis in the United States: a population-based study. J Clin Gastroenterol 2015;49(8):690–6.
2. Vernon G, Baranova A, Younossi ZM. Systematic review: the epidemiology and natural history of non-alcoholic fatty liver disease and non-alcoholic steatohepatitis in adults. Aliment Pharmacol Ther 2011;34(3):274–85.
3. D'Amico G, Morabito A, Pagliaro L, et al. Survival and prognostic indicators in compensated and decompensated cirrhosis. Dig Dis Sci 1986;31(5):468–75.
4. Jepsen P, Ott P, Andersen PK, et al. Clinical course of alcoholic liver cirrhosis: a Danish population-based cohort study. Hepatology 2010;51(5):1675–82.
5. Powell EE, Cooksley WG, Hanson R, et al. The natural history of nonalcoholic steatohepatitis: a follow-up study of forty-two patients for up to 21 years. Hepatology 1990;11(1):74–80.
6. Fattovich G, Giustina G, Degos F, et al. Morbidity and mortality in compensated cirrhosis type C: a retrospective follow-up study of 384 patients. Gastroenterology 1997;112(2):463–72.
7. Serfaty L, Aumaitre H, Chazouilleres O, et al. Determinants of outcome of compensated hepatitis C virus-related cirrhosis. Hepatology 1998;27(5):1435–40.
8. Sorensen TI, Orholm M, Bentsen KD, et al. Prospective evaluation of alcohol abuse and alcoholic liver injury in men as predictors of development of cirrhosis. Lancet 1984;2(8397):241–4.
9. Quigley EM, Stanton C, Murphy EF. The gut microbiota and the liver. Pathophysiological and clinical implications. J Hepatol 2013;58(5):1020–7.
10. Chen Y, Yang F, Lu H, et al. Characterization of fecal microbial communities in patients with liver cirrhosis. Hepatology 2011;54(2):562–72.
11. Farrell RJ, LaMont JT. Microbial factors in inflammatory bowel disease. Gastroenterol Clin North Am 2002;31(1):41–62.
12. Tamboli CP, Neut C, Desreumaux P, et al. Dysbiosis in inflammatory bowel disease. Gut 2004;53(1):1–4.
13. Schnabl B, Brenner DA. Interactions between the intestinal microbiome and liver diseases. Gastroenterology 2014;146(6):1513–24.
14. Bajaj JS, Heuman DM, Hylemon PB, et al. Altered profile of human gut microbiome is associated with cirrhosis and its complications. J Hepatol 2014;60(5):940–7.

15. Mariathasan S, Monack DM. Inflammasome adaptors and sensors: intracellular regulators of infection and inflammation. Nat Rev Immunol 2007;7(1):31–40.

16. Trinchieri G, Sher A. Cooperation of Toll-like receptor signals in innate immune defence. Nat Rev Immunol 2007;7(3):179–90.

17. Carvalho FA, Aitken JD, Vijay-Kumar M, et al. Toll-like receptor-gut microbiota interactions: perturb at your own risk! Annu Rev Physiol 2012;74:177–98.

18. Seki E, Schnabl B. Role of innate immunity and the microbiota in liver fibrosis: crosstalk between the liver and gut. J Physiol 2012;590(3):447–58.

19. Raman M, Ahmed I, Gillevet PM, et al. Fecal microbiome and volatile organic compound metabolome in obese humans with nonalcoholic fatty liver disease. Clin Gastroenterol Hepatol 2013;11(7):868–75.e1–3.

20. Mouzaki M, Comelli EM, Arendt BM, et al. Intestinal microbiota in patients with nonalcoholic fatty liver disease. Hepatology 2013;58(1):120–7.

21. Boursier J, Mueller O, Barret M, et al. The severity of nonalcoholic fatty liver disease is associated with gut dysbiosis and shift in the metabolic function of the gut microbiota. Hepatology 2016;63(3):764–75.

22. Younossi ZM, Stepanova M, Afendy M, et al. Changes in the prevalence of the most common causes of chronic liver diseases in the United States from 1988 to 2008. Clin Gastroenterol Hepatol 2011;9(6):524–30.e1 [quiz: e60].

23. Browning JD, Szczepaniak LS, Dobbins R, et al. Prevalence of hepatic steatosis in an urban population in the United States: impact of ethnicity. Hepatology 2004;40(6):1387–95.

24. Williams CD, Stengel J, Asike MI, et al. Prevalence of nonalcoholic fatty liver disease and nonalcoholic steatohepatitis among a largely middle-aged population utilizing ultrasound and liver biopsy: a prospective study. Gastroenterology 2011;140(1):124–31.

25. Caldwell S, Argo C. The natural history of non-alcoholic fatty liver disease. Dig Dis 2010;28(1):162–8.

26. Carter-Kent C, Zein NN, Feldstein AE. Cytokines in the pathogenesis of fatty liver and disease progression to steatohepatitis: implications for treatment. Am J Gastroenterol 2008;103(4):1036–42.

27. Ruiz AG, Casafont F, Crespo J, et al. Lipopolysaccharide-binding protein plasma levels and liver TNF-alpha gene expression in obese patients: evidence for the potential role of endotoxin in the pathogenesis of non-alcoholic steatohepatitis. Obes Surg 2007;17(10):1374–80.

28. Ley RE, Turnbaugh PJ, Klein S, et al. Microbial ecology: human gut microbes associated with obesity. Nature 2006;444(7122):1022–3.

29. Ley RE, Backhed F, Turnbaugh P, et al. Obesity alters gut microbial ecology. Proc Natl Acad Sci U S A 2005;102(31):11070–5.

30. Mouzaki M, Comelli EM, Arendt BM, et al. Intestinal microbiota in patients with nonalcoholic fatty liver disease. Hepatology 2013;58(1):120–7.

31. Jumpertz R, Le DS, Turnbaugh PJ, et al. Energy-balance studies reveal associations between gut microbes, caloric load, and nutrient absorption in humans. Am J Clin Nutr 2011;94(1):58–65.

32. Le Poul E, Loison C, Struyf S, et al. Functional characterization of human receptors for short chain fatty acids and their role in polymorphonuclear cell activation. J Biol Chem 2003;278(28):25481–9.

33. Baothman OA, Zamzami MA, Taher I, et al. The role of gut microbiota in the development of obesity and diabetes. Lipids Health Dis 2016;15:108.

34. Verdam FJ, Fuentes S, de Jonge C, et al. Human intestinal microbiota composition is associated with local and systemic inflammation in obesity. Obesity (Silver Spring) 2013;21(12):E607–15.

35. Miele L, Valenza V, La Torre G, et al. Increased intestinal permeability and tight junction alterations in nonalcoholic fatty liver disease. Hepatology 2009;49(6): 1877–87.

36. Pendyala S, Neff LM, Suarez-Farinas M, et al. Diet-induced weight loss reduces colorectal inflammation: implications for colorectal carcinogenesis. Am J Clin Nutr 2011;93(2):234–42.

37. Brignardello J, Morales P, Diaz E, et al. Pilot study: alterations of intestinal microbiota in obese humans are not associated with colonic inflammation or disturbances of barrier function. Aliment Pharmacol Ther 2010;32(11–12):1307–14.

38. Tiihonen K, Ouwehand AC, Rautonen N. Effect of overweight on gastrointestinal microbiology and immunology: correlation with blood biomarkers. Br J Nutr 2010;103(7):1070–8.

39. Ghoshal S, Witta J, Zhong J, et al. Chylomicrons promote intestinal absorption of lipopolysaccharides. J Lipid Res 2009;50(1):90–7.

40. Roh YS, Seki E. Toll-like receptors in alcoholic liver disease, non-alcoholic steatohepatitis and carcinogenesis. J Gastroenterol Hepatol 2013;28(Suppl 1): 38–42.

41. Henao-Mejia J, Elinav E, Jin C, et al. Inflammasome-mediated dysbiosis regulates progression of NAFLD and obesity. Nature 2012;482(7384):179–85.

42. Sabate JM, Jouet P, Harnois F, et al. High prevalence of small intestinal bacterial overgrowth in patients with morbid obesity: a contributor to severe hepatic steatosis. Obes Surg 2008;18(4):371–7.

43. Sajjad A, Mottershead M, Syn WK, et al. Ciprofloxacin suppresses bacterial overgrowth, increases fasting insulin but does not correct low acylated ghrelin concentration in non-alcoholic steatohepatitis. Aliment Pharmacol Ther 2005; 22(4):291–9.

44. Wigg AJ, Roberts-Thomson IC, Dymock RB, et al. The role of small intestinal bacterial overgrowth, intestinal permeability, endotoxaemia, and tumour necrosis factor alpha in the pathogenesis of non-alcoholic steatohepatitis. Gut 2001; 48(2):206–11.

45. Backhed F, Manchester JK, Semenkovich CF, et al. Mechanisms underlying the resistance to diet-induced obesity in germ-free mice. Proc Natl Acad Sci U S A 2007;104(3):979–84.

46. Day CP, James OF. Steatohepatitis: a tale of two "hits"? Gastroenterology 1998; 114(4):842–5.

47. Nair S, Cope K, Risby TH, et al. Obesity and female gender increase breath ethanol concentration: potential implications for the pathogenesis of nonalcoholic steatohepatitis. Am J Gastroenterol 2001;96(4):1200–4.

48. Zhu L, Baker SS, Gill C, et al. Characterization of gut microbiomes in nonalcoholic steatohepatitis (NASH) patients: a connection between endogenous alcohol and NASH. Hepatology 2013;57(2):601–9.

49. Spencer MD, Hamp TJ, Reid RW, et al. Association between composition of the human gastrointestinal microbiome and development of fatty liver with choline deficiency. Gastroenterology 2011;140(3):976–86.

50. Crespo J, Cayon A, Fernandez-Gil P, et al. Gene expression of tumor necrosis factor alpha and TNF-receptors, p55 and p75, in nonalcoholic steatohepatitis patients. Hepatology 2001;34(6):1158–63.

51. Aoyama T, Paik YH, Seki E. Toll-like receptor signaling and liver fibrosis. Gastroenterol Res Pract 2010;2010.
52. Begley M, Gahan CG, Hill C. The interaction between bacteria and bile. FEMS Microbiol Rev 2005;29(4):625–51.
53. Inagaki T, Moschetta A, Lee YK, et al. Regulation of antibacterial defense in the small intestine by the nuclear bile acid receptor. Proc Natl Acad Sci U S A 2006; 103(10):3920–5.
54. Ridlon JM, Kang DJ, Hylemon PB. Bile salt biotransformations by human intestinal bacteria. J Lipid Res 2006;47(2):241–59.
55. Kalhan SC, Guo L, Edmison J, et al. Plasma metabolomic profile in nonalcoholic fatty liver disease. Metabolism 2011;60(3):404–13.
56. Ferslew BC, Xie G, Johnston CK, et al. Altered bile acid metabolome in patients with nonalcoholic steatohepatitis. Dig Dis Sci 2015;60(11):3318–28.
57. Lake AD, Novak P, Shipkova P, et al. Decreased hepatotoxic bile acid composition and altered synthesis in progressive human nonalcoholic fatty liver disease. Toxicol Appl Pharmacol 2013;268(2):132–40.
58. Mouzaki M, Wang AY, Bandsma R, et al. Bile acids and dysbiosis in nonalcoholic fatty liver disease. PLoS One 2016;11(5):e0151829.
59. Neuschwander-Tetri BA, Loomba R, Sanyal AJ, et al. Farnesoid X nuclear receptor ligand obeticholic acid for non-cirrhotic, non-alcoholic steatohepatitis (FLINT): a multicentre, randomised, placebo-controlled trial. Lancet 2015; 385(9972):956–65.
60. Hartmann P, Chen WC, Schnabl B. The intestinal microbiome and the leaky gut as therapeutic targets in alcoholic liver disease. Front Physiol 2012;3:402.
61. Levene AP, Goldin RD. The epidemiology, pathogenesis and histopathology of fatty liver disease. Histopathology 2012;61(2):141–52.
62. Bode JC, Bode C, Heidelbach R, et al. Jejunal microflora in patients with chronic alcohol abuse. Hepatogastroenterology 1984;31(1):30–4.
63. Casafont Morencos F, de las Heras Castano G, Martin Ramos L, et al. Small bowel bacterial overgrowth in patients with alcoholic cirrhosis. Dig Dis Sci 1996;41(3):552–6.
64. Parlesak A, Schafer C, Schutz T, et al. Increased intestinal permeability to macromolecules and endotoxemia in patients with chronic alcohol abuse in different stages of alcohol-induced liver disease. J Hepatol 2000;32(5):742–7.
65. Bode C, Bode JC. Activation of the innate immune system and alcoholic liver disease: effects of ethanol per se or enhanced intestinal translocation of bacterial toxins induced by ethanol? Alcohol Clin Exp Res 2005;29(11 Suppl): 166S–71S.
66. Bjarnason I, Peters TJ, Wise RJ. The leaky gut of alcoholism: possible route of entry for toxic compounds. Lancet 1984;1(8370):179–82.
67. Keshavarzian A, Holmes EW, Patel M, et al. Leaky gut in alcoholic cirrhosis: a possible mechanism for alcohol-induced liver damage. Am J Gastroenterol 1999;94(1):200–7.
68. Bode C, Bode JC. Effect of alcohol consumption on the gut. Best Pract Res Clin Gastroenterol 2003;17(4):575–92.
69. Such J, Guardiola JV, de Juan J, et al. Ultrastructural characteristics of distal duodenum mucosa in patients with cirrhosis. Eur J Gastroenterol Hepatol 2002; 14(4):371–6.
70. Rao RK. Acetaldehyde-induced increase in paracellular permeability in Caco-2 cell monolayer. Alcohol Clin Exp Res 1998;22(8):1724–30.

71. Rao RK. Acetaldehyde-induced barrier disruption and paracellular permeability in Caco-2 cell monolayer. Methods Mol Biol 2008;447:171–83.

72. Nosova T, Jokelainen K, Kaihovaara P, et al. Characteristics of aldehyde dehydrogenases of certain aerobic bacteria representing human colonic flora. Alcohol Alcohol 1998;33(3):273–80.

73. Hartmann P, Seebauer CT, Schnabl B. Alcoholic liver disease: the gut microbiome and liver cross talk. Alcohol Clin Exp Res 2015;39(5):763–75.

74. Mutlu EA, Gillevet PM, Rangwala H, et al. Colonic microbiome is altered in alcoholism. Am J Physiol Gastrointest Liver Physiol 2012;302(9):G966–78.

75. Leclercq S, Matamoros S, Cani PD, et al. Intestinal permeability, gut-bacterial dysbiosis, and behavioral markers of alcohol-dependence severity. Proc Natl Acad Sci U S A 2014;111(42):E4485–93.

76. Kakiyama G, Hylemon PB, Zhou H, et al. Colonic inflammation and secondary bile acids in alcoholic cirrhosis. Am J Physiol Gastrointest Liver Physiol 2014; 306(11):G929–37.

77. Bajaj JS, Hylemon PB, Ridlon JM, et al. Colonic mucosal microbiome differs from stool microbiome in cirrhosis and hepatic encephalopathy and is linked to cognition and inflammation. Am J Physiol Gastrointest Liver Physiol 2012;303(6): G675–85.

78. Bajaj JS, Ridlon JM, Hylemon PB, et al. Linkage of gut microbiome with cognition in hepatic encephalopathy. Am J Physiol Gastrointest Liver Physiol 2012; 302(1):G168–75.

79. Bauer TM, Steinbruckner B, Brinkmann FE, et al. Small intestinal bacterial overgrowth in patients with cirrhosis: prevalence and relation with spontaneous bacterial peritonitis. Am J Gastroenterol 2001;96(10):2962–7.

80. Bauer TM, Schwacha H, Steinbruckner B, et al. Small intestinal bacterial overgrowth in human cirrhosis is associated with systemic endotoxemia. Am J Gastroenterol 2002;97(9):2364–70.

81. Bode C, Kugler V, Bode JC. Endotoxemia in patients with alcoholic and non-alcoholic cirrhosis and in subjects with no evidence of chronic liver disease following acute alcohol excess. J Hepatol 1987;4(1):8–14.

82. Fukui H, Brauner B, Bode JC, et al. Plasma endotoxin concentrations in patients with alcoholic and non-alcoholic liver disease: reevaluation with an improved chromogenic assay. J Hepatol 1991;12(2):162–9.

83. Kakiyama G, Pandak WM, Gillevet PM, et al. Modulation of the fecal bile acid profile by gut microbiota in cirrhosis. J Hepatol 2013;58(5):949–55.

84. Zein NN, Abdulkarim AS, Wiesner RH, et al. Prevalence of diabetes mellitus in patients with end-stage liver cirrhosis due to hepatitis C, alcohol, or cholestatic disease. J Hepatol 2000;32(2):209–17.

85. Elkrief L, Chouinard P, Bendersky N, et al. Diabetes mellitus is an independent prognostic factor for major liver-related outcomes in patients with cirrhosis and chronic hepatitis C. Hepatology 2014;60(3):823–31.

86. Bajaj JS, Betrapally NS, Hylemon PB, et al. Gut microbiota alterations can predict hospitalizations in cirrhosis independent of diabetes mellitus. Sci Rep 2015; 5:18559.

87. Jain L, Sharma BC, Srivastava S, et al. Serum endotoxin, inflammatory mediators, and magnetic resonance spectroscopy before and after treatment in patients with minimal hepatic encephalopathy. J Gastroenterol Hepatol 2013; 28(7):1187–93.

88. Bajaj JS, Betrapally NS, Hylemon PB, et al. Salivary microbiota reflects changes in gut microbiota in cirrhosis with hepatic encephalopathy. Hepatology 2015; 62(4):1260–71.
89. Zhang Z, Zhai H, Geng J, et al. Large-scale survey of gut microbiota associated with MHE Via 16S rRNA-based pyrosequencing. Am J Gastroenterol 2013; 108(10):1601–11.
90. Ahluwalia V, Betrapally NS, Hylemon PB, et al. Impaired gut-liver-brain axis in patients with cirrhosis. Sci Rep 2016;6:26800.
91. Bajaj JS, Gillevet PM, Patel NR, et al. A longitudinal systems biology analysis of lactulose withdrawal in hepatic encephalopathy. Metab Brain Dis 2012;27(2): 205–15.
92. Bajaj JS, Heuman DM, Sanyal AJ, et al. Modulation of the metabiome by rifaximin in patients with cirrhosis and minimal hepatic encephalopathy. PLoS One 2013;8(4):e60042.
93. Kristensen NB, Bryrup T, Allin KH, et al. Alterations in fecal microbiota composition by probiotic supplementation in healthy adults: a systematic review of randomized controlled trials. Genome Med 2016;8(1):52.
94. Dhiman RK, Rana B, Agrawal S, et al. Probiotic VSL#3 reduces liver disease severity and hospitalization in patients with cirrhosis: a randomized, controlled trial. Gastroenterology 2014;147(6):1327–37.e3.
95. Bajaj JS, Heuman DM, Hylemon PB, et al. Randomised clinical trial: lactobacillus GG modulates gut microbiome, metabolome and endotoxemia in patients with cirrhosis. Aliment Pharmacol Ther 2014;39(10):1113–25.
96. Bajaj JS, Betrapally NS, Gillevet PM. Decompensated cirrhosis and microbiome interpretation. Nature 2015;525(7569):E1–2.
97. Merli M, Lucidi C, Giannelli V, et al. Cirrhotic patients are at risk for health care-associated bacterial infections. Clin Gastroenterol Hepatol 2010;8(11):979–85.
98. Manges AR, Labbe A, Loo VG, et al. Comparative metagenomic study of alterations to the intestinal microbiota and risk of nosocomial Clostridum difficile-associated disease. J Infect Dis 2010;202(12):1877–84.
99. Bajaj JS, O'Leary JG, Reddy KR, et al. Second infections independently increase mortality in hospitalized patients with cirrhosis: the North American consortium for the study of end-stage liver disease (NACSELD) experience. Hepatology 2012;56(6):2328–35.
100. Moreau R, Jalan R, Gines P, et al. Acute-on-chronic liver failure is a distinct syndrome that develops in patients with acute decompensation of cirrhosis. Gastroenterology 2013;144(7):1426–37, 1437.e1–9.
101. Chen Y, Guo J, Qian G, et al. Gut dysbiosis in acute-on-chronic liver failure and its predictive value for mortality. J Gastroenterol Hepatol 2015;30(9):1429–37.

Fecal Microbiota Transplantation

Stephen M. Vindigni, MD, MPH[a],*, Christina M. Surawicz, MD[b]

KEYWORDS

- *Clostridium difficile* • Fecal microbiota transplant • Stool transplant • FMT
- Microbiome

KEY POINTS

- Fecal microbiota transplantation (FMT) is effective for treatment of recurrent *Clostridium difficile* infection (CDI) when standard therapy has failed.
- FMT may have a role in some patients with severe and complicated CDI.
- The following factors are important in selecting patients for FMT:
  - ○ Appropriate indications.
  - ○ Appropriate donor selection.
  - ○ Appropriate method of administering FMT.
  - ○ Appropriate follow-up.

INTRODUCTION

Fecal microbiota transplantation (FMT) is the transfer of stool from a "healthy" donor to a recipient believed to harbor an altered colonic microbiome resulting in disease. The goal is to restore eubiosis, or a "healthy" microbiome. Often referred to as stool transplantation, fecal transplantation, fecal flora reconstitution, or fecal bacteriotherapy, FMT has increasingly become a focus in both the public media and peer-reviewed literature. FMT is an effective treatment strategy for recurrent *Clostridium difficile* infection (rCDI) that has not responded to standard therapy. There is interest in using

Conflicts: None.
Disclaimer: The findings and conclusions in this editorial are those of the authors and do not necessarily reflect the views of the University of Washington. All authors declare: no support from any organization for the submitted work; no financial relationships with any organizations that might have an interest in the submitted work. The authors declare that they have no competing interests.
[a] Division of Gastroenterology, Department of Medicine, School of Medicine, University of Washington, 1959 Northeast Pacific Street, Box 356424, Seattle, WA 98195-6424, USA;
[b] Division of Gastroenterology, Department of Medicine, University of Washington, 325 9th Avenue, Box 359773, Seattle, WA 98104, USA
* Corresponding author.
E-mail address: vindigni@uw.edu

Gastroenterol Clin N Am 46 (2017) 171–185
http://dx.doi.org/10.1016/j.gtc.2016.09.012
0889-8553/17/© 2016 Elsevier Inc. All rights reserved.

FMT for other gastrointestinal (GI) and non-GI diseases, and multiple studies are under way to determine potential alternative indications.

HISTORY

FMT was first described in the fourth century Dong-jin dynasty. A Chinese doctor administered feces by mouth to patients with food poisoning or severe diarrhea with report of life-saving results.[1] There are also descriptions during the sixteenth century Ming dynasty whereby patients were prescribed fresh or fermented fecal suspensions for a range of GI conditions, including diarrhea, vomiting, constipation, and pain. Some reports also indicate the use of infant feces as therapy.[1] Subsequent accounts refer to Fabricius Aquapendente, an Italian seventeenth century anatomist who used FMT in veterinary medicine.[2] It was termed "transfaunation."[3]

More modern descriptions of use in humans were documented by Eiseman and colleagues[4] in 1958; 4 patients improved after they were given fecal enemas for treatment of staphylococcal pseudomembranous enterocolitis.

There has been considerable interest in FMT over the past decade. There have been multiple case reports and series describing differing FMT protocols, methods of stool administration, and variable patient responses. The highest success rates have been for rCDI with less robust findings, but active investigation, in other GI and non-GI diseases.[5]

GOAL AND EFFECTS OF FECAL MICROBIOTA TRANSPLANTATION

The main goal of FMT is to restore the "normal" population of bacteria in a dysbiotic colonic environment. Studies have examined the gut microbiome in patients with CDI before and after FMT. There is clearly a shift in the bacterial populations within the post-FMT gut that mirrors the donor stool. Gene-sequencing studies of stool samples have shown increases in the quantity of Firmicutes and Bacteroidetes and decreases in Proteobacteria and Actinobacteria following FMT, suggesting rapid donor engraftment.[6,7]

SCREENING AND PROCESS OF FECAL MICROBIOTA TRANSPLANTATION
Selection and Screening of Donor

The stool donor may be related or unrelated to the recipient. If related, the donor is typically a spouse or close relative. A systematic review by Gough and colleagues[8] showed resolution of CDI in 93.3% of studies with related donors (n = 19 studies) and 84% of studies with unrelated donors (n = 4 studies). Kassam and colleagues[9] similarly assessed the significance of donor type and found no difference in clinical outcome regardless if the donor was anonymous versus patient-selected. The investigators hypothesize that unrelated/anonymous donors likely harbor a completely different microbiome compared with related donors and thus may be more effective in "resetting" the microbiome of the recipients, although this has not been demonstrated in randomized studies. Furthermore, many patients prefer an anonymous donor to eliminate the sometimes awkward conversation requesting a stool sample from a family member.

With mild variation, donor screening protocols have been established to reduce the risks of transmission of an infection from the donor to recipient. Testing includes both stool and serum analysis as well as an extensive clinical and social risk assessment. A listing of donor assessment recommendations is included in **Box 1**. The inclusion of such a screening protocol is important to prevent transmission of infectious organisms

---

Box 1
Screening donors for fecal microbiota transplantation: exclusion criteria

History and chart review:

- Active infection

- Exposure to antibiotics in the prior 3 months

- Recent travel with exposure to epidemic diarrheal disease

- Significant gastrointestinal history, including inflammatory bowel disease, irritable bowel syndrome, chronic diarrhea/constipation, gastrointestinal malignancy

- Autoimmune or significant allergy history

- Other considerations: risk factors for Creutzfeldt-Jakob disease, diabetes, metabolic syndrome, chronic pain syndromes, and exposure to medications that may alter the gut microbiome

- Social factor considerations: high-risk sexual behaviors, drug use, incarceration or long-term care facility residence, and body piercing or tattoo in prior 6 months

Stool testing:

Bacteria
- *Clostridium difficile*
- Campylobacter
- *Helicobacter pylori* (if fecal microbiota transplantation administered via oral route)
- Salmonella
- Shiga-toxin producing *Escherichia coli*
- Shigella
- Other considerations: *Aeromonas, Plesiomonas, Listeria monocytogenes, Yersinia, Vibrio cholerae,* and *Vibrio parahaemolyticus*

Viruses
- Rotavirus
- Norovirus

Parasites
- *Cryptosporidium*
- *Cyclospora*
- *Giardia*
- *Isospora*

Blood testing:

Bacteria
- Syphilis

Viruses
- Hepatitis A, B, C
- Human immunodeficiency virus

Data from Refs.[54–56]

---

that may be harbored in donor stool. Additionally, we know little about the transmissibility of autoimmune diseases and other noninfectious conditions that may be influenced by changes in the microbiome. Although there have been instances of homeopathic or home-use of enemas to perform FMT without physician evaluation, this is strongly discouraged for the previously discussed reasons.

Some protocols will provide a laxative to the donor to assist with stool collection. We also recommend the donor avoid any foods (eg, nuts) to which the recipient has a known food allergy.

Regulations and Patient Consent

Currently, FMT is indicated for rCDI, although this application is still considered investigational. Despite Food and Drug Administration (FDA) oversight, physicians may perform FMT outside of a clinical trial (without an investigational new drug [IND] application and approval) for CDI that has not been responsive to standard antibiotic therapies; this has also been referred to as "enforcement discretion."[10] For non-rCDI applications, an IND must be submitted to the FDA.

From a clinical and research standpoint, any non-rCDI use of FMT is considered "off-label" and the evidence base of the benefits and risks should be strongly considered. In many cases, there are no data to justify its use. Following, we discuss the current evidence for CDI, inflammatory bowel disease (IBD), and other diseases in which FMT has been studied.

All patients should provide consent for FMT with the benefits, risks, process, and follow-up clearly explained to the patient. Some risks will be specific to the method of delivery. For example, with colonoscopy, we note the risk of reaction to anesthetic agents, discomfort during the procedure, gastrointestinal bleeding, and perforation. With regard to FMT, we also note the risk of transmission of an infectious agent or diseases/conditions for which the donor was not prescreened.

Screening of Recipient

There are no guidelines on screening requirements for FMT recipients. As noted previously, FMT is recommended for rCDI with less support for other disease indications currently. Although not standardized, we recommend baseline recipient testing for viral hepatitis, human immunodeficiency virus, and syphilis, because if the patient is diagnosed with one of these diseases post-FMT, further assessment can be performed to determine if the stool sample may have played a role.

Additional recipient screening considerations include comorbidities, such as immunocompromised status, which may increase the risk of adverse events.

Fecal Microbiota Transplantation Preparation and Administration

There is often some variation in FMT preparation across institutions where FMT is performed. The general process is the same, however, and involves mixing stool with a bacteriostatic liquid, removing particulate matter, and delivering donor stool to the patient. Patients should stop vancomycin (or any other antibiotic) at least 1 or 2 days before FMT administration.

Stool may be administered via several mechanisms, each with its own benefits and risks, as described in **Table 1**. These include the following:

- Oral (via nasogastric, nasoduodenal, or nasojejunal tube or capsule)
- Colonoscopy (stool deposited into right colon or terminal ileum)
- Enema

The process for performing FMT is described in **Fig. 1**. Currently, there are 3 main methods of obtaining the donor sample:

- Stool sample from unrelated or related local donor
- Stool sample from a stool bank, generally shipped frozen on dry ice overnight
- Frozen, encapsulated stool

Stool is prescreened as described previously, either locally or at a stool bank before shipment. The latter provides a unique identifier that can be tracked back to the donor if necessary. Additionally, stool banks may retain a sample of donor stool for freezer

Table 1
Advantages and disadvantages of various methods of fecal microbiota transplantation administration

Method	Advantages	Disadvantages
Oral/Nasogastric/ Nasoduodenal/ Nasojejunal	• Avoids sedation • Low cost	• Discomfort of tube placement • Risk of vomiting and aspiration • Inability to evaluate mucosa or take biopsies
Colonoscopy	• Ability to evaluate mucosa and take biopsies • Most effective route for treatment of recurrent *Clostridium difficile* infection (rCDI)	• Invasive • Generally requires sedation • Standard risks of colonoscopy (eg, discomfort, perforation, bleeding) • Expensive
Enema	• Less invasive • Can be administered in office setting or at home • No sedation risk • Low cost • Can more easily be repeated	• Donor stool does not reach the entire colon and limited to left-sided colon • Less effective than other routes for rCDI
Capsules	• Less invasive • Can be administered in office setting • No sedation risk	• Expensive, but eliminates cost of endoscopy • Less effective than colonoscopy for rCDI • Large capsule burden • Risks of vomiting and aspiration

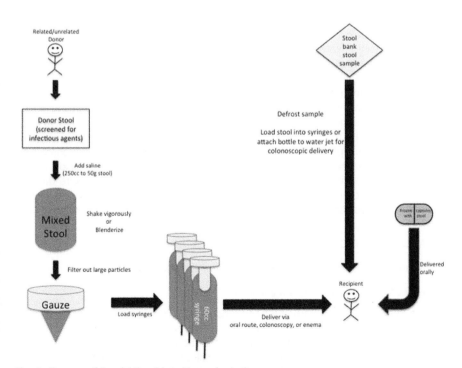

Fig. 1. Process of Fecal Microbiota Transplantation.

storage for future studies or if the recipient develops a rare infection following FMT. For local donors, stool is obtained with the plan to transplant in less than 8 hours. Stool is mixed with normal saline (although mixing with milk has also been described) and vigorously shaken to ensure good mixing. Blenders (either supplied by the health care facility or brought in by the patient) have also been used, but will likely need to be discarded following stool preparation unless there is a method of disinfection. Mixed stool is passed through a filter or gauze to remove large particulate matter that may clog the colonoscope channel. Stool is then drawn up into 60-mL syringes (generally 4–5) and administered to the recipient. There are no guidelines for how much feces to deliver, although many agree that at least 50 g (or 250 mL diluent) should be adequate.[11,12]

More recently, several stool banks have been formed. A stool bank collects stool from a set of prescreened donors, prepares and divides the donated stool, and freezes aliquots of screened stool that can then be shipped overnight to health care facilities. Samples are treated like a drug and frequently go through the institution's pharmacy. This frozen sample is defrosted and drawn up into 60-mL syringes for administration. Alternatively, the stool bottle can be attached to the colonoscope's water jet and sprayed into the colon rather than injecting syringes through the accessory channel. The use of a stool bank sample alleviates the need for mixing and filtering and is quite affordable (approximately $250 plus shipping). It also eliminates the need for the patient to ask a friend or relative to provide a stool sample. As that person would also need to be screened as described previously, a stool bank donor removes this step and associated cost.

Following FMT, we generally administer 1 dose of loperamide in the endoscopy recovery suite, although there are no clear data suggesting this alters outcomes. Some institutions will administer this medication before FMT. Additionally, we place the patient in reverse Trendelenburg for up to an hour with the goal of retaining stool in the colon as long as possible. At the time of discharge, we recommend home disinfection of all surfaces with a water-bleach cleaner (9:1 ratio) or sporicidal agent approved by the Environmental Protection Agency. We follow-up with the patient to assess for efficacy and adverse events.

There also has been the development of frozen, encapsulated stool. Capsules developed by OpenBiome (Medford, MA) use screened donor stool placed inside a size 0 capsule, which is then placed inside a size 00 capsule and frozen.[13] Studies have been performed with trypan blue demonstrating an average of 115 minutes elapsing before the capsule opens; enough time to pass through the acidic environment of the stomach.[14] The capsules are unique in the patented microbial emulsion matrix (MEM) technology using long-chain fatty acids as a carrier matrix to ensure delivery of live microbial communities.[13] FMT capsules must be stored at −20°C or below and must be swallowed by the patient in less than 90 minutes from freezer removal.

INDICATIONS FOR FECAL MICROBIOTA TRANSPLANTATION

The strongest evidence for efficacy of FMT is for the treatment of rCDI.

Recurrent Clostridium difficile Infection

Over the past 2 decades there has been a rise in CDI incidence, particularly among older adults.[15] There has been the emergence of the more virulent BI/NAP1/027 strain, a rise in community-acquired cases of CDI without prior antibiotic exposure, and the emergence of special populations at increased risk of CDI, such as patients with solid organ transplantation, patients with cancer receiving chemotherapy, and patients with

IBD.[16,17] The risk of recurrent CDI is high with at least 10% to 20% of patients developing a first recurrence within 8 weeks of treatment and 40% to 65% of patients with subsequent recurrences.[18] Frequently, these are patients who do not respond to traditional medical therapies with vancomycin or fidaxomicin; therefore, identifying therapies for these patients has been critical.

The greatest evidence for FMT is for treatment of recurrent CDI. These are patients with at least 3 episodes of confirmed CDI that has been unresponsive or refractory to current antibiotic therapies. The hypothesis is that through restoring normal colonic bacterial populations, there is more competition for nutrients and inhibition of C difficile growth. There also may be regulation of the immune system (a current area of research) and changes in bile acids that impair the C. difficile life cycle.[11]

The effectiveness of FMT for this indication has been impressive, with numerous studies demonstrating cure rates greater than 85% and many greater than 90%. Although many of these have been case reports or case studies with convenience samples, the first randomized controlled trial was performed by van Nood and colleagues[19] with FMT for rCDI through the nasoduodenal route. Given that 81% of patients with rCDI had resolution of C. difficile associated disease (CDAD) after 1 infusion compared with 31% of patients receiving vancomycin only (P<.001), the study was terminated early following interim analysis. There have been 2 randomized controlled trials showing efficacy of FMT via colonoscopy.[20,21]

Based on the success of FMT for rCDI, guidelines by the American College of Gastroenterology and the European Society of Clinical Microbiology and Infectious Diseases recommend this treatment option.[22,23]

As described previously, a more recent development has been the use of frozen, oral FMT capsules for treatment of rCDI. In one feasibility study of 20 patients with rCDI who had failed vancomycin therapy, 14 (70%) patients had resolution of diarrhea following capsule administration (15 capsules over 2 consecutive days).[14,24] Of the 6 nonresponders, 4 had resolution of diarrhea after a second administration of FMT capsules. There were no serious adverse events.

Among most studies for CDI, the highest cure rates are seen with colonoscopic administration of donor stool, generally greater than 90%. Oral administration is slightly less effective with resolution rates in the 76% to 79% range.[8] For recurrent CDI, Konijeti and colleagues[25] performed decision analysis to ascertain if FMT was a cost-effective strategy. Comparing various treatment strategies, FMT via colonoscopy was the most cost-effective initial strategy for rCDI with up to $17,000 in cost savings.

It should be noted that although there are case reports of successful treatment of severe and severe and complicated CDI, including in patients in the intensive care unit, this is not currently the recommended standard of care, but can be considered on a case-by-case basis remembering that patients should be treated aggressively with early surgical consultation for consideration of colectomy or loop ileostomy.

Inflammatory Bowel Disease

IBD includes both Crohn's disease (CD) and ulcerative colitis (UC). Similar to CDI, studies have shown dysbiosis with reduction in bacterial diversity (decreased Bacteroidetes and Firmicutes with increased Proteobacteria and Actinobacteria) in these patients.[26,27] There are also decreases in *Faecalibacterium prausnitzii*, which is thought to play a role in both decreasing inflammation and maintaining clinical remission.[28,29]

There are studies dating as far back as 1989 using FMT for treatment of IBD (mostly UC), all using a retention enema as the mode of administration.[30–33] In the first case report, Bennet self-administered an FMT enema following a diagnosis of UC 7 years prior that had been refractory to both steroid and sulfasalazine therapies.[31] Chronic inflammation remained, but active inflammation and symptoms improved. Follow-up studies by Borody and colleagues[32,33] of patients who had failed conventional IBD therapies (5-aminosalicylic acids [5-ASAs], steroids, azathioprine) documented variable periods of remission ranging from 3 months to 13 years. During this time, there were also numerous murine studies assessing microbiota transfer.[30]

A systematic review by Colman and Rubin[34] described 18 studies (122 patients) of FMT use in patients with IBD with an overall remission rate at only 36.2% among cohort studies; response was 22% when only patients with UC were subanalyzed compared with 60.5% in patients with CD. Among included studies, there was variation in donor stool source, stool preparation (frozen vs fresh) and method of FMT administration. At least 41% of patients received 2 or more FMTs, but there was no correlation with the frequency of FMT and response. There were no serious adverse events.

There are additional systematic reviews suggesting higher rates of efficacy, but with concerns of methodological study flaws and publication bias.[34,35]

A possible explanation for the less robust responses seen with FMT in patients with IBD is that there are other factors contributing to IBD exacerbations beyond the microbiome, such as leaky gut (impaired mucosal barrier function) and inflammation.[36] Multiple risk factors contribute to this dysbiosis, compromised mucosal integrity and inflammation, including genetics and environmental factors (eg, diet, tobacco, infection, stress, surgery, and medications). FMT is a potential treatment focused on microbiome reconstitution, but the effects on the immune system and mucosal integrity are less clear.

In summary, despite the dysbiosis in patients with IBD, FMT studies have been less robust with mixed results. In some cases, there is evidence of remission induction; however, this effect is frequently not seen in all patients, nor is it sustained.

Other Potential Indications

Beyond rCDI and IBD, there is great interest in other applications for FMT. These include both GI and non-GI diseases, such as chronic fatigue syndrome, Parkinson disease, obesity and the metabolic syndrome, and multiple sclerosis.[11]

Among the lay public, there is particular interest in the use of FMT for functional disorders, such as irritable bowel syndrome (IBS). It remains unclear if there is a dysbiotic contribution to IBS, although some studies do show differences in bacterial populations among patients with IBS.[37,38] A single-center experience of 13 patients with IBS nonresponsive to medical therapies who received FMT demonstrated resolution or improvement of symptoms in 70% of patients with most improvement in abdominal pain, dyspepsia, bloating, and flatus.[39] Additional studies in patients with IBS and chronic constipation showed some short-term improvement in symptoms, but fewer than 50% of patients had long-term improvement.[40] Related, there may be a role for postinfectious IBS and small intestinal bacterial overgrowth, but these areas need to be further explored.[38]

One of the greatest areas of research revolves around obesity and the metabolic syndrome, given the growing number of patients who are developing this disease process, particularly in the United States. Studies have suggested a potential intestinal microbiome role in the development of obesity, and microbial analysis demonstrates significant differences in the microbiome of lean versus obese individuals.[41,42] Additionally, in initial murine FMT studies when stool from an obese mouse was transferred to germ-free mice, it led to increased adiposity when compared with lean donor transplants.[43] Follow-up studies have been performed in humans, although on a small scale. Obese recipients with "lean" donor stool FMTs had improved insulin sensitivity, increased diversity of the gut microbiome and increased *Roseburia intestinalis*, a butyrate-producing bacteria.[44] Although more studies need to be performed to determine if there are long-term benefits, these findings do raise the concern of using obese FMT donors (for any indication, including rCDI), as a lean recipient may develop unintended outcomes: an increase in adiposity.

Other potential FMT applications are less well studied, but there are case reports describing individual successes, particularly with autism, chronic fatigue syndrome, fibromyalgia, idiopathic thrombocytopenic purpura, multiple sclerosis, myoclonus dystonia, and Parkinson disease; none of these have been evaluated in randomized clinical trials.[11,45–48]

ADVERSE EFFECTS OF FECAL MICROBIOTA TRANSPLANTATION

FMT delivers a foreign compound (or a mixture of various microorganisms) into the recipient. Similar to any drug, we must consider possible adverse events that may result from this introduction, particularly as the use of FMT continues to increase. The most common adverse events are described in **Box 2**. Typically, any adverse events are mild and transient, such as abdominal discomfort, nausea, vomiting, bloating, or flatulence. It is often difficult to know if these symptoms are related to the underlying disease that triggered the need for FMT (such as postinfectious IBS), the sedative medications received during endoscopy, the use of air or $CO2$ during colonoscopy, or a true result of the infused donor stool. More serious complications are rare and often relate to the well-established risks of endoscopy and sedation. Development of a new infection is rare. Most FMT efficacy studies have examined adverse events as a secondary outcome with overall minimal findings.

Box 2
Potential adverse events of fecal microbiota transplantation

Minor (and common):

- Nausea/vomiting (particularly with oral FMT route)
- Abdominal discomfort or pain
- Bloating
- Flatulence
- Diarrhea/constipation
- Low-grade fever

Severe:

- Sedation related (eg, aspiration)
- Endoscopy related (eg, bleeding, perforation)
- Infection ± sepsis (infection may be a long-term sequelae)
- Inflammatory bowel disease flare
- Postinfectious irritable bowel syndrome

Potential:

- Risk of chronic disease development related to changes in gut microbiome
- Other unknown?

There has been ongoing concern that immunocompromised patients may be at greater risk for infection and sepsis following FMT. A multicenter, retrospective study examining post-FMT adverse events in 80 immunocompromised patients showed high CDI cure rates following a single FMT (78%).[49] Two patients died (one from unrelated pneumonia and the other following an aspiration event during sedation for colonoscopy). There were no infections linked to FMT. Among mild adverse events, 3 patients reported abdominal discomfort post-FMT.

Among patients with IBD, also considered to be immunocompromised, there is a subset of patients that will develop an IBD flare. Of the patients with IBD included in the study of immunocompromised patients by Kelly and colleagues,[49] 14% experienced a flare post-FMT. These flares frequently manifest with fever and increases in inflammatory markers along with typical flare symptoms of irregular bowel habits and abdominal pain. We have also witnessed several cases of postinfectious IBS in patients, although it is unclear if these are related to FMT versus prior infection, such as CDI.

Less well known are the long-term risks of FMT, particularly on the development of chronic diseases that may be related to alteration of the gut microbiome or be unknowingly harbored by the donor stool. Although donor screening testing protocols are quite extensive, it is impossible to check for all organisms and there is always a risk of transmitting an untested infectious agent to the recipient.

Based on the evidence, FMT is an overall safe therapy with minimal adverse effects. Despite this, we urge caution in the use of FMT in severely immunocompromised patients, as there are isolated reports of sepsis, possibly related to bacterial translocation in the setting of impaired gut mucosal integrity and inflammation. Nonetheless, for patients with rCDI that have not responded to other therapies, this may be the best option.

SPECIAL POPULATIONS

In addition to immunocompromised patients, there are other groups that warrant special attention when FMT is being considered. These include the following:

- Elderly
- Pediatric populations

Elderly

The increased prevalence of CDI in the elderly population (older than 65) has been well established; mortality is also greatest in this cohort with more cases of severe, severe and complicated, and rCDI. Given this older population often has a number of serious comorbidities, there is increased scrutiny in performing FMT in these patients. Agrawal and colleagues[50] performed a multicenter, retrospective study evaluating the efficacy and safety of FMT in 146 patients aged 65 or older. There was a mix of patients with recurrent, severe, or severe and complicated CDI. Primary cure was established in 82% of patients with recurrent CDI, 91% in patients with severe CDI and 66% in patients with severe and complicated CDI. There were no adverse events, but there were a total of 6 hospital admissions for diarrhea recurrence.

Although FMT appears safe in these populations, there are several concerns to note, including the risks of performing an invasive procedure (although with an overall good safety profile), increased comorbidities making anesthesia of higher risk, greater difficulties performing adequate bowel preparation, current medications that may include blood-thinning or antiplatelet agents, and decreased anal sphincter tone that may make it more difficult to retain infused stool for an extended period of time.[51] These factors raise the question if donor stool administration via an upper GI route may be safer, although likely slightly less effective. Frozen encapsulated stool also may be an option, although as elderly patients more frequently experience dysphagia, capsules may be administered only in patients with normal swallowing.

Pediatric Population

There is substantially less evidence for the use of FMT in pediatric populations. There are reports of FMT use for both CDI and IBD with varying results.[52] Additionally, there is more concern for adverse events in children. In the short-term, there are the risks of performing any invasive procedure and related anesthesia, but in children who have many years of life ahead of them, there are also the fears of the long-term effects of microbiome manipulation.

FUTURE CONSIDERATIONS/NEXT STEPS

The goal of FMT is to alter the gut microbiome (ideally back to the preinfection state) and we have evidence suggesting clear changes in bacterial populations and an overall increase in the diversity of species following FMT. As described previously, there does not appear to be any significant short-term adverse events following FMT, although we must acknowledge that long-term outcomes related to changes in the microbiome are less clear and will require ongoing, prospective review to assess. An FMT registry to collect long-term data has just been funded and will provide important data on outcomes and complications.

Despite the absence of major adverse events, there remains the potential for infection, the development of donor diseases (such as metabolic syndrome), and dysregulation of the immune system; there are multiple reports of autoimmune diseases post-FMT, although the causality of this is less clear. Therefore, we must consider donor stool a "drug" and subject to regulation by the FDA. There needs to be standardization regarding the screening of donor stool and a clear protocol for the monitoring of adverse events.

Over the past several years, we have learned a lot more about the bacterial populations within our gut; however, we know very little about the function of these bacteria. We know bacteria have the ability to produce and secrete bioactive compounds ranging from antimicrobial agents to neurotransmitters to quorum-sensing molecules that influence and communicate with nearby bacteria. We also know very little about the gut's virome or mycome. Research needs to shift from identifying the bacteria present in the gut to determining the function of these bacteria.

Finally, there is ongoing interest in the broader application of FMT for other diseases beyond rCDI and there are dozens of studies ongoing to determine if there are benefits both for infectious and noninfectious conditions. Additionally, there remains the question if alternatives to donor stool are effective, such as synthetic stool formulations. There is an active clinical trial (NCT01372943) using a purified mixture of donor bacteria for treatment of rCDI with the hypothesis that this probiotic approach would provide a "more controlled, reproducible, cleaner and more aesthetically acceptable method of administration" that is "a safer strategy than using freshly defecated donor fecal matter." Preliminary proof-of-principle data in a very small sample (n = 2) demonstrate effectiveness in treating rCDI, and improvement in patient symptoms.[53] We anticipate ongoing focus on the development of alternatives to stool transplantation, although any competing therapy will need to demonstrate efficacy rates as robust as FMT, which will be challenging.

In conclusion, FMT is clearly a highly effective therapy for management of rCDI with ongoing studies to determine if there is a role in other diseases. The rise in the popularity of FMT and newly found focus on the microbiome and its role in health and diseases make for an exciting future in the field of gastroenterology and infectious disease.

REFERENCES

1. Zhang F, Luo W, Shi Y, et al. Should we standardize the 1,700-year-old fecal microbiota transplantation? Am J Gastroenterol 2012;107:1755 [author reply: 1755–6].
2. Brandt LJ, Aroniadis OC, Mellow M, et al. Long-term follow-up of colonoscopic fecal microbiota transplant for recurrent *Clostridium difficile* infection. Am J Gastroenterol 2012;107:1079–87.
3. Borody TJ, Warren EF, Leis SM, et al. Bacteriotherapy using fecal flora: toying with human motions. J Clin Gastroenterol 2004;38(6):475–83.
4. Eiseman B, Silen W, Bascom GS, et al. Fecal enema as an adjunct in the treatment of pseudomembranous enterocolitis. Surgery 1958;44(5):854–9.
5. Vindigni SM, Broussard EK, Surawicz CM. Alteration of the intestinal microbiome: fecal microbiota transplant and probiotics for *Clostridium difficile* and beyond. Expert Rev Gastroenterol Hepatol 2013;7(7):615–28.
6. Hamilton MJ, Weingarden AR, Unno T, et al. High-throughput DNA sequence analysis reveals stable engraftment of gut microbiota following transplantation of previously frozen fecal bacteria. Gut Microbes 2013;4:125–35.
7. Khoruts A, Dicksved J, Jansson JK, et al. Changes in the composition of the human fecal microbiome after bacteriotherapy for recurrent *Clostridium difficile*-associated diarrhea. J Clin Gastroenterol 2010;44(5):354–60.
8. Gough E, Shaikh H, Manges AR. Systematic review of intestinal microbiota transplantation (fecal bacteriotherapy) for recurrent *Clostridium difficile* infection. Clin Infect Dis 2011;53:994–1002.
9. Kassam Z, Lee CH, Yuan Y, et al. Fecal microbiota transplantation for *Clostridium difficile* infection: systematic review and meta-analysis. Am J Gastroenterol 2013; 108(4):500–8.
10. Food and Drug Administration Center for Biologics Evaluation and Research. Guidance for industry: enforcement policy regarding investigational new drug requirements for use of fecal microbiota for transplantation to treat *Clostridium difficile* infection not responsive to standard therapies. Silver Spring (MD): Food and Drug Administration; 2013.
11. Choi HH, Cho YS. Fecal microbiota transplantation: current applications, effectiveness, and future perspectives. Clin Endosc 2016;49(3):257–65.
12. Brandt LJ, Aroniadis OC. An overview of fecal microbiota transplantation: techniques, indications, and outcomes. Gastrointest Endosc 2013;78(2):240–9.
13. OpenBiome. OpenBiome FMT capsule G3 clinical primer. Medford (MA): OpenBiome; 2016.
14. Youngster I, Russell GH, Pindar C, et al. Oral, capsulized, frozen fecal microbiota transplantation for relapsing *Clostridium difficile* infection. JAMA 2014;312(17): 1772–8.
15. Lessa FC, Gould CV, McDonald LC. Current status of *Clostridium difficile* infection epidemiology. Clin Infect Dis 2012;55(Suppl 2):S65–70.
16. Lessa FC. Community-associated *Clostridium difficile* infection: how real is it? Anaerobe 2013;24:121–3.

17. Khanna S, Pardi DS. The growing incidence and severity of *Clostridium difficile* infection in inpatient and outpatient settings. Expert Rev Gastroenterol Hepatol 2010;4(4):409–16.
18. McFarland LV, Surawicz CM, Rubin M, et al. Recurrent *Clostridium difficile* disease: epidemiology and clinical characteristics. Infect Control Hosp Epidemiol 1999;20(1):43–50.
19. van Nood E, Vrieze A, Nieuwdorp M, et al. Duodenal infusion of donor feces for recurrent *Clostridium difficile*. N Engl J Med 2013;368(5):407–15.
20. Cammarota G, Masucci L, Ianiro G, et al. Randomised clinical trial: faecal microbiota transplantation by colonoscopy vs. vancomycin for the treatment of recurrent *Clostridium difficile* infection. Aliment Pharmacol Ther 2015;41(9):835–43.
21. Kelly CR, Khoruts A, Staley C, et al. Effect of Fecal Microbiota Transplantation on Recurrence in Multiply Recurrent Clostridium difficile Infection: A Randomized Trial. Ann Intern Med 2016. [Epub ahead of print].
22. Surawicz CM, Brandt LJ, Binion DG, et al. Guidelines for diagnosis, treatment, and prevention of *Clostridium difficile* infections. Am J Gastroenterol 2013; 108(4):478–98 [quiz: 499].
23. Debast SB, Bauer MP, Kuijper EJ, et al. European Society of Clinical Microbiology and Infectious Diseases: update of the treatment guidance document for *Clostridium difficile* infection. Clin Microbiol Infect 2014;20(Suppl 2):1–26.
24. Youngster I, Sauk J, Pindar C, et al. Fecal microbiota transplant for relapsing *Clostridium difficile* infection using a frozen inoculum from unrelated donors: a randomized, open-label, controlled pilot study. Clin Infect Dis 2014;58(11):1515–22.
25. Konijeti GG, Sauk J, Shrime MG, et al. Cost-effectiveness of competing strategies for management of recurrent *Clostridium difficile* infection: a decision analysis. Clin Infect Dis 2014;58(11):1507–14.
26. Ott SJ, Musfeldt M, Wenderoth DF, et al. Reduction in diversity of the colonic mucosa associated bacterial microflora in patients with active inflammatory bowel disease. Gut 2004;53(5):685–93.
27. Frank DN, St Amand AL, Feldman RA, et al. Molecular-phylogenetic characterization of microbial community imbalances in human inflammatory bowel diseases. Proc Natl Acad Sci U S A 2007;104(34):13780–5.
28. Fujimoto T, Imaeda H, Takahashi K, et al. Decreased abundance of *Faecalibacterium prausnitzii* in the gut microbiota of Crohn's disease. J Gastroenterol Hepatol 2013;28(4):613–9.
29. Sokol H, Pigneur B, Watterlot L, et al. *Faecalibacterium prausnitzii* is an anti-inflammatory commensal bacterium identified by gut microbiota analysis of Crohn disease patients. Proc Natl Acad Sci U S A 2008;105(43):16731–6.
30. Damman CJ, Miller SI, Surawicz CM, et al. The microbiome and inflammatory bowel disease: is there a therapeutic role for fecal microbiota transplantation? Am J Gastroenterol 2012;107:1452–9.
31. Bennet JD, Brinkman M. Treatment of ulcerative colitis by implantation of normal colonic flora. Lancet 1989;1(8630):164.
32. Borody TJ, George L, Andrews P, et al. Bowel-flora alteration: a potential cure for inflammatory bowel disease and irritable bowel syndrome? Med J Aust 1989; 150(10):604.
33. Borody TJ, Warren EF, Leis S, et al. Treatment of ulcerative colitis using fecal bacteriotherapy. J Clin Gastroenterol 2003;37(1):42–7.
34. Colman RJ, Rubin DT. Fecal microbiota transplantation as therapy for inflammatory bowel disease: a systematic review and meta-analysis. J Crohns Colitis 2014;8(12):1569–81.

35. Anderson JL, Edney RJ, Whelan K. Systematic review: faecal microbiota transplantation in the management of inflammatory bowel disease. Aliment Pharmacol Ther 2012;36(6):503–16.
36. Vindigni SM, Zisman TL, Suskind DL, et al. The intestinal microbiome, barrier function, and immune system in inflammatory bowel disease: a tripartite pathophysiological circuit with implications for new therapeutic directions. Therap Adv Gastroenterol 2016;9(4):606–25.
37. Kassinen A, Krogius-Kurikka L, Makivuokko H, et al. The fecal microbiota of irritable bowel syndrome patients differs significantly from that of healthy subjects. Gastroenterology 2007;133(1):24–33.
38. Simren M, Barbara G, Flint HJ, et al. Intestinal microbiota in functional bowel disorders: a Rome foundation report. Gut 2013;62(1):159–76.
39. Pinn DM, Aroniadis OC, Brandt LJ. Is fecal microbiota transplantation the answer for irritable bowel syndrome? A single-center experience. Am J Gastroenterol 2014;109(11):1831–2.
40. Pinn DM, Aroniadis OC, Brandt LJ. Is fecal microbiota transplantation (FMT) an effective treatment for patients with functional gastrointestinal disorders (FGID)? Neurogastroenterol Motil 2015;27(1):19–29.
41. Nicholson JK, Holmes E, Kinross J, et al. Host-gut microbiota metabolic interactions. Science 2012;336(6086):1262–7.
42. Ley RE, Turnbaugh PJ, Klein S, et al. Microbial ecology: human gut microbes associated with obesity. Nature 2006;444(7122):1022–3.
43. Turnbaugh PJ, Ley RE, Mahowald MA, et al. An obesity-associated gut microbiome with increased capacity for energy harvest. Nature 2006;444(7122): 1027–31.
44. Vrieze A, Van Nood E, Holleman F, et al. Transfer of intestinal microbiota from lean donors increases insulin sensitivity in individuals with metabolic syndrome. Gastroenterology 2012;143(4):913–6.e7.
45. Ananthaswamy A. Faecal transplant eases symptoms of Parkinson's. New Sci 2011;209:01.
46. Borody T, Leis S, Campbell J, et al. Fecal microbiota transplantation (FMT) in multiple sclerosis (MS). Am J Gastroenterol 2011;106:S352.
47. Borody T, Campbell J, Torres M, et al. Reversal of idiopathic thrombocytopenic purpura [ITP] with fecal microbiota transplantation [FMT]. Am J Gastroenterol 2011;106:S352.
48. Finegold SM, Molitoris D, Song Y, et al. Gastrointestinal microflora studies in late-onset autism. Clin Infect Dis 2002;35(Suppl 1):S6–16.
49. Kelly CR, Ihunnah C, Fischer M, et al. Fecal microbiota transplant for treatment of Clostridium difficile infection in immunocompromised patients. Am J Gastroenterol 2014;109(7):1065–71.
50. Agrawal M, Aroniadis OC, Brandt LJ, et al. The long-term efficacy and safety of fecal microbiota transplant for recurrent, severe, and complicated Clostridium difficile infection in 146 elderly individuals. J Clin Gastroenterol 2016;50(5):403–7.
51. Vindigni SM, Surawicz CM. Stool transplant for the senior citizen: is it safe? Maturitas 2016;88:23–4.
52. Kelly CR, Kahn S, Kashyap P, et al. Update on Fecal Microbiota Transplantation 2015: indications, methodologies, mechanisms, and outlook. Gastroenterology 2015;149(1):223–37.
53. Petrof EO, Gloor GB, Vanner SJ, et al. Stool substitute transplant therapy for the eradication of Clostridium difficile infection: 'RePOOPulating' the gut. Microbiome 2013;1(1):3.

54. McCune VL, Struthers JK, Hawkey PM. Faecal transplantation for the treatment of *Clostridium difficile* infection: a review. Int J Antimicrob Agents 2014;43(3):201–6.
55. Bakken JS, Borody T, Brandt LJ, et al. Treating *Clostridium difficile* infection with fecal microbiota transplantation. Clin Gastroenterol Hepatol 2011;9:1044–9. United States: 2011 AGA Institute. Published by Elsevier Inc.
56. Brandt LJ. *American Journal of Gastroenterology* Lecture: intestinal microbiota and the role of fecal microbiota transplant (FMT) in treatment of *C. difficile* infection. Am J Gastroenterol 2013;108:177–85.

Index

Note: Page numbers of article titles are in **boldface** type.

A

Achlorhydria, 131–132
Acid suppression, gastric microbiome effect of, 130–133
Acute-on-chronic liver failure and death, 163–164
Adaptive immune system, 23–26
Alcoholic-related fatty liver disease, pathophysiology of, 161–164
Ampicillin, impact of, on microbiome, 64
Antibiotics, impact of
    on microbiome, 62–67
    on necrotizing enterocolitis, 64–67
Atrophic gastritis, 130
Autism, in brain gut-microbiota axis dysfunction, 82–83
Autophagy, 23

B

B lymphocytes, 25–26
Bacterial overgrowth. *See* Small intestinal bacterial overgrowth.
Bacterial peritonitis, spontaneous, 163
Barrett's esophagus, 122–123
Bile acids, 42–43, 68–69
Brain-gut-microbiota axis, **77–89**
    at extremes of life, 80
    communication in, 78–79
    dysfunction of
        autism in, 82–83
        depression in, 80–81
        irritable bowel syndrome in, 80–81
        Parkinson disease in, 83
        psychobiotics for, 84–85
Breath tests, for SIBO, 110–113

C

Cancer
    esophageal, 122–123
    gastric, 128–130
Carbon isotope breath tests, for SIBO, 111, 113
Chemotherapy, immune system interactions with, 21–22
Ciprofloxacin
    for SIBO, 113–115
    impact of, on microbiome, 62

Gastroenterol Clin N Am 46 (2017) 187–193
http://dx.doi.org/10.1016/S0889-8553(17)30008-0
0889-8553/17

gastro.theclinics.com

Cirrhosis, **155–169**
    incidence of, 155
    pathophysiology of, 155–164
Clindamycin, diarrhea due to, 6
Clostridium difficile infections
    antibiotic-associated diarrhea due to, 67–71
    fecal microbiota transplantation for, 171–177
Colonization, of microbiome, 62, 68–69
Colonoscopy, for fecal microbiota transplantation, 174–177
Communication, in brain-gut-microbiota axis, 78–79
Cotrimoxazole, for SIBO, 113–115
Crohn's disease. *See* Inflammatory bowel disease.
Culture-based studies, 10–11, 110

D

Databases, 40
Dendritic cells, 20–22
Depression, in brain-gut-microbiota axis dysfunction, 80–81
Diarrhea, antibiotic-associated, 67–71
Diet, **49–60**
DNA sequencing, **9–17**
Doxycycline, for SIBO, 113–115
Dysbiosis, in liver disease, 156
Dyspepsia, postinfectious, 130

E

Eicosanoids, 42–43
Elderly persons
    brain-gut-microbiota axis in, 80
    FMT for, 180–181
Encephalopathy, hepatic, 162–163
Enema, for fecal microbiota transplantation, 174–176
Enteral feeding, of liquid diet, 53–54
Environmental factors, in IBD, 144–145
Eosinophilic esophagitis, 122–123
Epithelial cells, 23
Escherichia coli infections, 79
Esophagus, microbiome of, **121–141**
    in disease, 122–123
    in health, 122

F

Fecal microbiota transplantation, 149–151, **171–185**
    adverse effects of, 179–180
    definition of, 171–172
    donor for, 172–173
    effects of, 172
    for special populations, 180–181

    goals of, 172
    history of, 172
    indications for, 176–179
    process for, 174–176
    screening for, 172–174
    stool bank for, 174–176
Fermentation, 26–28
Fibromyalgia, 109
Flora, definition of, 2
Fluoroquinolones, for SIBO, 113–115
FMT. *See* Fecal microbiota transplantation.
FODMAP diet, 51–55, 115
Functional bowel disorders, **91–101**
Fungi, in IBD, 149

G

Gas chromatography, 39–44
Gastritis, 130
Gastroesophageal reflux disease, 122–123
Genetic factors, in IBD, 144, 146, 149
Gentamicin, impact of, on microbiome, 64–65
Glucose breath tests, for SIBO, 111, 113
Gnotobiotic animals, 41–42
Granulocyte macrophage colony-stimulating factor, 23
Gut microbiome
    antibiotics and, **61–76**
    composition of, 2–3, **9–17,** 11–12, 92–93
    definition of, **1–8,** 49–50
    diet and, **49–60**
    esophageal, **121–141**
    fecal microbiota transplantation, 149–151, **171–185**
    functional bowel disorders and, **91–101**
    functions of, 2–3, 12–13
    gastric, **121–141**
    host immune response interactions with, **19–35,** 95–96
    in inflammatory bowel disease, 51–58.**143–154,** 177–178
    irritable bowel and, 80–81, **91–101,** 178
    metabolites and, **37–47**
    necrotizing enterocolitis and, 46–47
    organization of, **1–8**
    small intestinal bacterial overgrowth and, **103–120**
Gut-associated lymphoid tissues, 20–21

H

Helicobacter pylori, 122–132
Hepatic encephalopathy, 162–163
Histamine, 26–28
Histone deacetylases, 26–28
Host response. *See* Immune system.

Hydrogen breath tests, for SIBO, 110–113
Hypochlorhydria, 108, 131–132
Hypothalamic-pituitary axis, 78–79

I

IBD. *See* Inflammatory bowel disease.
Immune system, **19–35**
    adaptive, 23–26
    bacterial interactions with, 26–28
    dysfunction of, in irritable bowel syndrome, 95–96
    in early life, 28–29
    innate, 20–23
Immunoglobulins, 25–26
Infants, brain-gut-microbiota axis in, 80
Inflammation
    biomarkers of, 81
    SIBO in, 108–109
Inflammatory bowel disease, 51–55, **143–154**
    environmental factors in, 144–145
    FMT for, 177–178
    microbiome of, 147–148
    mycobiome of, 149
    pathogenesis of, 144–149
    risk factors for, 144–146
    treatment of, 149–151
    virome of, 148–149
Innate immune system, 20–23
Interleukins, 22, 26–28
Intestinal barrier
    in irritable bowel syndrome, 95
    in liver disease, 159–161
Irritable bowel syndrome, **91–101**
    FMT for, 178
    in brain-gut-microbiota axis dysfunction, 80–81

J

Jejunal culture, for SIBO, 110

K

Kanamycin, impact of, on microbiome, 65–66

L

Lactase deficiency, in SIBO, 115
Lactobacillus, 127–128
Liquid chromatography, 39–44
Liver disease, **155–169**
    pathophysiology of, 155–158

alcoholic-related, 161–164
nonalcoholic, 159–160
Lymphoid cells, innate, 22

M

Macrophages, 22
Malabsorption, SIBO in, 108–109
Mass spectrometry, 38–40
Metabiomics, definition of, 2
Metabolic syndrome, FMT for, 178–179
Metabolomics, **37–47**
   analytical methods for, 38–40
   functional studies in, 40–44
   importance of, 38
Metagenomics, 2, **9–17**
Microbiome. *See also* Gut microbiome.
   definition of, 2
Microbiota, definition of, 1–2
Migratory motor complex, abnormal, 94–95
Monocytes, 22
Motility, abnormal, SIBO in, 108
Mucosal immune system. *See* immune system.
Mycobiome, in IBD, 149

N

Natural killer T cells, 25
Necrotizing enterocolitis, 64–67
Neomycin, for SIBO, 113–115
Neurohormones, in irritable bowel syndrome, 9
Neurotransmitters, in brain-gut-microbiota axis, 78–79
NOD2 protein, 23
Nonalcoholic fatty liver disease, 159–160
Norfloxacin, for SIBO, 113–115
Nuclear magnetic resonance spectroscopy, 38–44

O

Obesity, FMT for, 178–179
Oral administration, for fecal microbiota transplantation, 174–176
Overgrowth, bacterial. *See* Small intestinal bacterial overgrowth.
Oxytocin, 83

P

Paneth cells, 107
Parkinson disease, in brain-gut-microbiota axis dysfunction, 83
Pediatric patients, FMT for, 181
Peritonitis, spontaneous bacterial, 163
Phagocytes, 22

Polymerase chain reaction, **9–17**
Prebiotics
    for brain-gut-microbiota axis dysfunction, 84–85
    for IBD, 149–150
Pregnancy, immune system development in, 28–29
Preterm infants
    brain-gut-microbiota axis in, 80
    necrotizing enterocolitis in, 64–67
Probiotics, 66–67, 70–71, 84–85, 149–150
Psychobiotics, 84–85
Psychological factors, in irritable bowel syndrome, 96–97

R

Rifaxamin, for SIBO, 113–115
Ruminococaccea, 63

S

Second hit hypothesis, in liver disease, 160
Sensorimotor dysfunction, 94–95
Serotonin
    in brain-gut-microbiota axis, 78–79
    in irritable bowel syndrome, 96
Shannon index, 82
Short-chain fatty acids, 26–28
Shotgun metagenome sequencing, 50
SIBO. *See* Small intestinal bacterial overgrowth.
16S rRNA profiles, 50–51
Small intestinal bacterial overgrowth, **103–120**
    definition of, 104
    diagnosis of, 110–113
    etiology of, 104–108
    liver disease and, 159–160
    pathogenesis of, 104–108
    predictors of, 109–110
    symptoms of, 109
    treatment of, 113–115
Spontaneous bacterial peritonitis, 163
Steatohepatitis
    alcoholic, 161–164
    nonalcoholic, 159–160
Stomach, microbiome of, **121–141**
    acid suppression effects on, 130–133
    in disease, 128–130
    in health, 123–128
Stool transplantation. *See* Fecal microbiota transplantation.
Stress, 81
SULT1A1 protein, 43–44

T

T lymphocytes, 24–25
TARGET studies, 115
Tetracycline, for SIBO, 113–115
Tolerance, immune, 20
Transplantation, fecal microbiota, 149–151, **171–185**
Trimethylamine, 43

U

Ulcerative colitis. *See* Inflammatory bowel disease.

V

Vancomycin, impact of, on microbiome, 62, 65–66
Virome, in IBD, 148–149
Vitamin A, metabolism of, 21
Vitamin B12 deficiency, 109
Vitamin deficiencies, in SIBO, 115

W

Walkerton catastrophe of water contamination, 79

Printed and bound by CPI Group (UK) Ltd, Croydon, CR0 4YY

07/10/2024

01040502-0019